CAMBRIDGE LIBRARY COLLECTION

Books of enduring scholarly value

History of Medicine

It is sobering to realise that as recently as the year in which On the Origin of Species was published, learned opinion was that diseases such as typhus and cholera were spread by a 'miasma', and suggestions that doctors should wash their hands before examining patients were greeted with mockery by the profession. The Cambridge Library Collection reissues milestone publications in the history of Western medicine as well as studies of other medical traditions. Its coverage ranges from Galen on anatomical procedures to Florence Nightingale's common-sense advice to nurses, and includes early research into genetics and mental health, colonial reports on tropical diseases, documents on public health and military medicine, and publications on spa culture and medicinal plants.

A Practical Essay on the History and Treatment of Beriberi

Reissued here together are two medical works, both published in 1835, by John Grant Malcolmson (1803–44), a British surgeon based in India. His extended essays explore the symptoms, diagnosis and treatment of beriberi and rheumatism, conditions which were widespread in Asia at the time. Also describing the contrasting effects that the illnesses had on India's native population and on European colonials, Malcolmson draws on his first-hand experience to speculate on the underlying causes. His analysis of beriberi, forming the larger of the two components here, discusses a disease which had perplexed doctors in the early nineteenth century. Beginning with numbness and spasms in the legs, and eventually rendering the patient completely bedridden, beriberi was frequently fatal, and physicians frequently confused it with other rheumatic disorders. It is now known to be caused by a deficiency of thiamine (vitamin B_1).

Cambridge University Press has long been a pioneer in the reissuing of out-of-print titles from its own backlist, producing digital reprints of books that are still sought after by scholars and students but could not be reprinted economically using traditional technology. The Cambridge Library Collection extends this activity to a wider range of books which are still of importance to researchers and professionals, either for the source material they contain, or as landmarks in the history of their academic discipline.

Drawing from the world-renowned collections in the Cambridge University Library and other partner libraries, and guided by the advice of experts in each subject area, Cambridge University Press is using state-of-the-art scanning machines in its own Printing House to capture the content of each book selected for inclusion. The files are processed to give a consistently clear, crisp image, and the books finished to the high quality standard for which the Press is recognised around the world. The latest print-on-demand technology ensures that the books will remain available indefinitely, and that orders for single or multiple copies can quickly be supplied.

The Cambridge Library Collection brings back to life books of enduring scholarly value (including out-of-copyright works originally issued by other publishers) across a wide range of disciplines in the humanities and social sciences and in science and technology.

A Practical Essay on the History and Treatment of Beriberi

With Observations on Some Forms of Rheumatism Prevailing in India

J.G. Malcolmson

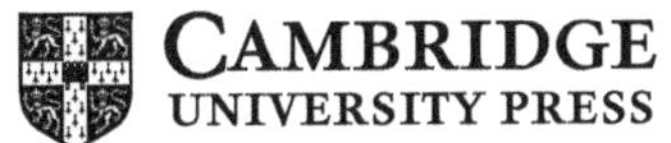

CAMBRIDGE
UNIVERSITY PRESS

University Printing House, Cambridge, CB2 8BS, United Kingdom

Published in the United States of America by Cambridge University Press, New York

Cambridge University Press is part of the University of Cambridge.
It furthers the University's mission by disseminating knowledge in the pursuit of education, learning and research at the highest international levels of excellence.

www.cambridge.org
Information on this title: www.cambridge.org/9781108068932

This edition first published 1835
This digitally printed version 2014

ISBN 978-1-108-06893-2 Paperback

A

PRACTICAL ESSAY

ON THE

HISTORY AND TREATMENT

OF

BERIBERI.

BY ASSISTANT SURGEON JOHN GRANT MALCOLMSON,

MADRAS MEDICAL ESTABLISHMENT.

" The same disease yields diversity of symptoms; which howsoever they be diverse, intricate and hard to be confined, I will adventure yet, in such a vast confusion and generality to bring them into some order." *Burton's Anatomy of Melancholy.*

" The use of remedies one does not know is very warily to be done, and can have no other reasonable foundation, but the truth, memory and judgment of him that vouches the experience of it." *Locke.*

MADRAS:

PRINTED BY ORDER OF GOVERNMENT.

VEPERY MISSION PRESS.

1835.

FORT ST. GEORGE GAZETTE, *No.* 38, *dated* 12*th May,* 1832, *Saturday.*

"ADVERTISEMENT."

"MEDICAL PRIZE ESSAYS."

"With a view to aid the advancement of medical science, and to communicate useful medical knowledge, the Medical Board, under the sanction of Government, announce to the medical officers under this Presidency, whether of his Majesty's or the Honorable Company's service, that a prize of Rupees 500, or a gold medal of that value with a suitable inscription, will be awarded, in the course of the year 1833, to the best dissertation on each of the two following subjects:

1st. On the disease called "Beriberi."

2d. On Rheumatism, and the neuralgic affection, occasionally a sequela of it, which is termed among natives "Burning in the feet."

Every essay, on each of these subjects, is to comprise a full and accurate history of the disease, as it affects Europeans and Natives, its varieties, and terminations; the diagnosis; an account of the morbid appearances observed on examination after death; an enquiry into the predisposing, exciting, and proximate causes; the prognosis; and the most successful mode of treatment.

Beriberi being known to be endemic in certain parts of this country, and having hitherto been but imperfectly discussed by European authors, the practice of the more intelligent native doctors deserves to be deliberately investigated: and two native remedies, in particular, which have been frequently prescribed with advantage in this disease, and are known in the northern division, by the names "Treeak Farook" and "Oleum Nigrum," should be made the subject of examination and report. The same observation, as to the expediency of inquiring into the treatment adopted by native practitioners, is equally applicable to "Burning in the feet."

The dissertations are to be transmitted to the Secretary of the Medical Board, on or before the 1st of May, 1833; and the adjudication of the prizes will take place in the month of July following.

To each dissertation must be prefixed a motto, which must likewise be written on the outside of a sealed packet, containing the name and address of the author. No dissertation will be received with the author's name affixed; and all dissertations, except the successful one, will be returned, if desired. Such as may not be desired to be returned will be retained in the Medical Board office, and published, should that be considered expedient.

Although only one dissertation on each subject can be successful, others may possess great, and indeed nearly equal, merit: and the Medical Board will have much satisfaction in bringing the names of the authors of such dissertations to the favourable notice of the Right Honorable the Governor in Council.

Fort St. George,
Medical Board Office,
3*d May*, 1832.

By order,
(Signed) H. S. Fleming,
Secretary Medical Board."

Fort St. George Gazette, *No.* 187, *dated* 25*th September* 1833, *Wednesday.*

No. 155.

"To

The Right Honorable Sir Frederick Adam,
Governor in Council,
&c. &c. &c.
Fort St. George.

Sir,

With reference to our letter, dated the 3rd of May, 1832, No. 68, submitting the draft of an advertisement inviting prize essays on certain medical subjects, we have now the honor to report the result of that invitation.

2. Within the period fixed by the advertisement, four essays on "Beriberi," and three on "Rheumatism" and "Burning in the feet," were received; and it affords us much gratification to be enabled to state, that, although there could be no difficulty in determining those entitled to the prizes, all of them possessed very considerable merit.

3. On examination of the sealed packets, corresponding with the essays,* which we had unanimously adjudged to be the most meritorious, it was found that Assistant Surgeon J. G. Malcolmson, of the Madras European regiment, is the author of both dissertations.

* Herewith forwarded for inspection.

4. This officer's essay on Beriberi, contains a very able and laborious investigation of the causes, nature, and treatment, of that disease; and is, in our opinion, eminently calculated to impart just views of its nature, and to render its treatment more discriminating and successful.

5. In the essay on Rheumatism, it has been the author's chief object to direct attention to such practical observations, on the varieties of that disease prevalent in India, as may not readily occur to a medical practitioner on his first arrival; to practical remarks on various disputed points in its history and treatment; and to a few novel observations, which, if confirmed by the experience of others, are calculated to advance our knowledge of the disease, and to lead to some valuable practical inferences.

6. After the observations just submitted, we need scarcely add, that we consider it highly desirable that the essays should be published, and distributed among the medical officers of this establishment; and we beg to recommend, that authority may be given for discharging the amount of the prizes.

7. We cannot conclude this letter without bringing particularly to notice the indefatigable zeal, which has enabled Mr. Malcolmson, while discharging arduous professional duties, and exposed to the disadvantages incident to military movements, to produce two dissertations not less remarkable for laborious research, than for original and comprehensive views.

8. As the authors of the unsuccessful essays, some of which possess a high degree of merit, might be unwilling that their names should be publicly known, we will report, in a separate communication, our opinion as to the merits of their respective dissertations.

We have the honor to be,

SIR,

Your most obedient humble servants,

THOMAS H. DAVIES, *1st Member,*
JOHN HAY, *2nd Member,*
K. MACAULAY, *Acting 3d Member.*
Medical Board.

FORT ST. GEORGE,
Medical Board Office,
16th September, 1833.

To

The Medical Board.

Gentlemen,

I am directed to acknowledge the receipt of your letter of the 16th instant, and to state that the Right Honorable the Governor in Council has perused with great satisfaction the report which it contains upon the result of your examination of the Prize Essays on certain medical subjects described in the notice published in the Fort St. George Gazette of the 12th May, 1832. That result is considered to be highly creditable to all the gentlemen who have submitted essays, and especially to Assistant Surgeon Malcolmson of the Madras European regiment, to whom both the prizes have been awarded.

Agreeably to your recommendation, the Right Honorable the Governor in Council is pleased to direct that the amount of the prizes be discharged, and the essays published and distributed among the Medical Officers of this Establishment.

The Right Honorable the Governor in Council observes with great gratification the highly favorable terms in which the zeal, talents and acquirements of Mr. Malcolmson are mentioned in the 7th paragraph of your letter under acknowledgement.

The Right Honorable the Governor in Council considers the report submitted in the separate communication referred to in the concluding paragraph of your letter to be highly creditable to the authors of the essays therein brought to the notice of Government.

I have the honor to be,

Gentlemen,

Your most obedient servant,

(Signed) Henry Chamier,

Chief Secretary."

Fort St. George,
24th September, 1833.

When the paper on beriberi was submitted to the Medical Board, they were informed in a note attached, that so much time had been occupied in preparing the materials, that the author was obliged to write it at once and to have it copied without correction, and that in consequence, many inaccuracies in the expression and arrangement of the sentences could not be avoided, but that, should the essay meet with the approbation of the Board, these would be corrected and some additional observations communicated. The subsequent appointment of the author as secretary to the Medical Board, having entailed on him the duty of carrying the papers through the press, it has been considered best, carefully to distinguish from the original essays, the additional observations referred to, and such others as his own experience had in the interval suggested, and as have been communicated by his friends or extracted from the records of the Medical Board.

Since the paper on beriberi was printed, the account of the examination of the malkungnee seeds and black oil has been submitted to the distinguished chemist, Mr. O Shaughnessy of the Bengal medical establishment, who concurs entirely in opinion, as to the nature of the oil and of the process by which it is prepared. *Note by the Author.*

ERRATA.

Page 199, line 15, *for* 'whethter' *read* 'whether.'
,, 232, line 16, *for* 'beriberi' *read* 'barbiers.'
,, 268, line 45, *for* 'Though' *read* 'Through.'
,, 321, line 8, *for* 'œdma' *read* 'œdema.'

A

PRACTICAL ESSAY

ON THE

HISTORY AND TREATMENT

OF

BERIBERI.

INTRODUCTION.

ALTHOUGH I am sensible that he serves medical science poorly, who encumbers it with ill digested matter, and that the frequent, unexpected and distant movements to which I have been subject, have deprived me of leisure for careful condensation, and broken off some of the most interesting observations and experiments, when they seemed about to establish important facts; I am encouraged to lay before the Board the following paper, from a hope, that it will be found to establish some important facts in the history, causes and treatment of Beriberi, and direct the attention to many obscure but important phenomena, hitherto little noticed or altogether overlooked. I shall attempt no systematic treatise on beriberi in its general history, but confine myself to an account of my own experience, borrowing from books only occasional illustrations of the disease known in the Northern Circars * under that name.

There is no disease regarding which our knowledge is more defective; and in which practice has been more injuriously directed by wrong theory; and the most valuable remedies more abused, by being recommended in improper stages or forms of one of the most complicated maladies to which the animal economy is liable. A few scattered essays seldom met with; a very small number of detailed cases, and scanty accounts of others in systematic works, by authors who have never seen the disease, are all that have yet been given to the public; and therefore one "cannot wonder that an experience "so contracted should have left some symptoms of "the disease unnoticed and much uncertainty with "regard to the distinctions and pathology."† My object shall therefore be, far more, to afford the profession copious materials than to build up a system, and to bring forward no opinions either in the pathology or treatment without the grounds for them, being fully stated; and having done this faithfully, I shall have less fear of expressing my opinions freely even when I am sensible that they can be of no further use than to direct enquiry.

Prize essays are principally useful by affording opportunity of recording collections of facts, which however important they may be to the advancement of knowledge, are yet too voluminous, minute, and

* A province extending along the west side of the Bay of Bengal, from 15 to 20 degrees N. L.

† Parry on Angina Pectoris.

uninteresting to the general reader to admit of publication in a separate form; and with this conviction, I shall not hesitate to notice such inferences as the singular phenomena of the disease suggest, regarding other obscure affections and actions of the frame.

My personal experience in the disease has extended to most of the military stations in the Circars, at a time when it was peculiarly prevalent, and the records of several of the hospitals have since been kindly communicated to me, and according to a plan of study I have long practised in other diseases, the cases were individually carefully studied; when they illustrated any fact satisfactorily or suggested new enquiries, they were copied or abridged for future reference, and the inferences suggested by each recorded and gradually generalized. The general facts thus obtained were afterwards subjected to comparison with a vast number of other cases, and corrected, enlarged or limited in their application by their evidence and that of clinical observation. This plan almost excludes bias from preconceived opinions; and the study of the genuine records of the practice of other medical men, affords a body of unprejudiced evidence of great importance in giving stability and universality to individual observations, and showing the effects of various plans of treatment. I have found some of the journals of less use, from the superficial way, many of the most interesting cases are recorded, and the almost total neglect of important circumstances, evidently present, but only noted accidentally; which must excuse the incompleteness of some of the following histories, which are in other respects too important to be rejected.

Under the name of Beriberi it is proposed to include all the cases, whether acute or chronic, of that peculiar affection of the lower extremities, chest and other parts, which prevails in certain Indian provinces near the coast and is known by that name amongst Europeans and is usually confounded by the Mussulmauns (like gout by the ancients) with rheumatism. The disease is named by the Telingees "timmeree waivo," but the term is not in universal use, the disease being by them also, confounded with other complaints. It has been adopted (after enquiry) on my information, by a distinguished Teloogoo scholar who gives the translation of the former word, "palsy, numbness, tingling" and of the latter "rheumatism."[1]

General account of the Symptoms.

The disease presents such a variety of symptoms that it will be more instructive to consider them in detail, than to attempt any elaborate general description. It will be sufficient to describe the most remarkable characters.

It usually commences gradually, with a feeling of numbness, sense of weight and slight weakness and stiffness below the middle of the thighs, some-

[1] Dr. Pearse in a valuable paper on Beriberi presented to the Medical Board mentions that it is called in Teloogoo ఉబ్బు వాయువు-or తిమిరి వాయువు- Ooboo waivoo or Timmery waivoo which terms signify rheumatism combined with dropsy or swellings; and Messrs. W. Geddes and G. B. Macdonell state "that the Telingees call it "wayawah," and when there "is swelling it is called "ooboo vayavah" and when this disappears "timeri "wayawah."

The Rev. Mr. Howell of Cuddapah informs me that వాయువు-voyuvu (which may be written either with a *w*, or *v*, although the latter is nearer the English sound) is a word frequently added to the names of diseases signifying both "wind" and "disease;" the received medical theories amongst the Gentoos ascribing most diseases to "wind." The proper name of Rheumatism is వాయునొప్పులు-voyuvu nopalu; the latter word means pains. "In తిమిరి- timmeri there are two kinds. 1st. When cramp or numbness arises from sitting in one posture it is simply called timmeri, but when

times preceded by muscular pains. There is slight œdema of the feet and legs, especially along the tibiæ, often found to come on after the other symptoms. The walk is unsteady and tottering even when the patient is not aware of weakness in the limbs, which are occasionally tremulous; spasms occur in the calves and soles of the feet sometimes becoming general and occasionally shooting to the chest and larynx, obstructing respiration and speech. The want of power often rapidly increases to almost total palsy, especially of the extensor muscles, and in a few cases, the patient after slight indispositi-

"it is a distemper it is called timmeri voyuvu. In dropsical cases ఉబ్బు — "ooboo is never used; it signifies the uneasy sensations with swelling of the "belly from indigestion. Oodara Pandoova వుదరపాండువ is dropsy."

"It is called by the Mussulmauns of Southern India سوج بائی Soojh Ba'ee (Hindee.)" *Dr. Pearse's paper.*

"Among the Mussulmauns Soond which means (in Duccanee) "numbness "is the general term used and under the supposition that it is connected "with rheumatism they sometimes call it Soond Ke Ba'ee." *Messrs. Geddes and Macdonell.*

The late Dr. Herklots author of the Qanoon i Islam, gives in his report to the Medical Board for the 2d half year of 1823 the following account of the Hindoostanee terms used for this disease.

"In Bengal, denominated by the Mohummudan practitioners Soon B'hay- "ree, and on the Peninsula Soond B'hay-ree, Soondee, or Soond Ka Murz, "(vulgo Soon Ka azar;) but which might with greater propriety be termed "Paralysis Orientalis."

"As to the appellation Beriberi, it appears to me perfectly unaccountable "how it could ever have crept into such general use as it has; for it is per- "fectly unintelligible to the Natives from whom it is said to have originated. "Though the word B'hay-ree does really mean a sheep in the Hindoostanee "dialect, and by repeating it (making allowances for the orthographical "error, in persons unacquainted with the language and consequently of the "proper sound of the word), we may form such a name as Beriberi; yet "after the most particular enquiries on the subject, I find the natives are to- "tally ignorant of any disease under that title."

"On the Peninsula then, (which has been more particularly the sphere of "my observations) the disease is not called B'hay-ree Bhay-ree (sheep sheep) "but Soond B'hay-ree, signifying numbness and sheep; the latter in re- "ference to the gait of that animal, which some, (not all), patients afflicted "with this disease, have. The Hakeems make a further distinction in the "designation of this disease; and that is, when loss of power of motion in "the limbs is the most prominent feature, they do not call it by any of the "names before mentioned (which though commonly applied to the disease in "general, is more correctly made use of when numbness is the principal "symptom), but term it J'ho-la (a swinging); and in like manner when "œdema is the predominant symptom, they denominate it Sooj (swelling)."

On the whole I am of opinion, notwithstanding these general statements by

on suddenly loses the use of his legs. Rigidity and various painful affections of the nerves accompany the paralytic symptoms; and there is sometimes pain along the spine, commonly at the two last lumber vertebræ. In some cases the disease goes no further and a cure is effected: but more frequently, the numbness extends upwards towards the abdomen, there is general sense of lassitude and aversion to motion, and the hands, arms, and chest, (and in a few cases even the neck and lips) are gradually benumbed. There is oppression and weight at præcordia, dyspnœa on slight exertion, diffused

gentlemen so well versed in Hindoostanee, that the disease is not accurately or usually distinguished in the South of India by these or any other names. How much caution is necessary in adopting inferences founded on similarity of sound, will appear to any one who looks over a page of a dictionary of Hindoostanee. He will find بهربهري Bhárbhári "a swelling, a sore" more near the word in question than those in either Good or Mr. Marshal's work on Ceylon: and a comparison of the Nosology P. 346 and Study of Medicine Vol. 3 P. 451 (Edition of 1822) of the former author, with each other, and with Mr. Marshal's work P. 208—210 will show still more strongly the uncertainty of such enquiries. It is necessary also to guard against accepting as a specific name of the disease, that applied to the symptom which attracts most of the patient's attention. The following extract on this subject is the more valuable as Mr. Geddes has been long engaged in the Study of the Medical works of the best Persian authors.

"In the Mussulmaun system, it is not to be expected that a disease similar "to beriberi should be found, peculiar as it is to a part of the world so distant "from that, from whence this people acquired their learning, and from the "same cause it is believed, as well as from the obscurity attending their des- "cription of disease it is either not mentioned by the Hindoo systematic me- "dical authors, or in so vague a manner as not to be discovered as an idio- "pathic disease. In the empirical works again, and among those also whose "information has been acquired without the aid of books, the medical know- "ledge does not seem to have sufficed for the distinction of a peculiar disor- "der different from those which had been already named and classified, and "the result in all these accordingly is the same, that with some, the case is "considered as paralysis, and in others, as dropsy, and that as far as can be "discovered there is no peculiar name or description applicable to beriberi "as a distinct disease, in those parts of India where it prevails. It appears "fortunate however, that the usual theories of the above symptoms, or other "circumstances should have led to a treatment, which is found useful in this "disease, and accordingly European practitioners have been induced to "adopt some portion of the native practice and with advantage, although "perhaps without being fully aware to what part of the treatment the bene- "ficial effects were to be ascribed. Of the natives' opinions in Ceylon and the "eastern islands where beriberi exists, no account has as yet been given, "but there appears no reason to believe that medical learning is more ad- "vanced in those countries than on the continent of India. *Messrs. Macdo-* "*nell and Geddes.*

and irregular pulsation in the cardiac region, and the face and hands are puffy and œdematous. The patient is often found dead in bed or sinks after several fainting fits or throbbings at the heart; or the œdema rapidly increases and extends up the trunk, violent dyspnœa and inability to lie down in bed comes on, with anxiety, cold sweats, cold extremities, rapid feeble pulse, urgent thirst and partial suppression of urine.[2] At the commencement the urine is always scanty, of a deep red colour without cloud or sediment and possessing very peculiar properties; in some old cases it becomes copious, turbid, and pale with a large white deposit, and is passed with pain, from an irritable bladder. The stomach is irritable in many bad cases, and pain and tenderness in the epigastrium is sometimes complained of; there is in a few, pain in the abdomen, or a sense of heat is diffused over it and the chest. Effusion takes place into the chest and more rarely into the abdomen, and there are now and then some signs of inflammation of the pleura or bronchi. In the early stage, the pulse may be full hard and frequent or little altered; when the face is puffy and there is weight and oppression at the præcordia it is quick, often irregular and usually small, although it is occasionally strong.

Various dyspeptic symptoms occur, the bowels are often costive, the stools green and variously disordered and the eyes are often tinged yellow. The skin is rather cold, unless there is pyrexia which is often present in the evening. The disease

[2] Lividity of the lips is only observed when the dyspnœa is extreme. Restlessness is an important but not very common idiopathic symptom. As in many diseases of the nerves there is a tendency to intermission of the painful symptoms. *Original note.*

is sometimes fatal in a few hours, but is often chronic, and in these, the patient is liable to sudden death, to rapid aggravation of the symptoms, or supervention of new and more formidable ones, by which he is soon carried off; and if he survives these, he may live for a long time bedridden, dropsical, and a true paralytic.[3]

Extent to which Beriberi prevails in the Circars.

The general abstract returns of the Northern Division afford valuable information regarding the prevalence of this disease; the influence of residence, season and situation; and forcibly point out its great importance in relation to the most fatal diseases.

[3] Although beriberi may with practical advantage be divided into a sthenic and asthenic form, I trust that it will appear in the sequel, that there are strong reasons for avoiding making a division of the symptoms in this stage of the enquiry and with our present knowledge. The following extracts will illustrate this imperfect description.

Extract from the 1st half yearly report of 1823 of the 1st Battalion 17th Regiment Native Infantry stationed at Masulipatam, by Assistant Surgeon A. Campbell.

"Two men died of beriberi. One of them was admitted with ulcers on his "feet, and was taken ill of beriberi, after being some time in hospital, which "is the reason that his death is placed under the head of ulcers. His com-"plaint commenced with thirst, lassitude, dyspnœa, slight swelling all over "his body particularly of his legs which pitted on pressure, his tongue was "white, pulse 100 pretty strong but intermitting, his lower extremities were "affected with palsy or loss of voluntary motion; and he complained of a hea-"viness all over him. Those symptoms became severe, particularly the dif-"ficulty of breathing; and he died the day after he was seized. His death "appeared to proceed immediately, from the action of the lungs and heart be-"ing impeded in consequence of effusion. On being taken ill 16 ounces of "blood were abstracted, and a large blister applied to his chest; calomel and "squills united given in pretty large and frequently repeated doses, and "purgatives administered occasionally; but I must say with little or no ap-"parent benefit, indeed, I am not acquainted with any disease unless per-"haps cholera, over which medicine appears to have so little control, or to "exert so little of a beneficial influence."

Extract from the second half yearly report of 1825 of the 37th Regiment Native Infantry stationed at Masulipatam, by Assistant Surgeon George Pearse M. D.

"The only remaining casualty which I have to notice is the death of a se-"poy belonging to the Grenadier company, a remarkably stout man, who was "admitted into hospital on the morning of the 21st October, complaining of "urgent dyspnœa, total inability to move his body or limbs, which as well as "his face were much swollen, with a sensation of fulness and tightness of "the skin, pulse 90, full, and firm: no sickness at stomach or complaint of "pain in any part of the body. Said he went to bed quite well last evening "after having eaten a hearty supper of rice as usual, and this morning early,

Those of the 2d half year of 1826 are less instructive, in consequence of the name "Beriberi" having been seldom used, the disease being classed under the heads of dropsy, rheumatism, or palsy, agreeably to the orders then in force requiring the use of the names in Cullen's nosology. Still some valuable information may be gleaned.

"was suddenly seized with the present symptoms. 16 oz. of blood were immediately taken from his arm, and a dose of pulv. jalap. comp. ℥i administered, which produced several fluid evacuations during the day; towards evening the dyspnœa was much diminished, and two pills consisting of calomel. gr. ij, pulv. scillæ gr. iij, were ordered; (to be repeated twice a day).—During the following night difficulty of breathing again returned and continued till morning, when he expired rather suddenly, about 24 hours after the commencement of the attack."

Extract from the 2d half yearly report of 1824 of the 11th Regiment Native Infantry stationed at Vizianagram, by Assistant Surgeon George Rose.

"The stout and healthy seem to be equally susceptible of it (beriberi) as those who have suffered from disease or dissipated habits and the rapidity of its progress is somewhat singular. A numbness about the ancles is the first symptom, which is generally thought nothing of till the 2d or 3d day, when the patient finds he is unable to walk or even stand without assistance, this is followed by an œdematous swelling and leucophlegmatic countenance, the pulse is feeble, the skin cold, the urine scanty, and the person sometimes as soon as the 7th or 8th day is suddenly seized with oppression at the præcordia and dyspnœa and carried off. I have never in any instance seen it attended with pain and seldom with swelling in any part of the trunk. The mode of treatment which I have followed consists in giving small doses of the hydrarg. submuriat. combined with the pulv. scillæ maritimæ 3 or 4 times a day, in conjunction with other diuretics, frictions, blisters, &c. but in most cases which have occurred, the progress of the disease seemed to be very little affected by any remedy, and in the few which appeared to recover, relapses took place soon after and proved fatal."

Extract from Dr. Pearse's Essay.

"A man who has been ill a few hours with febrile symptoms under which he may still labour, is brought into hospital by his friends, who perhaps state that he was perfectly well the day before, and that after having had a febrile attack his feet became swollen, and that the œdema extended quickly over the body, limbs, face, and even to the scalp. The pulse as in the first variety mentioned is strong and vibrating, but fuller, beating from 100 to 130 in a minute, the eyes and tongue are exsanguineous, the latter clean and moist, and the countenance leucophlegmatic. The peculiar circumstances, which taken with its being of a more urgent form, and which appear to me to constitute this as a distinct variety of beriberi, are the patient being altogether free from pain, numbnesss or paralysis of the limbs, and that there is a certain hurriedness of manner, and feeling of anxiety about the præcordia, causing restlessness, and apparent uneasiness, although if questioned there will be no particular complaint made either of pain or uneasiness of any kind. If the system be not speedily relieved by active depletion, dyspnœa arising from effusion into the thorax rapidly follows, and death more or less suddenly is the certain consequence. The urine is high coloured and scanty, but there is little or no complaint of derangement of the other functions."

"Should a case of this description take a favourable turn, and the arterial excitement and other urgent symptoms become moderated, a slight degree

In the jail at Masulipatam, two brothers from Rajahmundry were admitted with beriberi and both died, being one third of the total deaths; and in the prison at Chicacole where there were in all 11 deaths, 5 were of this disease viz.

Diseases.	Admitted.	Discharged.	Died.	Remaining.
Dropsy..........	6	1	2	3
Palsy...........	7	2	3	2
Total.	13	3	5	5

These cases I know from personal observation to

" of numbness, known by the peculiarity in the manner of walking, may then " be discernible, though no complaint is made by the patient of such an affec- " tion."

Extracts from the Essay of Messrs. W. Geddes and Macdonell.

" Those who have once had the disease are extremely subject to a relapse. " Sometimes this takes place, when the symptoms of the first attack had not " entirely been removed; numbness of the limbs, and the tottering in the " gait continuing on the patient and inducing the medical attendant of the " individual in hospital, to place him on the convalescent list for the advan- " tage of air and exercise. In these circumstances a return of the former " symptoms, or the accession of a new form of the disease is after a certain " period not unusual, and the patient is frequently brought again to hospital, " in a state which no medical means can relieve. At other times, the " symptoms become entirely removed and continue so for one or more years, " when the disease recurs, most generally under a new and that an aggra- " vated form, for it is to be remarked, that each succeeding relapse seems " to present an increase of severity and this often under another variety of " the disease."

* * * * * * *

" Shaik Hoosan, sepoy, ætat. 27. Admitted 27th December, 1828. " Had been affected for 15 days with dropsical swelling in both legs, face " rather puffed, no dyspnœa or pain in the chest. Pulse 90, skin cold and " damp, bowels costive. Had a purgative of jalap and calomel on this day, " and the day following. On the 29th the report is " complained of severe " oppression in the chest and dyspnœa since last night. Had this morning " much thirst, called for cold drink and expired immediately after he took " it."

" Seethah Ram, ætat. 50, artificer. Admitted 1st November, 1830, " 3 p. m. Had been affected for seven days with considerable swelling " of the lower limbs, attended with numbness and difficulty of respiration " on any exertion. These had been partly removed by native medicines, " the swelling having left his limbs about three days before, but the numb- " ness continued and considerable dyspnœa had seized him in the morning " of the day he came in. He also vomited his food tinged with bile once " or twice. On admission his pulse is not to be felt, his skin cooler than " natural, countenance puffed with much anxiety and restlessness, tongue " covered with a brown fur and his bowels had been bound for two days. " Calomel ℈i was given and a purging enema; in two hours had a dose of " jalap and a blister was applied to his chest, but he died at 6 p. m.

have been beriberi; 5 of the others were doubtful and 1 was shot by accident, so that half or more of the whole deaths were from it. At Rajahmundry where beriberi does not occur, there was no death.

Most of the regiments in the division arrived by sea from Rangoon the middle of the year, and their state of health compared with other corps is very remarkable. Thus the 11th regiment, 1,100 strong, for a long time stationed at Vizianagram did not lose a man, while the 22d recently arrived at Samulcottah from Ava lost 25 from dysentery, fever, &c.; and the 34th which arrived at Vizagapatam in July and at Chicacole in August, lost no man from beriberi, although otherwise sickly, 13 having died of ulcers, low remittent, diarrhœa, and dysentery. Burning of the feet prevailed in these two regiments on their arrival, but by the time beriberi began to appear, had become very uncommon. Had any cause which did not require a long time to produce its effects given rise to beriberi, it most assuredly would have appeared amongst the worn out veterans and emaciated lads of these regiments. The disease prevailed in the division at this time: in the 47th regiment N. I. at Berhampore, which lost 16 of whom apparently one half were of beriberi; at Ellore of 11 deaths 7 seem to have been from the same disease, and of the 200 veterans at the same station with the 34th, 3 died of it, or 3-5ths of the total deaths.

Of one hundred and forty-two deaths which occurred out of 7023 native troops in the division, 33 died of fever, and 25 of beriberi; a much lower proportion of the latter than would have happened in the ordinary course of the service, when a greater proportion of the men had been a sufficient time, exposed to the causes which produce the disease in these districts.

The European regiment which arrived at Masulipatam in June lost 10 men of other diseases, out of 314; while the veteran battalion at Vizagapatam lost 18 out of 303, and several of them from beriberi: but no conclusion can be drawn from this as the disease is more prevalent at Vizagapatam, and the men are more liable to it, from their broken constitutions and intemperate habits; however I can state, on the authority of the late Mr. Bond, that several deaths arose the following season from this disease in the European regiment, although one only appears in the returns.

1827.

1st and 2d half year.

JAILS.

At Chicacole during the 1st half year, 6 died of beriberi and 2 of dysentery. In the 2d half year, 5 deaths from beriberi occurred, and one of other disease, so fatal is it and not confined to any season. These were men mostly sent the preceding year from Ganjam. Four men died at Masulipatam and 3 of them of beriberi, while there was no death in the jail at Rajahmundry.

RETURNS OF NATIVE TROOPS. 1st HALF YEAR.

Total strength 8596.

The native troops were all healthy, the effects of the campaign having diminished, the season being favourable, and the corps either habituated to the country or not yet sufficiently long exposed to its morbid influence; however of 6 deaths in the 34th, three were from beriberi which had already begun to prevail, and a few cases occurred at other stations.

2D HALF YEAR.

Total strength 8600.

Notwithstanding that beriberi is now found generally in the returns, many cases of the disease still appear under other heads, and I do not think I shall lessen their value, by endeavouring to restore these to their proper place. Having seen many of the cases in most of the stations, and having compared the journals with the returns in others, I find almost every death from rheumatism, dropsy, or palsy, to have been examples of beriberi, classed under either of these heads according to the greater developement of particular symptoms, or sometimes according to the theory of this disease adopted by the surgeon. When I did not possess *accurate* information, I have ventured to alter little without noting the particulars. I found the attempt to ascertain the number of cases which did not prove fatal, admitted under other heads, to require more time than I could command; as it was necessary to read the *whole* of the journals of practice to which I had access, at a season when the ordinary duties of the regiment, and the preparation, at one time for embarkation for foreign service and at another for a march to a distant station, left no leisure which could be spared from the examination of the histories of the cases returned as beriberi, and into the cause of death in the fatal examples of diseases commonly confounded with it. The real numbers of admissions are in consequence necessarily underrated. Any excess in the deaths which might be supposed to arise, is more than compensated for by a considerable number of the fatal fevers, having been beriberi complicated with or mistaken for the prevailing remittent. A still more important source of error in estimating the comparative fatality of this disease, arises from the numbers who died in the villages, when allowed to go on leave for the recovery of their health, or were pensioned or discharged the service.

At Vizianagram the 12th regiment N. I. about 10 months from Rangoon, began to suffer from beriberi in June. Of 14 deaths, 10 were of beriberi, 2 of fever, 1 cholera, 1 dropsy (beriberi also). Two other men died of the disease who were on sick leave from Chicacole.

Samulcottah.—22d regiment N. I. from Rangoon. The first case occurred in July in rainy raw weather. Admitted 17, died 5, discharged 5. Three died of rheumatism and about 20 were admitted with dropsy of whom 2 died ; some of these were beriberi, others depending on other disease. On the whole it appears that of 13 deaths 9 or 10 were from beriberi.

Chicacole.—34th regiment N. I. from Rangoon. The returns show that 1 remained ill of beriberi on the 1st July. Admitted during the 6 months 51, discharged 19, many of whom relapsed or died on leave ; died 10, remained on the 31st December 23. Of 19 deaths the total casualties in the regiment, 12 were of beriberi[4]. The native veterans sufferred less but the cases were rapidly fatal.

Rheumatism prevailed to a great extent in the 34th but less than in the 37th at Berhampore which had yet little beriberi, having lost 15 men in the 6 months, of whom more than two cannot be referred to that disease. Eight died of cholera. It is remarkable that this corps had recently moved from Masulipatam, where the disease also prevails, and suffered after the usual period of residence at Berhampore, a fact analogous to the deaths at Chicacole, of the prisoners from Ganjam, and must be carefully attended to in considering the causes of the disease.[5]

Masulipatam.—38th regiment N. I. from Rangoon a year. Admitted with beriberi 15, of whom 6 died. Besides these 2 died of dysentery and 1 of fever.

30th regiment N. I. long at Masulipatam. It had formerly suffered and had the usual proportion of fever, but no beriberi, from which it appears that the men get enured to the cause.

Ellore.—2d extra regiment, raised in the beginning of the year 1826. Six cases of beriberi and no

4 I must remind the reader, that these statements are drawn up from the figured returns compared with the hospital journals, the results of personal observation, and other authentic sources. I returned from Rangoon in medical charge of the 34th, and the severity with which beriberi attacked the regiment having forcibly attracted my attention, the returns show more nearly the real number of cases treated than those of any other corps whose history I had an opportunity of investigating, yet two deaths occur under other heads which were really examples of beriberi. I have been recommended to give the information of these pages in a tabular form, but this could not be done in any convenient shape, without in a considerable degree sacrificing truth. Tables are only adapted for general statements involving few circumstances and not resting on evidence of various degrees of probability. See appendix A.

5 From 1820 to 1824 many prisoners died at Masulipatam from beriberi and these were mostly from Ganjam. Berhampore is 16 miles from Ganjam. Mr. Stevenson ascribes the prevalence of intermittent fever and beriberi amongst the hill and Ganjam prisoners sent to Masulipatam to change of climate and food.

deaths ; the disease being generally mild when subsiding, or when it is from other causes of rare occurrence.

The pioneers employed on the military road were very healthy, of which hereafter.

General results.

Died 88. Of beriberi 28 ; dropsy 7 ; rheumatism 17 ; in all 52 deaths undoubtedly referrible to beriberi, being $\frac{5}{8}$ths of the total mortality and 5 times more than the deaths either from cholera (10), or from fever (10). Of 114 cases *returned* as beriberi 52 are marked as being discharged and 36 remaining ; of the former I ascertained the deaths of many in the villages and garrison hospitals ; and as has been already noticed, of those occurring under other names, it is imposible to say what proportion were of this disease, as the deaths and some partial examination of journals, only give any light. One fourth of the cases *returned* as beriberi die : of fever 1 in 12 only are fatal ; of dysenteries $\frac{1}{3}$d die in natives, and $\frac{1}{4}$th in Europeans. The deaths from beriberi in this half year exceed that of ordinary years, in consequence of the much larger portion of the troops having arrived together, in a state predisposed to disease, and at a season which brought them under the influence at the same time, of the period of residence and the season of the year most favourable to the production of the complaint.

It is of the highest importance to the health of the troops, that movements should be so timed as to avoid this unfavourable coincidence. I know of no other means of prevention, at once practicable and effectual.

The following table will afford a clear view of the influence of the seasons, but as the disease depends so much on length of residence, it must be compared with a similar one for the succeeding year (page 18) to afford certain conclusions. To avoid any chance of error, when the documents did not afford the means of accuracy the spaces are left blank, and these tables are not intended to show the proportion of deaths to admissions, many of the latter which ended favourably, not being returned or ascertained to be beriberi.

Table shewing the comparative prevalence of beriberi in different months of the year amongst the Native Troops serving in the Northern Division.

Months.	Remaining.	Admitted.	Died.	Remarks.
1827.				During September three deaths occurred, of intermittent fever, of which however the admissions do not exceed those in July when none died. And in December there were three deaths from fever, and one from mercury taken to excess for the cure of beriberi.
January	7	12	6	
February	8	10	3	
March	7	3	1	
April........	6	5	1	
May		5 or 6	1	
June		Several	1	
July		8	6	
August		30	8	
September ..		40 to 50	16	
October	23	47	10	
November ..	53	17	7 or 8	
December ..	37	23	3 or 4	

From this it would appear, that the disease in some instances gets milder without any reduction in the numbers attacked. I have not been enabled to procure satisfactory evidence of the reason of the difference observed above (page 16) in this respect, but a number of observations render it probable, that while predisposition remains amongst a body of men and the season is favourable, the cases will be numerous and mild; and that on the decline or commencement of the endemic they will be few and often without dangerous consequences, if the season is not unfavourable.

The greatest number of admissions was in October, the second greatest in December.

The greatest number of deaths was in September, the second greatest in October.

Table of monthly admissions, deaths &c. of beriberi in 1828.

Months.	Remained.	Entered.	Died of beriberi.	Died of other diseases.	Remarks.
January ..	36	8	4	5	
February ..	15	5	1	3	
March.. ..	14	8	0	2	
April......	18	6	1	6	
May	13	5	2	1	
June	6	3	0	6*	* Probably one or two of beriberi.
July	5	11	4	3	
August.. ..	10	18	4	6	
September. .	19	16	3	5	
October ..	23	39	7	4	
November..	43	22	7	7	
December	27	33	8	9	See note [6].

1828.

JAILS.

1st and 2d half year.

Of 7 deaths which occurred in the jails of Chicacole and Masulipatam during the 1st half year, 3

[6] The following table will confirm the inferences drawn from those in the text; and from the length of time embraced in it, during which increased attention was paid to this disease and to the correctness of the individual returns from which it is taken, there is no reason to fear any serious error.

Abstract of admissions of beriberi, among the native troops in the Northern Division under the Madras Presidency, for 3 years, commencing 1st January 1831. See Appendix A.

1st Half Year.

January.	February.	March.	April.	May.	June.	Total.
25	17	19	27	13	27	128

2d Half Year.

July.	August.	Sept.	Oct.	Nov.	Dec.	Total.
34	68	99	90	99	54	444

Additional valuable information is contained in the following extract from the late Dr. Herklots' report for the 2d half of 1823, which contains the result of much accurate observation.

were from beriberi; and of 9 the 2d half year, 2 were from the same complaint. Three died at Ra-

Table shewing the number of cases of beriberi, which were admitted into the hospital of the 1st batt. 19th regt. N. I. since the arrival of the corps at Chicacole from Chandah (viz. March 1822) with the proportional cures, deaths, &c.

Year.	Months.	Admitted.	Cured.	Relieved.	Discharged on sick certificate.	Died.	Remaining 1st January 1824.	Remarks.
1822	March	,,	,,	,,	,,	,,	,,	
,,	April	,,	,,	,,	,,	,,	,,	
,,	May........	,,	,,	,,	,,	,,	,,	
,,	June	,,	,,	,,	,,	,,	,,	
,,	July........	,,	,,	,,	,,	,,	,,	
,,	August	3	,,	,,	,,	2	,,	
,,	September ..	,,	,,	,,	,,	,,	,,	
,,	October	3	,,	,,	,,	3	,,	
,,	November ..	5	2	,,	2	1	,,	
,,	December ..	6	5	,,	1	,,	,,	
1823	January	4	4	,,	,,	,,	,,	
,,	February ..	2	1	,,	,,	1	,,	The deceased was treated by the garrison surgeon during my absence.
,,	March	,,	,,	,,	,,	,,	,,	
,,	April	,,	,,	,,	,,	,,	,,	
,,	May........	,,	,,	,,	,,	,,	,,	
,,	June	,,	,,	,,	,,	,,	,,	
,,	July........	2	2	,,	,,	,,	,,	
,,	August	6	2	3	,,	1	3	The only death that occurred under native treatment.
,,	September ..	3	2	1	,,	,,	1	
,,	October	4	1	3	,,	,,	3	
,,	November ..	2	,,	2	,,	,,	2	
,,	December ..	6	,,	6	,,	,,	6	
	Total	46	20	15	3	8	15	

Abstract of diseases which terminated in beriberi.

	Cases admitted with	Admitted.	Cured.	Relieved.	Discharged on sick certificate.	Died.	Remaining 1st January 1824.	Remarks.
1822 and 1823.	Febris	5	3	2	0	0	2	Of the 19 cases admitted included in this table, only one was attacked with the beriberi in June, the remaing 18, between the months of August and January of both years.
	Phlogosis......	2	0	2	0	0	2	
	Rheumatismus...	5	2	1	1	1	1	
	Diarrhœa......	1	1	0	0	0	0	
	Tetanus	1	1	0	0	0	0	
	Anasarca......	3	1	0	0	2	0	
	Syphilis	2	1	0	0	1	0	
	Total	19	9	5	1	4	5	
	Grand Total	65	29	20	4	12	20	

jahmundry from dysentery, and the same number at Masulipatam. In the former there was no beriberi.

EUROPEAN TROOPS.

Total strength 944.

1ST HALF YEAR.

Twenty four deaths occurred in the European regiment at Masulipatam, none of which can be referred to beriberi, the diseases having been dysentery 5, liver 6, fever 5, thoracic disease 2. At Vizagapatam 8 died out of 262.

Total strength 1002.

2D HALF YEAR.

The European regiment lost 26: 8 dysentery, 5 liver, and 5 fever. No beriberi.

At Vizagapatam 13 died, of which 4 were from beriberi, being 2-3ds of the admissions. A number of strangers had joined the battalion. Two pensioners died of the disease in the garrison hospital of Masulipatam, shewing how much the decay of constitution from age and excess, predisposes to the disease.

NATIVE TROOPS. 1ST HALF YEAR.

Total strength 8416.

Vizianagram.—12th regiment N. I. Lost one of beriberi and 1 of fever.

Samulcottah.—22d regiment N. I. Lost 6 of beriberi and 2 of other disease.

Chicacole.—34th regiment N. I. had 23 remaining, and admitted 9; of these none died and the regiment was otherwise so healthy as to have lost but one man. The disease was evidently far milder, but much of the success in the treatment, was ascribed to the black oil having been generally used.

Masulipatam.—The 38th regiment N. I. lost 3, one of them from beriberi. The 30th regiment N. I. lost 5 from other complaints.

Ellore.—2d extra regiment lost one man only, who died of apoplexy. After long residence the men are less subject to the disease, hence the mortality in prisons [7] and corps is no index of its fatality amongst the inhabitants.

2D HALF YEAR.

Total strength 7044.

Vizianagram.—12th regiment N. I. Six deaths of beriberi, 3 being marked beriberi and 3 rheumatism ; of the former, all those admitted die.

Samulcottah.—22d regiment N. I. had 1 remaining, 23 admissions and 6 deaths of beriberi, out of 10 casualties.

Chicacole.—34th regiment N. I. Thirty-eight admissions, but only 2 deaths out of 8 casualties, (fever 2, cholera 3, and dropsy 1).

Masulipatam—38th regiment N. I. Two deaths of beriberi out of 7 admissions. No other casualty.

The pioneers and 2d extra regiment were at this time broken up.

I am afraid I shall be blamed for tediousness, in giving the facts taken from the returns of 1829 and 30, but they are necessary to complete the history

[7] Besides the circumstance here mentioned and the remark on the sickness in the jail at Masulipatam in a preceding note, it is necessary to observe that "all disorders among the prisoners are much more intractable than they are among sepoys." Mr. G. Thomson, the medical officer of the zillah of Masulipatam whose words I have quoted, and to whom I am under great obligations for his communications, professes himself unable to account for this, in a satisfactory manner. He observes that their food although any thing but luxurious is quite sufficient for them, but yet the mortality is great in proportion to other classes of natives, and he expresses regret at the disappointment frequently experienced in the sudden death at noon, of a man admitted perhaps in the morning, without any symptom which could be considered of a fatal character.

of these corps, and to show that the same influence of climate acts in all years and on men in no way peculiarly circumstanced. For this purpose it will not be necessary to go into much detail.

1829.

NATIVE TROOPS. 1st HALF YEAR.

Total strength 6867.

	Admissions with beriberi.	Deaths from beriberi.	Deaths from otherdiseases.	Total casualties.
12th Regiment N. I.	1	1	2	3
22d " "	9	2	2	4
34th " "	11	1	"	1
38th " "	"	"	2	2

The 38th had marched from Masulipatam to Berhampore in the month of January, when the weather is very favourable, to relieve the 37th regiment N. I. The 37th left 14 men ill of beriberi on marching from that station to Nagpore, where the regiment continued to suffer from the disease for some time.[8]

[8] Three or four cases occurred in the regiment during each of the years 1829 and 1830, and ten or eleven in 1831, and in 1832, whilst the regiment remained at Nagpore. In January 1833 the corps marched to Hyderabad and during that year five cases of beriberi occur in the returns. The subject of the prevalence of the disease in the interior will be noticed at some length in the Appendix B, but the following observations by Dr. Pearse of the 37th regiment are too important to be omitted in this place. After stating that beriberi is confined, for the most part, to low and damp situations on the sea coast, he observes that the neighbourhood of the sea is not necessary to its production and that "the complaint is not uncommon at Nagpore nearly in "the centre of the Indian peninsula far beyond the reach of sea influences." * * * * "And though cases of beriberi may be met with at all seasons of the "year, and in a variety of situations, they are far from being common, or of "an equal degree of severity with those which occur where the disease breaks "forth in its true epidemic form, during the continuance of a monsoon sea- "son; and it will often be found if strictly enquired into, that when it does "occur under other circumstances, and in other situations than those in which "it is endemic, that they are merely relapses, or that the individuals had "previously suffered from the complaint under other circumstances, or in a "different part of the country; no disease that I am acquainted with, inter- "mittent fever excepted, being more liable to relapse from the least ex- "posure to any of its exciting causes, such as cold, damp air, and fatigue,

Masulipatam.—49th regiment N. I. which arrived from the southern Mahratta country the beginning of the year, lost 5 from fever, dysentery, &c. but had no case of beriberi.

General results.

There were 44 cases of beriberi of whom 7 died, besides 6 or 8 under other names, being 12 or 14 out of 41, the total deaths in the half year.

2d HALF YEAR.

Total Strength, 6700.

12th regiment N. I. Three admissions and 3 deaths of beriberi. No other casualty.

22nd regiment N. I. Seventeen admissions and 1 death. Two other men died apparently of beriberi.

34th regiment N. I. Lost 1 of small pox, 2 of fever, and a 4th of dropsy.

" and I have met with one instance in which it returned every rainy season " for three, or four successive years, and with several who have suffered from " repeated attacks within the space of a few years."

To the same effect are the following valuable observations by Messrs. Geddes and Macdonell.

" Another circumstance respecting the prevalence of beriberi is, that al- " though it does not affect the natives of the country, at a greater distance, " it is said than 60 miles from the sea coast, it nevertheless attacks indivi- " duals even in the centre of the peninsula of India whose native country is " along the sea coast where it prevails, or who have been resident there for " some time and perhaps suffered from some modification of the disease on " the coast. Thus it seems to be met with in this class of persons at Seringa- " patam, and in the last year it has shewn itself with considerable frequency " among the sepoys at Kamptee (near Nagpoor), whose native villages are in " the Northern circars, or in the Carnatic; Dooly's case is also an instance of " its affecting an European at that place, he having formerly had a modifica- " tion of the disease at Masulipatam. It may be remarked at the same time, " that no instance of beriberi has fallen within the experience of the resi- " dency surgeon at Nagpore, during a period of 14 years' practice, amongst " the inhabitants of the place or natives of Hindostan residing there, and " few or no cases of this disease are to be seen among the Hindostanees of our " native corps, even when stationed in that part of the country where it is " chiefly prevalent." The extract also from the same paper given in the note at page 10 may be referred to. A servant of the author whose case is briefly noticed in the text, has suffered a relapse while these sheets are in the press, two years after apparent recovery, but he informs me, that the sense of numbness in the toes and fingers had never entirely left him.

38th regiment N. I. at Berhampore. Lost 1 of beriberi, 1 diarrhœa, 2 jaundice, 1 cholera, and 1 of fever.

The 49th regiment N. I. had yet no beriberi.

It is instructive to observe that the fluctuating population of the prisons, have their usual proportion of cases of beriberi when the corps for several years at the station are almost free from it. A few cases indeed occur amongst them but I believe principally of men returned from leave, or recruits. [9]

1830.

NATIVE TROOPS. 1st HALF YEAR.

Total strength 7752.

12th regiment N. I. Three admissions, no death.

22nd regiment N. I. Seven admissions and 1 death from beriberi.

[9] I have however known it, in a good many instances, attack permanent residents both European and native.—*Original note.*

Several observers whose opinions are of great weight, state that the disease prevails more extensively amongst the fixed inhabitants, than I have found it to do. Messrs. Geddes and Macdonell observe that " there is every rea- " son to believe, that with the exception of one class of prisoners in the jail, " the inhabitants at large suffer equally from the disease with those who " more immediately come to the notice of the European practitioners, and the " general result is, that when cholera is not prevalent, this class of diseases " forms one of the most common causes of death throughout those parts of " the country in which it is endemic. This will appear still more conspicuous " if we take into consideration the numerous chronic disorders, which in " these places end in symptoms analogous to some varieties of beriberi."

Mr. Wright of the 8th regiment N. I. in a very valuable dissertation on beriberi makes a similar statement, but in a report submitted to the Medical Board since that was written, he remarks, that he has lately observed that it prevails more amongst troops and temporary residents after being for a certain period within the sphere of action of the general cause, than amongst the resident inhabitants. No person was better qualified to investigate this question than Dr. Herklots who possessed an intimate knowledge of the language and habits of the people and of the history and characters of the disease. The following extract therefore from his report for the 2d half of 1823, confirmed as it is by the facts in the text and those mentioned by authors, is entitled to every confidence. " It appears to occur more frequent- " ly among new comers in the district, than among those who have resid- " ed in it for many years; and accordingly, it is comparatively more com- " mon among the sepoys than the villagers."

The 38th regiment N. I. at Berhampore had 14 cases of beriberi, and lost 3 of that disease, out of 7 the total casualties ; almost the greatest proportion I have met with during the 1st half year, although the corps was long in the division, which is explained, by its having moved from Masulipatam a little more than a year before ; an additional proof that a change *within the endemic boundary* has the same effect as from other provinces ; and also, when compared with the less number of cases in the succeeding and unfavourable half year, demonstrates that those liable will be attacked with the disease at any season. The period of greatest danger is between the 10th and 18th month of residence and this and other facts prove, that by moving corps so that these months may fall as nearly in a good season as possible, a number of lives would be saved.

The 41st regiment N. I. which arrived at Chicacole the preceding April or May lost 2 from beriberi ; and none from cholera.

2d HALF YEAR.

Total strength 7283.

12th regiment N. I. Three cases of beriberi and 1 death, out of 4 total casualties.

22nd regiment N .I. Fourteen cases of beriberi and 2 deaths, out of 7 total casualties.

38th regiment N. I. at Berhampore, had 17 cases, and it is remarkable that there were no deaths.

41st regiment N. I. Chicacole. Had 47 cases and lost 5 from beriberi and 6 from other diseases. During the 1st half year while this corps had suffered little, 2-5ths of the fatal cases in the jail of the station were from beriberi, and in the 2d half year, there were 16 admissions and 9 deaths in that prison, the complaint being more destructive, amongst the prisoners than the sepoys; which is not to be ascribed to the diet to which they are restricted, few of this class of people having been accustomed to such good food as they are supplied with in the jails; nor from exposure to the dews and winds at night, they being locked up in close wards from 8 P. M. till morning.

The 21st regiment N. I. at Ellore and 42d regiment N. I. at Masulipatam also suffered, and the 49th regiment N. I. I am informed, had the usual porportion of cases, but the history of these corps need not be entered on, as they exhibited no phenomena different from those already described.

General results.

Of 52 deaths during the half year, 20 appear to have been of beriberi, 12 of fever, and 4 of dysentery.

It does not seem necessary to follow up in the same manner the history of the European troops. A good many cases of beriberi occurred in the Carnatic European veteran battalion, but dropsies and palsies from organic disease are so common, that the diagnosis must be difficult, and the constant additions they receive of new subjects preclude any instructive deductions. I have reason to believe that some cases occurred in the European regiment, but if so, they are returned under other names.

Of the supposed causes of Beriberi.

It will now be convenient to enquire, if there are any circumstances in these districts, which may justly be supposed to influence the constitution, so as to produce so peculiar a train of symptoms, and such disastrous results. Laennec observes, that there are few diseases of which the cause is known, and of these beriberi is assuredly not one, notwithstanding the positive opinions on the subject given by most writers on the disease. My enquiries will demonstrate the inaccuracy of these, but will establish nothing in their room, unless the necessity of more accurate investigations, of full statements of every circumstance in the state of corps, and if the peculiarities of the station, seasons &c. however little connection they may be supposed to have with the disease; as in the investigation of all new phenomena, the essential ingredient will probably be found in some slight peculiarity, only to be discovered, by carefully removing from the enquiry, as many accidental combinations as possible. For this purpose, much more extensive acquirements and opportunities than I possess will be necessary; something however will be done to facilitate the investigations of others.

The disease is known to prevail from Ganjam to Masulipatam; and on native information it appears to occur, although rarely, at Nizamapatam 40 miles south, and instances are seen occasionally at Madras and Saint Thomas's Mount. Accurate enquiries are much wanted as to the circumstances in which it occurs in the stations along the coast south of the Kistnah, as the causes of disease, like those of other natural phenomena are investigated with the greatest prospect of success, where they can be traced gradually to cease to operate. North of Ganjam it appears to be little known, or the Medical and

Physical Society of Calcutta would not have left its history unexamined ; but explicit accounts are wanted, and especially, whether the forest tracts near the sea (see Asiatic Researches vol. xv.) by removing the population from its shores, save them at the same time from beriberi.

The district between Masulipatam and the Chilca lake, extends about 400 miles along the coast and is bounded by the sea to the S. E. and to landward by deeply wooded hills, which, except in the height of the hot weather, are the most destructive to health of any in India. They approach sometimes within less than twenty miles of the shore, but are in general upwards of 30 or 40, and near Masulipatam where the disease is comparatively mild they are at a much greater distance. From the mountains lesser hills extend into the plain country, forming beautiful and fruitful valleys ; and the whole face of the extensive flat country near the sea is studded with insulated hills or ranges of barren primitive rocks, and in various parts of the district the granite is penetrated and apparently heaved up by injected veins or great masses of trap, and dykes of green stone. There is much alluvial soil along the whole range of the coast, except where the sea encroaches on the rocky headlands; and immediately within the sea barrier of low sand hills, there are many belts of salt and fresh water swamp, which are flooded by the rains and high tides ; affording at other times excellent pasturage and a large revenue from salt. These tracts however are not often productive of disease, the soil is usually sandy, and appears frequently to have been formed by the gradual encroachment of the land on the sea, and the drifting inland of the sand thrown up by the surf. The level of the swamps is sometimes below that of the sea, from which they are separated by a narrow bank of sand hills, and the grass is always short and of a description to which injurious influences cannot be ascribed. Rice grounds (watered by tanks and cuts from the numerous rivers) abound, and there is also a considerable portion of dry cultivation and waste. Fever prevails a good deal over the district, sometimes in a malignant remittent form, which is exceedingly fatal in the jungles and the neighbouring towns. The back waters, formed by the overflowing tides and floods within the mouths of the streams, are also productive of severe disease, as at Ganjam, and during some seasons at Vizagapatam; which last is generally healthy, as Ganjam is said to have formerly been, and as Masulipatam is, although surrounded by brackish swamps, often under water but entirely destitute of vegetation.[10] The causes of these differences are little known. Dysentery and hepatic diseases are not more prevalent than in other parts of India, and affections of the spleen and severe fever are rare, compared with Bengal and the northern parts of the Dekkan.[11] Rheu-

---

[10] Since this was written His Majesty's 62d regiment has suffered to a nearly unprecedented extent at this station, but the labours of the committee appointed by the Commander in Chief to investigate the cause of the severe sufferings of that regiment, have not led to the conclusion that Masulipatam is an unhealthy station. The sickness in that regiment appears to depend on other causes, which predisposed the men to suffer from the unusual heats of 1833. It is remarkable that the present great sickness in that garrison, occurred after two years of scarcity from failure of the rains, and that in 1793 two years of famine from drought were followed by fatal fevers, attacking individuals who could have suffered no want of the comforts of life. The extensive surface of mud to the south of the fort, generally under water, will probably be found to be the source of deleterious exhalations during such seasons. The malignant fever which raged at Ganjam and led to its being deserted as a civil and military station in 1816 and 17, was ascribed by the Medical Board, to the exhalations from a similar spot to the south of the town and exposed to a powerful sun during unusually dry seasons.

[11] Of the diseases of Bengal I have no personal knowledge, but Mr. Twin-

matism is a common complaint in the northern stations, but has prevailed much where there was little beriberi, and little when that endemic was most destructive, and in few stations in India is it less known than at Masulipatam.

Of the meteorology of the circars, I am able to communicate few accurate observations. The chief distinction between their climate and that of the Carnatic, is their partaking more of the S. W. monsoon, and in the rains commencing in June and July with considerable violence. At Berhampore at the northern extremity, the hot season is very violent, but for the rest of the year, the temperature is moderate and the variations not so great as at many other stations. The following extract shows the variations of the thermometer for 5 months

"August 78° to 92°. September 79° to 86°. October (rains break up) 70° to 89°. November 64° to 84°. December 58° to 80°."[12]

---

ing's papers afford every information required. Of those of the Dekkan my own experience has been ample. *Original note.*

[12] The following extract from a report by Mr. G. Dunbar, garrison surgeon of Ganjam, on the malignant remittent fevers, dysenteries, and ulcers which proved destructive to 172 of the 1st and 2d battalions of the 6th regiment of Bengal Native Infantry, employed from June 1801 till February 1802, in the hills of the interior of the northern part of the province of Ganjam, will be read with interest. The report is dated 3d May, 1802.

" The town of Ganjam exposed on one side to the immediate influence of " the sea ; on the other, washed by the river of Aska, enjoys a perennial " salubrity which, far from extending to a great distance, scarcely affects " even its vicinity, and the opinion of an elegant historian *Mr. Orme* that " the climate of Goomsur and of the neighbouring country, during a certain " season of the year, may be ranked among the hottest of Asia, succeeding " experience and more familiar knowledge manifestly confirm."

" From different registers of the weather kept in the months of May and " June, while a detachment consisting of Bengal and Madras troops was on " service in those countries, it was accordingly found that the range in Fah- " renheit's thermometer, in the officers' tents, was from 110° to 118° ; seldom, " in the course of the twenty four hours, falling below the first mentioned " gradation. At present, the thermometer at Ganjam stands at 84°; where- " as at Aska it is as high as 102°, and will at the latter station considerably " ascend as the season advances ; although the atmosphere there be account- " ed milder than in Goomsur. Thus it clearly appears that in the months of " April, May, and June, the climate of the interior of this province is distin- " guished by intense heat, not much alleviated by the heavy showers of rain " that occasionally fall during the season now the object of attention."

* * * * * * * * * *

At Chicacole the thermometer in January varies from 62° to 86°. February 65° to 87°. During these months fogs prevail before 10 A. M.—March 72° to 90°. April 72° to 96°, winds S. W. and slight fevers prevail. May 80° to 97°. It fell in the sun on the occurrence of a shower from 126° to 80°. June 88° to 90°. These statements are taken from reports by Mr. Desormeaux then zillah surgeon of Chicacole. The following remarks on the state of the weather at that station from July till December 1822, will give a sufficiently accurate view of the climate of Chicacole for the remainder of the year, and of the prevailing diseases. This valuable document was not in the original paper, but it cannot be conveniently introduced in the form of a note. It is extracted from one of Dr. Herklots's reports on the 1st battalion 19th regiment N. I., which arrived at that station in March 1822.

"July. No. of rainy days....13
" " dry " 18
Wind most prevalent S. E. and S. W.
Thermometer, greatest cold at 6 A. M. 78°.
" " heat at 2 P. M. 90°.
" " greatest diurnal range during 24 hours 12°.

" Of the inland parts of the province of Ganjam it may be affirmed, that " there are perhaps few countries more diversified by unconnected hills and " intermediate valleys; the one clothed with wood, the other enriched with " cultivation, so that in the months of November and December the whole " presents a landscape on which the eye delights to dwell, at once adorned " by the wildness of uncultivated nature and the regularity of industrious " art; yet as good both physical and moral is generally mixed with some al- " loy, so is this beautiful and varied aspect connected with the principles of " sickness and of death."

" The showers which fall in the months of May and June and the heavy " and incessant rains in August, September, and October, precipitate from " the hills vast quantities of vegetable and probably some portion of animal " matter; which being distributed over the lower grounds, either resting in " the marshes or accumulating in the tanks commonly small, dirty, and neg- " lected, in time and by the influence of the heats of the succeeding sea- " son, undergo the ultimate decomposition of organized matter."

Diseases. Total admitted 36. Fevers, the only disease prevalent; 21 cases having been admitted during the month; of these 17 were of the quotidian type.

Of dysentery 3 cases.

N. B. None of beriberi.

August. No. of rainy days....11

„ „ dry „ ....20. During a few of these, the atmosphere was overcast and gloomy; but no rain.

Wind S. W. occasionally towards the middle of the day, shifted to S. E.

Thermometer, greatest cold at 6 A. M. 78°.

„ „ heat at 2 P. M. 93°.

„ diurnal range......... 11°.

No thunder and lightning.

Diseases. Total admitted 25. Number of fever cases diminished. Only 9 entered during this month; and the first 3 cases of that species of palsy denominated beriberi, and which has since proved so fatal, were admitted; also a 4th placed under the head of rheumatism, changed into this disease and terminated unfavourably.

September. No. of rainy days.....15

„ dry „ 15

Wind S. W. towards noon, occasionally shifted to S. E.

Thermometer, greatest cold....78°.

„ „ heat....95°.

„ diurnal range....12°.

Slight thunder and lightning occurred 3 or 4 days in the month.

Diseases. Total admitted 7. An extremely healthy month. Of only seven cases which entered the hospital during the whole month, six were trifling ones. Not a single case of fever. No beriberi One of cholera.

October. No. of rainy days......10
,, dry ,, ...21

Wind N. E. Now and then about the period of new and full moon N. westers at 5. P. M.

Thermometer, greatest cold at 6 A. M. 70°.
,, ,, heat at 2 P. M. 92°.
,, diurnal range........ 20°.

Little thunder and lightning two days within the first fortnight. New moon occurred on the 14th. From the evening of the 13th till the morning of the 17th a very heavy rain continued without intermission, accompanied with a most dreadful gale. River very full. After the 17th the weather during the rest of the month was most beautifully clear, fair, and dry.

Diseases. Total admitted 11. Not one case of fever, 3 cases of beriberi, and the first and only one case of guinea worm that has occurred since the arrival of the corps here (near 10 months).

November. No of rainy days...... 4
,, dry ,, ...26, including 6 gloomy days.

Wind N. E. with scarcely any variation. No thunder and lightning. Several mornings and evenings piercingly cold.

Thermometer, greatest cold at 6 A. M. 60°.
,, ,, heat at 2 P. M. 89½°.
,, diurnal range........ 22°.

Diseases. Total admitted 16. Fever 4; beriberi 6, including one marked anasarca in the monthly returns; and 1 cholera.

December. No. of rainy days...... 3
dry ,, ...28.

Wind, a steady N. E. wind the whole month.

Thermometer, greatest cold at 6 A. M. 65°.

,, ,, heat at 2 P. M. 82°.

,, diurnal range.. ...16°.

Delightful weather the whole month; but what is somewhat singular, it has generally not been near so cold as the preceding month.

Diseases. Total admitted 17. Four with ague, seven with that unmanageable disease beriberi, including one placed under the title of anasarca in the returns."

Masulipatam at the other extremity of the division is not in ordinary seasons so hot as Madras, as will appear by the following abstract I have drawn up, from a series of observations with which I have been favoured from the 1st July 1831 to 30th June 1832.

	Thermometer.					Barometer.			Remarks.
	Average height.			Greatest height observed.	Lowest height observed.	Average height of barometer.	Greatest height observed.	Lowest height observed.	
	At 10 A. M.	Noon.	3 P. M.						
1831.									
July......	72	87	88	97	81	29° 49′	30° ,,	29° 45′	S. W. Wind with rain and clouds.
August ..	83	85	85	91	80	29° 49′	30° ,,	29° 40′	S. W. heavy rains and clouds.
September	83	84	85	89	80	29° 47′	30° ,,	29° 40′	S. W. much rain.
October ..	82	83	83	88	79	29° 55′	30° 6′	29° 40′	N. to E. rain on 6 days.
November	79	81	80	86	73	30° 8′	30° 20′	29° 55′	N. E. no rain, fresh breezes.
December.	97	80	80	82	79	30° 17′	30° 24′	30° 10′	N. E. fine.
1832.									
January ..	77	78	78	80	76	30° 19′	30° 25′	30° 10′	N. E. to S. & E. S. E. fresh breezes.
February ..	79	80	79	86	70	30° 8′	30° ,,	30° ,,	N. E. variable—one day of heavy rain.
March....	82	83	83	86	82	30° 7′	30° 15′	30° ,,	N. to S. & S. W.
April	85	87	87	93	84	30° 4′	30° 15′	29° 55′	S. E. to S. S. W. one day rain.
May......	89	90	88	97	81	29° 54′	30° 1′	29° 40′	S. W.
June	90	85	93	100	82	29° 50′	30° ,,	29° 40′	Westerly winds. Rain from 23d to 30th.

The barometric observations were made with two barometers; I do not believe however that they are quite correct, but they will equally show the relative states of the atmosphere at different times. The moisture on the coast is always in a much more sensible state and the dew more profuse than inland; but the circars do not seem to differ from other provinces in this respect, further than their intermediate situation between the Carnatic and Bengal would lead us to expect, and neither this, nor a comparison of the preceding table with similar observations at Calcutta, Delhi, &c. published in the Journal of the Asiatic Society, will in the present state of our knowledge, afford us any insight into the cause of the disease.

After this very general outline of the Medical Topography of the division, it will be useful to enquire if there are any peculiarities in the several stations to which the returns refer, from which any inferences may be drawn.

It appears that Chicacole and Samulcottah suffered most. Chicacole is 6 miles from the sea, standing on the lower and north bank of a considerble river never completely dry, and surrounded on the north east and west by extensive flats of rice fields, of rich very retentive black soil, (commonly called cotton ground and formed from the decomposition of trap rocks), watered by nullahs cut from the river. The winds from the north are cold and those from the E. and S. E. which prevail a considerable part of the year, coming from the sea and along the wide sandy bed of the river, are generally cool. They carry much sand from the sea and channel of the river, which has accumulated in loose sand hills about the town. From one of them, the top of the minaret of a buried mosque is seen to project a few feet. The country on the opposite bank of the river rises gradually, the soil is red, dry and little adapted for cultivation. There are no remarkable hills within 10 miles. The sepoys are hutted near the river and amongst the town population, affording temptation and facility for all kinds of dissipation.

This description may be transferred to Samulcottah, without taking in any essential particular from its correctness. The cantonment of Vizianagram, on the other hand, 36 miles distant from Chicacole, is beautifully situated on the brow of a rising ground, 12 miles from the sea, and a mile from the town; and over the neighbouring country, high rocky hills rise out of rich flats or gentle slopes partly under wood or dry grain, but principally under rice. The winds are drier, fogs are less common, and from the greater distance of the sea and the nearness of the low rocky hills, both the days and nights are hotter and the daily variations less; and cases of fever are less numerous and violent. To which of these local differences the comparative health of the troops at Vizianagram is to be attributed, or whether it was in part owing to the hard drills at Chicacole usual in Light Infantry regiments, and the less robust frames of the southern sepoys of the 22d regiment N. I. at Samulcottah, much more extended observations can alone determine. Berhampore is a few miles further from the sea and I believe is more surrounded by rice fields than Vizianagram, although in other respects similarly situated, and the cases of beriberi are more numerous. Ellore is 25 miles from the sea, but the extensive inundation in its immediate neighbourhood, the flatness of the surrounding country and the abundance of wet cultivation, place it in nearly the same circumstances as Chicacole, and together with the neighbourhood of the jungles sufficiently account for the prevalence of fever at this station.

There certainly appears to be some connection between the moisture of the surrounding country and the prevalence of beriberi; but much more complete and accurate series of observations are necessary, to show to what extent this acts, in how far it is necessarily present, and by combination with what other influences it produces effects so different from those of similar or greater degrees of the same cause.

Beriberi then, prevails at all the stations on the coast and within 25 miles of it; but the town of Rajahmundry situated on the bank of the Godavery 40 miles from the sea, with little wet cultivation in the neighbourhood, and nearer the jungles, escapes the disease although suffering from the usual pro-proportion of fevers, &c. A still more remarkable instance presents itself in the Pioneers who arrived at Masulipatam with the other corps from Rangoon, and continued there for some time. They were remarkably healthy and had no cases of beriberi; a fact so singular arrested my attention and several explanations suggested themselves, but all were unsatisfactory until it was discovered, that a few months after their landing, they marched to Beizwarrah, on the Kistnah, 40 miles from the sea and were there employed in making the military road.[13]

[13] In Ceylon men of the class from which the Pioneers are recruited suffered less than others, but neither this, their hardy constitution and more stimulating diet would have protected them entirely from influences, which I have often seen to affect men, hardly differing in any respect from them.

The country in the neighbourhood is dry, and the granitic felspar rocks of the same kind as at Vizagapatam. We may therefore adopt the common opinion, that the disease does not prevail 40 miles inland. Two exceptions however present themselves. It has already been observed that the 37th regiment N. I. (and it might have been added the 47th regiment N. I. also), continued to have cases occasionally at Nagpore for some time after leaving the circars. I have seen cases at Hyderabad of the same kind, and I have also been informed, that sepoys returning on leave from the circars to Bellary and the Southern Mahratta country, are occasionally found to have the disease; probably in many instances formed before they left the Northern division.[14] The second exception is presented in Kandy in Ceylon, which is 60 miles from the nearest shore, but its insular situation and the intensity of the cause in that island, accounts for the circumstance, and will not alter in any great degree the general law which we are now prepared to state; viz. that beriberi prevails in certain districts, within 40 miles of the sea and at no great distance from mountainous forest tracts, and in which the rains commence early, are of considerable violence, and the face of the country much flooded, affecting chiefly adults and strangers from other districts and other parts of the same, who have resided from 8 to 20 months in the place.[15] This law will, I have no doubt, require to be greatly modified as our inform-

[14] I have seen one or two men long in the interior, ill of a disease difficult to be distinguished from beriberi. *Original note.*

[15] I have seen it attack two persons in one family three months after their arrival from the interior, and a serjeant of one of His Majesty's regiments had a disease very like beriberi from exposure to night air at Hyderabad. It is said that no persons under 18 years suffer from the disease; I have

ation is extended, but it will be useful at present in directing our enquiries.[16]

On examining my notes taken, when engaged in enquiring into the history of the disease at different stations, I find that the prevalence of fever and beriberi at the same time, and at Ellore very frequently in the same patient, and the constant neighbourhood of jungle tracts to the place where the complaint prevails, had led me to conclude that there was a very intimate connection between them. But on enquiry how far this was an accidental circumstance, it was found, that at Ellore, almost all rheumatic, venereal and local complaints became complicated with fever while in hospital, and that the men received from the field detachment at Ragapore, situated in the jungles, suffered much from fever, but seldom from beriberi. At Rajahmundry also, where there is no beriberi, fever is common enough,[17]

seen it in boys of 14. *Original note.* Dr. Herklots saw a case in a child 4 or 5 years old. My opinion was asked regarding a disease in a boy 3 years old who was considered to have beriberi. There was some loss of power of the lower limbs with dropsy, but the child was stated to have had a sight eruption over the body and a tumid belly, and to have been relieved by purgatives. I did not see the patient, but I do not think the disease was beriberi.

[16] Since this was written, many cases of beriberi or of diseases resembling it have occurred in the interior, and numerous histories of such cases have been furnished me by the kindness of various friends. I have not yet completed an analysis of these histories, but after deducting those alluded to in note 8, and others which are obviously improperly styled beriberi, some will remain which I could not on careful personal examination distinguish from genuine examples of that disease. The truth of the general law as stated in the text is however, not affected by these exceptions, which are rare and many of them will, I have reason to believe, be hereafter found to be examples of some of the allied classes of ill understood affections which prevail at certain times in this country. It is stated by several to whom these cases occurred, that they never before met with any thing of the kind. If the disease is beriberi, the neighbourhood of the sea cannot be considered necessary to its production, although it must still be viewed as greatly favouring the generation of its cause. Most of the supposed cases have occurred in seasons of great drought, which is singular, as it is so much under the influence of moisture. In two instances some of the troops suffered much from low forms of fever, but in others this was not the case.

[17] The returns to which I had access, showed no beriberi in the jail at Rajahmundry. I have since learned that sepoys, on detachment duty at this station from the regiment at Samulcottah, have occasionally suffered. In the medical report on the Zillah jail for the 1st half of 1830 by Mr. Macdonell, he history of a fatal case of acute rheumatism which ended in beriberi is

and in many other stations and at different seasons, there was no correspondence in the prevalence of these diseases, and both intermittent and remittent fevers, when they attack beriberi patients, generally go through their usual course and are cured by the same remedies as if that disease did not exist. We must therefore conclude, that there is something more than the influence of febrile causes concerned.

A similar train of reasoning applies to the effect of sea air and moisture, the disease being rare north of Ganjam where the rains are heavy, and the climate moist, and south of Masulipatam, where the hill tracts are distant, the soil light and the rains more scanty. Nor with the singular fact before us, of strangers from places even in the same collectorate, on residing for a time in another town where the disease is not more prevalent than in that they have left, being equal sufferers with those from the most distant places, will we be justified, in ascribing the disease to any of those great agents *alone*. The damp weather of the rainy season, while it favours the occurrence of the disease is not essential to its appearance, as it occurs in the height of the hot weather, as at Berhampore and other stations, and in Ceylon (see Dublin Hospital Reports Vol. 2d). In Malabar, Ceylon and the circars, it is frequently ascribed to exposure at night in the open air, to moist cold winds ; and most writers even assert, that new arrivals suffer from being unguarded in this respect, and Mr. Hamilton concludes from

given, but the man stated that he had previously suffered from the disease, and his liver was found enlarged and tuberculated. During the succeeding year one or two cases of dropsy allied to beriberi are noticed by Mr. Macdonell, but he states, that almost all the cases of dropsy which have come under his observation in the jail proved fatal, and that those cases which he examined after death, had been affected with extensive organic disease of the principal viscera of the chest or abdomen, principally of the latter. No case of beriberi appears in the returns of the jail for the last two years and a half

this supposed cause, that the disease consists in internal congestion. But we have seen the prisoners at Chicacole and Masulipatam, who are regularly locked up all night in close wards and are allowed sufficient clothing, suffer as much as any other class of men; and who, as well as the sepoys who have suffered at other stations, have had sufficient experience of the disease. On this principle too, it is impossible to explain the necessity of a long residence for its production.

Confusion has arisen in this enquiry, from not discriminating between beriberi and what is called "a stroke of the landwind," which is always a local affection confined to one limb, generally the forearm, or the side of the face or neck, and sometimes, but not always, attended with pain and followed by emaciation of the limb. This is obviously a palsy, arising from an injury of the functions of the particular nerves of the part, and is caused by cold and usually dry winds, from mountainous tracts. It does not prevail more in the circars than in many other provinces, nor it is ever endemic, and the method of treatment is different, consisting of stimulating frictions and blisters, and where these fail, electricity often effects a cure.

Much has also been said of the effects of various kinds of food, and Dr. Herklots enumerates a number of articles whose use he considers injurious; but when we reflect that these are standard aliments all over India, we cannot carry our deference to his experience so far, as to admit, that they can produce in these districts only, so singular a train of symptoms.

What effect the extensive use of fish may have, in

combination with other influences, I am not prepared to say; but the comparative cheapness of all kinds of grain in the circars, and the easy circumstances of many of the native soldiers who suffered, are fatal to any supposition of the disease depending on deficient and unhealthy diet.[18]

Diseases having many symptoms like those of beriberi, have been caused by the use of grain which had become diseased by the attack of parasites, either of the animal or vegetable kingdom, and attention should be directed to this, as the ears of corn are in this country much infested by them.

[19] (The following important observation by Dr. Pearse of the 37th regiment N. I. will perhaps assist in the prosecution of this enquiry. "Europeans " and the natives of inland countries of India, are " less liable to this disease than natives of the coast; " although numbers of men from the upper provin- " ces of Bengal were residing in the same situations, " and in every respect subject to the same influ- " ences as coast men, in a native corps in which " beriberi was prevailing extensively at the time, " they all escaped." At page 96 of Hunter on diseases of Lascars, the same fact is stated by Mr. Colhoun (afterwards Stirling), late first member of the Madras Medical Board, who was at that time (1800) assistant surgeon to a battalion of Madras sepoys serving in Ceylon. As this work is so scarce, that I

[18] It is mentioned in Christison's work on poisons, that a disease, of which puffiness of the face and feet, and palpitation, were amongst the symptoms, arose in some parts of France, from salt being accidentally adulterated with iodine or hydriodate of potass. I have examined some specimens of salt from the coast, and could not discover any of either of these substances; but since I met with the remark, I have not been able to procure any, which I could ascertain, to have been brought from a district where beriberi was prevailing. *Original note.*

[19] The paragraphs within brackets were not in the original paper.

could not, until these sheets were in the press, obtain a copy in Madras or Calcutta, I shall give the extract at length.

" That temperance is a probable preventive of " beriberi, cannot be questioned; yet, I have found " on inquiry, that amongst the sepoys of the parria " caste, by far the most debauched of the natives, " only one case of this disorder has occurred; " probably from their having no religious prejudices " with respect to food, and from the labour of their " families affording them the means of living better " than the other castes. I cannot as yet speak from " my own experience, as to the general proportion " of cases of beriberi, to the number of men, of each " caste, present with the corps; an inquiry into " which, may, I think, throw light on this sub- " ject; but according to the information I have re- " ceived, from my black doctor (a very intelligent " man) the proportions have been as follows. The " greatest number amongst the Mussulmauns. The " next amongst the Gentoos and Malabars; the next " amongst the Rajpoots; and lastly of all amongst the " Parrias. The two last castes have almost entirely " escaped the disease: only one woman of the corps " has been affected. Perhaps these remarks, if accu- " rate, might be explained as follows:—A certain " quantity of some stimulus (perhaps especially oxy- " gen) becomes habitual; the abstraction of a certain " proportion of which predisposes to, or produces beri- " beri. The Mussulmauns are, of all the natives, the " most addicted to luxurious living on the coast: and " have been accustomed to the use of much animal " food, and spices; which they are prevented from pro- " curing on this island, by the dearness of all kinds of

" food, by the remittances they make to their families, " by the still greater expense of supporting their fami- " lies here, or in some instances by their own parsimo- " ny. For, inadequate as the allowances of a sepoy " are, to supplying him with perhaps even the ab- " solute necessaries of life, three out of the four " deaths, last month, happened to men of some " property.

" The Malabars and Gentoos, being seldomer af- " fected than the Moors, may depend on the follow- " ing circumstances. The labour of the families of " many of them is turned to account, while those " of Mussulmauns are an invariable burthen to them; " and the poor living they are here subjected to, " has not been preceded by the use of so much sti- " mulant food, as in the case of the Mussulmauns. " The Rajpoots, who have suffered very little in- " deed from the disease, are a temperate people, " accustomed to only one meal a day, which they " can even here afford themselves, particularly as " I believe they are less generally burthened with " families, than the other castes of the corps."

To the same effect, Messrs. Geddes and Macdonell observe, that " these peculiarities have been " remarked rather more distinctly among the Mus- " sulmauns than in other casts of natives, and tak- " ing into consideration the relative proportion of " individuals of this religion, to the Hindoos; there " seems some ground for supposing, that the Mus- " sulmauns suffer more generally from this disease " than those of the Hindoo religion." I had observed the same fact regarding the Mussulmauns, but as there is much uncertainty in general impressions of this kind, I examined the journals of two corps for a period of between two and three years; and the number of sick of beriberi of each class, compared with their average numbers during the period, gave the following results.

38th regiment N. I. Average number of Hindoos for 4 years.......................... ...365
Average number of Mussulmauns.............309

61 cases of well marked beriberi occured in the following proportions.

12. 5 per cent. Mussulmauns.
6. 27 per cent. Hindoos.

34th regiment N. I. Average number of Hindoos for 4 years... 563
Average number of Mussulmauns..... 144

75 cases of well marked beriberi, occurred in the following proportions.

21 per cent. Mussulmauns.
8 per cent. Hindoos.

These statements, together with the opinions above given, fully establish the fact of the Mussulmauns suffering more than the Hindoos. The Rajpoots are not included with the other Hindoos, and in these two corps were too few in number, to warrant any positive inference; but there having been, but one admission out of 56, the average strength of the Hindoostanees in both corps, confirms the remark of Dr. Pearse, in whose corps no case of the disease was seen in that class, although they constituted, according to the information kindly communicated by Captain Haig, one sixth of the strength of the regiment. In ascertaining facts of this kind, caution is very necessary, as in small numbers accidental sources of error will constantly occur; thus one gentleman reports, that the disease seems to be confined to the Hindoos, and the books of the 38th Regiment N. I. show no case amongst the Indo Britons, whom I have found very subject to the disease. Women are also by no means so exempt from beriberi as has been stated, and I have known many of the lowest castes suffer. A fatal case, has also lately occurred in a gentleman who resided long in the Northern division.

Leaving out of view the peculiar notions, at that time fashionable, of Mr. Stirling regarding deficiency of oxygen being the cause of disease, the circumstances he mentions demand a few observations. The exemption of the lowest class of natives is not sufficiently established, and if it were, the explanation given would not be admissible, these people being seldom so dissolute as to induce disease; and from their greater poverty, when not in the public service, they suffer more than others from many diseases, to which deficient nutriment is believed to predispose. The cause assigned for the greater prevalence of the disease amongst the Mussulmauns, is shown to be insufficient by the fact, that they suffer more, not in Ceylon only, but also on the coast, where they are accustomed, as Mr. Colhoun correctly remarks, to live more luxuriously and to use a more stimulating diet than any of the other classes. The fact noticed in a following page, that the young Mussulmauns, who are mostly unencumbered with families, suffered greatly, also supports this view; and the same remarks apply to the causes to which the comparative exemption of the Malabars and Telingees is ascribed. The important fact of the exemption of the Rajpoots, will not be explained by their being accustomed to only one meal a day, (which they could afford themselves in Ceylon), and their being less encumbered by families. They are notoriously parsimonious in their habits, their whole object being to save money with which to return to their native provinces; and no class of troops suffer so much from diseases arising from hardship and deficient nutriment.

Mr. Dunbar, in the report on the dreadful mortality in the Bengal battalions, already quoted, notices as follows, the exemption of the Madras sepoys from the fatal diseases which raged amongst the Bengal troops.

" Having thus endeavoured, shortly to delineate " the more prominent features, by which the dis" eases among the Bengal sepoys were distinguish" ed ; the singular contrast to those diseases pre" sented by the native troops of the Madras estab" lishment, who were uuder the influence of the " same climate, exposed to the same fatigue, " deserves particular notice. The sick of both esta" blishments had my attendance in the course of the " same day, and the almost total exemption of the " one from the sufferings of the other, forcibly, ob" truded itself on my attention, the sick of the " Madras corps being only affected with slight fe" vers of the intermittent or remittent type, which " speedily gave way before the operation of a few " evacuants and the subsequent administration of " Peruvian bark.

" The Bengal sepoy not only shunned the use of " animal food, with the religious abhorrence inspir" ed by the prejudices of his cast; but was, during " the campaign, addicted to live principally on " gourds and pompions and other vegetable pro-

" ductions of that kind; with which the country, " abounds. The coast sepoy, on the contrary, free- " ly indulged in the use of animal food and seemed " to regard those moist and cold fruits as destruc- " tive of health.

" The Bengal sepoy was under the dominion of " that peculiar depression of mind known by the " name of the *Maladie de pays:* his fellow soldier of " the coast, influenced by no such sensation, was " generally full of alacrity and ardour. Of these " contrarieties of habit and disposition, the impor- " tance towards a more copious elucidation of the " nature of the diseases under review, will presently " appear."

There is nothing then in their previous habits, which exempt the natives of Hindoostan from diseases arising from new modes of life, poor diet, and other ordinary causes of disease.

The great contrast in mental and physical qualities, between the natives of Hindoostan and of the coast must not be overlooked in this enquiry, but one very important difference in the food of these classes, requires especial notice. The greater portion of that of the Bengal sepoys, is composed of wheat made into cakes and otherwise prepared, and they use little either of rice or any other of the grains produced in the circars; the wheat being brought, for the most part, from the interior provinces of Berar and Gondwana, by the Bringaries who resort to the coast for salt. The diseases of grain, which have given rise to epidemics in Europe, have been caused by a damp warm atmosphere, to which a low moist soil and surrounding woods have greatly contributed.* Such influences

* Christison on Poisons. Chap. 39.

are in operation in the districts where this disease prevails, but in the absence of observations bearing directly on this question, it would be premature to draw any conclusion from these facts, which however, if taken in connection with the injunction of the native practitioners to patients labouring under beriberi, to restrict themselves to a wheaten diet, are sufficient to afford encouragement, to the careful observation of the causes of disease, to which they seem to point.)

The severe sufferings from other diseases, experienced by corps which had been for years on bare rations and had been long at sea, after their arrival in the northern division; and beriberi having only appeared when the health of the men had become re-established, by quietness and abundance, would seem to refute the notion, of its depending on causes such as give rise to scurvy.[20]

[20] An observation of the same kind is made by Dr. C. Rogers, late a Superintending Surgeon on this establishment, in his thesis published at Edinburgh in 1808. Referring to the opinion of Dr. Hunter, that scurvy and beriberi were the same disease, he observes, that the characteristic symptoms of the former were wanting in the latter, and that the men of a regiment which arrived in Ceylon from England, suffered much from scurvy on their arrival, but had no case of beriberi till they had resided six months on the island. The former disease was easily cured by acid fruits, &c. which were tried without any success in the latter.

Dr. Christre also remarks (Hunter on Diseases of Lascars, page 82), probably in reference to the same fact, that " notwithstanding the similiarity of " the causes of the two diseases, it certainly is not the same disease with scur- " vy. Besides the absence of some of the most characteristic symptoms of " scurvy, and the difference in the mode of cure; the existence of scurvy " in the 80th regiment, and of beriberi amongst the Company's *European* re- " giment; when doing duty together in the garison of Trincomalie, and the " entire exemption of each corps from the other disease, is certainly suffi- " cient proof of this."

The correspondence of these opinions, with those drawn in the text from a different series of facts, when I had not seen either of the publications, strongly corroborate their truth. Several writers have ascribed the occurrence of beriberi to indolence and want of exercise, and when conjoined with the unfavourable circumstances described by Dr. Dick, their powerfully injurious effects on the constitution of bodies of men cannot be doubted. Mr. Geddes lays great weight on this circumstance and adduces various facts in proof of it. Some of them admit of a different explanation, and the assertion that beriberi is unknown amongst troops on the march, is not quite correct. Cases have occurred to myself, and the disease has prevailed both in the circars and Ceylon amongst troops very actively employed.

The qualities of the water have also been adduced as a cause, and Mr. Ridley in Ceylon and Dr. Herklots at Chicacole, found that some of the wells were impregnated with saline matter, and in Malabar similar facts are appealed to. This opinion prevails much amongst the natives, and I have been informed by intelligent men, that they had found great benefit in abstaining as much as possible from its use, and substituting milk in different forms. The known effects of different waters too, in principally affecting those unaccustomed to their use, seemed to confirm the opinions of these intelligent surgeons, and rendered it desirable to obtain precise information. It is true that many of the wells in Chicacole, as in many other districts, are brackish, but the water of the river is mostly used by the sepoys and is, in sensible qualities, unobjectionable. The following facts will set this question at rest in the negative, and show the necessity of caution in drawing inferences from imperfect and limited information.[21]

Two specimens of water, principally drank at Chicacole, were both remarkably pure. The first examined, was drawn from a well near the jail, used by the prisoners, which from being kept for some time, had a disagreeable smell, probably from animal matter. It contained no sulphuretted hydrogen. Its specific gravity before boiling was 1.0004; after boiling nothing beyond 1.0000 could be shown by the instrument. It contained a very minute portion of muriate of lime and probably of soda.

[21] J. H. Smith Esq. of the Madras Engineers, at whose request this paper was written, and to whom I am under the greatest obligations, for the many valuable remarks and suggestions with which he favoured me, took a great interest in the examination of the various specimens of water, and to his enquiries, whatever value they possess is entirely owing.

Water from river; spec. gravity before boiling 1 001.
Do. „ after „ 1.0003.

On boiling, carbonate of lime was precipitated, being probably held in solution by carbonic acid, which was driven off. The water contained a little of the carbonates of lime and of soda, and no sulphates or muriates were shown by the appropriate tests, even after concentration to one third. Eight fluid ounces evaporated to dryness, did not leave half a grain.

I obtained in November two small specimens of the water used by the troops at Ellore; the first from a well near the octagon bungalow; the other from the river,—a mere mountain torrent, usually nearly dry, which arises in the hills and 30 miles from the town, before it passes into the plains, flowing through blocks of granite. They are both exceedingly pure.

Water from well in octagon bungalow compound, spec. gravity 1.00075. Ditto from bed of river 1.0004.[22]

Two specimens of water from Vizianagram were also obtained, and carefully examined for me, by Mr. Smith, in whose accuracy I have the most implicit confidence.

They were so nearly perfectly pure, that it will not be necessary to detail the experiments by which the following results were obtained; and some minute error in the spec. gravity must be allowed for, when the quantity to be estimated was so exceedingly small, and the instrument used not a very fine one.

1st specimen. Water from a well (on the parade) generally used by the men.

Spec. gravity before boiling 1.0005.

[22] These were not minutely examined. Muriates and carbonates existed in them, but in very minute quantity. *Original note.*

Spec. gravity after being boiled and filtered, little more than 1.0000.

Six ounces were evaporated, and the salts which were in very minute quantity, proved to be carbonate of lime which had been dissolved by carbonic acid, a little muriate of soda and probably of lime. The absence of iron and the sulphates was positively ascertained.

The second specimen, from a tank near the lines of the 8th regiment N. I., was still more pure, the spec. gravity before and after boiling being only 1.0002, and the salts contained in it, in the most minute quantity, were carbonate and muriate of soda and possibly a trace of carbonate of lime dissolved in carbonic acid; so small were the quantities of these, that the usual tests hardly acted on them, previous to concentration.[23]

The water of the Godavery at Rajahmundry has a specific gravity of nothing beyond 1.0008. No trace of iron or of the muriates or sulphates were afforded by nitrate of silver, nitrate of baryta, and prussiate of potass, but a very faint indication of lime and of carbonic acid was apparent. This great river carries down during the floods which commence early in June, the debris of the trap rocks, and decayed vegetable matter derived from the forests, through which it flows for great part of its course, and has formed an alluvial delta at its mouth, similar to that of the Kistnah.

[23] A somewhat different account of the contents of the Vizianagrum water, was given by a medical friend, but the record of the experiments of which the results are given in the text are so minute and explicit, that I took the liberty of requesting the gentleman to re-examine the subject; which he kindly did, and informed me, that the water he had examined was taken from a new well, into which the rain had washed various impurities, from the building materials and plaster, and that he considered the water was too pure, to have any effect in the production of disease.

The water of the fort of Masulipatam is little used by the troops, or by any but the poorer inhabitants. A specimen obtained from a well opposite the Engineer's office, after rain, had a spec. gravity of 1.0018. Sixteen fluid ounces evaporated to dryness, left a residuum of 21 grains. The contents appeared from the results of a great many experiments, to be carbonate of lime held in solution by carbonic acid, a considerable quantity of muriate of soda, with a very little of the sulphate of soda and a trace of magnesia. The water of the various wells differ much in quality, and that of one belonging to Tungiah, said to be the best within the walls, contains only $\frac{1}{500}$ part of its weight of muriate of soda. They are, I believe, most pure during the dry weather. The water brought from Goodoor, several miles distant, for the use of the troops, is limpid, clear, without sensible taste or smell and had a spec. gravity of 1.0005. Mr. Smith found from the results of numerous tests, as well as from the small quantity of residuum after evaporation, amounting only to 4. 3 grains in 10.000,[24] that the water is of excellent quality. The few substances in it, with the exception of the muriate of soda, do not affect the tests even when the liquid is concentrated to one half, and only become visible, after evaporation to dryness, and solution of the residuum in a small quantity of rain water. Besides the muriate of soda, the salts consist of a small quantity of carbonate and a very minute portion of sulphate of lime.

From these facts, it is evident that no relation

[24] When water contains more than 5 grains in a pint of saline matter, it is generally regarded as too hard for many economical and manufacturing purposes. Bostock on the spontaneous purification of Thames' water. Phil. Trans. 1829, page 289.

exists, between the quality of the waters and the prevalence of the disease; and on the whole it is probable, that the elucidation of the causes of this singular complaint, will long continue to exercise the industry of the profession; but however unpromising and difficult the enquiry may be, every fact should be carefully recorded. Labour thus bestowed will not be wasted, even if the principal object should not be obtained, the circars affording the very best opportunities of investigating may difficult questions, connected with the production of remittent fever and other tropical diseases.

It was frequently noticed, that several members of the same family fell victims to the disease. Three brothers from Ganjam died in the prison at Chicacole, in the course of a few weeks; and many of the finest young Mussulmauns who died, were brothers or near relations of others, who had previously suffered. No one thought it contagious, but the circumstance deserves to be observed.

Ratio Symptomatum.

"Gout affords a striking proof, of the long experience and wary attention, necessary to find out the nature of diseases and their remedies, for though this distemper be older than any medical records and in all ages so common, we are still greatly in the dark about its causes and effects, and the right method in which it should be treated."* It is not probable then, that the present writer will succeed in fully illustrating the phenomena of beriberi, a disease as complicated in its nature as gout: but by cautiously distrusting conclu-

* Heberden's Commentaries.

sions which rest on this or that individual case, and by carefully combining those of many, so as to separate accidental conjunctions from established connections, he believes he will be able in some degree to advance the knowledge of the complaint; and afford an explanation of part of the confused mass of symptoms and morbid appearances, related in the reports of the Ceylon surgeons, and in other writers. Had the former of these,[23] who enjoyed such extensive opportunities of dissection, been less easily satisfied with inferences, drawn from striking but not necessary appearances, there would have been no necessity for dwelling long on this part of the subject.

I shall endeavour to establish the proposition, that the spinal cord is primarily disordered, and that through actions induced by the affections of its nerves, the other organs suffer secondarily. The very imperfect and unsettled state of our knowledge, of the pathology of the most carefully studied diseases of the spinal cord and its investing membranes, as given in the best recent works, as well as the probable inference, from the success of certain remedies to be hereafter noticed, that there is for the most part, rather a functional than an organic affection in the first instance, will lead us to expect, that an accurate survey of the symptoms, and a comparison of these with affections whose pathology is best known, will throw more light on the early morbid actions, than even accurate dissections, by individuals accustomed to observe and record carefully.

In the Medico-chirurgical Review of January 1830,

[23] I allude to the reports quoted in the last edition of Good's Study of Medicine. The papers of Messrs. Christie, Colhoun, and Ridley, are full of valuable information.

there is an interesting case, which in many of its symptoms, bears a resemblance to beriberi; and together with a survey of the symptoms of palsy, will be a proper introduction to the consideration of its nature.

Case 1st. A French soldier found his legs weak, especially the extensor muscles, numbness affected ed his feet and gradually extended upwards, while the muscles were painful to the touch. In a month his hands got numb and palsy gradually spread over his body, he had no pain of head or spine and made his urine voluntarily. The numbness declined from above downwards while in hospital, but difficulty of breathing with a quick pulse came on and he died. The spinal cord was very firm and the nerves congested. But in a celebrated case recorded by Dr. Bostock, where there was irregularity and difficulty of motion affecting only the voluntary muscles; rigidity and pricking sensations of the limbs, and affection of the larynx, no appearance of disease existed in any part.*

Palsy is little dependent, directly, on the circulating system, and nervous debility alone will often give rise to it. Its approach is frequently insidious, a portion of the body, usually the most distant supplied by the affected nerves, will be found a little numb and weak, and from this, as the disease advances, the palsy ascends. (*Abercrombie.*) The nerves of sensation and voluntary motion suffer more than those of the involuntary muscles, which however, when some parts of the brain (*Dr. Duncan, jun. Clinical lectures in the Lancet*), or much of the spinal

* See Medico-chirurgical Transactions Vol. 9. and Good's Study of Medicine: article, beriberi.

cord are injured (*W. Philip*), partake in the disease. The motory and sensitive nerves suffer in very different degrees in different cases, and occasionally, the sensibility is greatly increased when power of motion is nearly lost. Formication and pricking sensations, occur equally in simple palsy and where it depends on chronic inflammation of the spinal cord (*Good by Cooper, and Martinet's Pathology*). Spasms, ascribed to weak and consequently irregular distribution of nervous power, occur in the affected limb, which is often cold or œdematous; and in the worst cases the skin is dry and withered. There are other symptoms peculiar to paraplegia, which is usually insidious in its progress, and affects chiefly men of middle age. The lesion of the spine, whether in the boney case, the membranes, or the nervous matter, may exist long without any external signs; these are at first, only a little numbness with an appearance of awkwardness or stiffness in the motions, by degrees walking and preserving a balance become difficult, the legs cross each other and the patient requires the assistance of a stick or arm. When the disease is high in the spine, the organs of digestion and respiration suffer, the various symptoms of which may exist long before the palsy appears.[26] The urine becomes copious, pale, and turbid, its smell is ammoniacal and it deposits the

[26] See Abercrombie on diseases of the Brain and Spinal cord, 2nd edit. pp. 383, 400, 401, &c. Amongst the symptoms observed to accompany diseases of the spinal cord, he mentions the following; "difficulty and loss of speech, loss of voice, contraction of the jaw, resembling trismus, and difficulty of swallowing." "In the viscera of the thorax, there have been observed oppression, palpitation, and strong and irregular action of the heart; painful sense of stricture in the region of the diaphragm, and difficulty of breathing, which, in some cases, has been permanent, and in others, has occurred in paroxysms resembling asthma. In the organs of the abdomen and pelvis we find vomiting," &c. page 410.

earthy phosphates. Whether this happens equally, where paraplegia arises from disease of the brain, as when it is a consequence of injury or disease of the back, I am not aware that there are any observations, which would enable us to determine. Paraplegia has been, till of late, generally considered as most frequently arising from the former, no accurate diagnosis is yet established, and the deposition of the phosphates has but recently attracted much attention. However, as the urine undergoes this change, whenever the loins are injured by violence, so as to cause palsy, I am of opinion that it will be found essentially to depend on disease of the cord.[27]

If the above summary, of the most remarkable phenomena of palsy, be compared with those which are found essentially to belong to beriberi, the difference will appear so slight, that no doubt will remain, of both depending on a modification of the same proximate cause.

The disease however is peculiar in many of its features, especially in the singular affections which arise in various organs. There are nevertheless, none of these, ordinarily enumerated, which are not frequently absent during the whole course of the disease, or they appear at no fixed period, or not till the patient has suffered several relapses, and are

[27] At the time of writing the paper, I had not Dr. Abercrombie's work to refer to, although as a pupil of that eminent pathologist, his opinions were familiar to me. The following remark is of great importance. " In several cases to be afterwards described, it will be found that though there was disease in the brain, the real cause of the paraplegia appeared to be in the spinal cord; and, perhaps, it may be considered as a point not yet ascertained, whether paraplegia ever arises from disease confined to the brain." Page 337. See also Mr. Earle's valuable paper in Medico-chirurgical Transactions, vol 13. He endeavours to distinguish between paraplegia, from disease of the brain and of the cord, but the fact of both being diseased at the same time was not attended to, and in other respects his observations are objectionable.

very often cured permanently or for a time, while the original symptoms remain unmitigated. In the commencement and decline of the malady, and when it is mild, this is very evident; and even in Ceylon, where its attack is usually violent and its progress rapid, the same may be gathered from the conflicting reports and opinions of Mr. Collier and of Drs. Farrell and Dwyer; the latter of whom expressly mentions, that the thorax becomes affected, only in the latter stages.

The widely different statements of Dr. Hamilton are also important, in affording additional proof, that there is no viscus, which necessarily takes on diseased actions, although some are more liable to them than others. As the subject is intricate, minuteness in the detail and examination of symptoms will be necessary, and when no direct pathological inference can be safely drawn, it will be useful to class particular facts with similar ones, occurring in other diseases.

In several of the cases I have lately met with, there was acute pain, not increased on pressure, at the sacro-lumbar junction or last lumbar vertebra, which is explained in part by the following highly important case, to which I shall have frequent occasion to refer.

Case 2d. On the night of the 24th May, 1832, I was asked to see J. D. aetat. 50, an European pensioner* born in India. He had been 3 days ill of fever, which excited no alarm, and he had taken a purgative in the morning. In the evening, skin got hot with low delirium and insensibility. Pulse was quick and large but feeble.

* He was an Indo-briton.

A blister and cold applications were applied to the scalp, twelve leeches to the temples, and a scruple of calomel was administered. He died at 1 A. M.

Of his previous history the following is an abstract. He was ill during June, July, and August, 1830, of beriberi, attended with loss of power of the lower extremities, and on partial amendment was allowed to remain out of hospital, and used nux vomica without benefit. On 15th January, 1831, he was readmitted with pains, numbness, and swelling from abdomen downwards, and voided his urine with difficulty. Nux vomica gr. iv daily was omitted, on his complaining of startings in his legs. Nitrate of potassa, gum, and gin were prescribed, and his urine became free and the symptoms were mitigated.

February 3d. Complained of tightness in epigastrium and hurried breathing. Took acet. potassæ and spirit. ather. nitros. He derived benefit from a blister to the chest and anodyne draughts; on the 11th, pain, swelling, and numbness were greatly relieved and he derived much benefit from blisters applied to the calves of legs. He now proceeded on a journey in a dooly. The anasarca returned, and he was admitted into the hospital of Ellore, with palsy and spasms of the lower extremities, anasarca, some swelling of abdomen, thirst, interrupted sleep, cough, slight dyspnœa, and sense of load at præcordia. He passed six ounces of high coloured clear urine in the day, the conjunctiva was yellow, and the stools bilious. Pulse 88, full, and firm. He was treated with purges, cream of tartar, and treeak farook in doses of eight grains four times a day.

On the 11th he was easier at præcordia and urine was ℥ 8 in the night. 16th. Stools often exhibit a peculiar appearance, being yellow and mixed with tenacious yellow lumps, speckled white, or entirely colourless. Cough prevents sleep, spits a little and urine has increased regularly to 42 ounces. 19th. Anasarca gone, abdomen rather hard, no dyspnœa. Pulse 84 ; skin soft ; tongue moist and little furred ; pains of back and thighs towards evening ; urine ℥ 40 in 24 hours. He then proceeded to Masulipatam and on his arrival had slight afternoon exacerbations, and complained much of pains of loins, which were relieved by hip baths and warm frictions. The heat and sensibility of legs were in some degree restored by sinapisms ; mustard and the root of the horse radish tree were taken internally. In June, he had an attack of dyspnœa, oppression at chest, and throbbing of the chest. Pulse 160 full, spasms aggravated, vertigo, and slimy stools ; notwithstanding the advanced stage of the disease, bleeding did good. Till his death, he suffered from palsy and cramps of his legs and thighs, especially at night ; he had occasional dropsical symptoms and distressing flatulence ; and his urine was copious, pale, turbid, and ammoniacal. The febrile attack of which he died, probably arose from the state of the urinary secretion. The following is an account of the post mortem appearances, taken before I had obtained the above abstract of his case, and the opinion of his early medical attendants, that the disease was beriberi.

Dissection ten hours after death. *Head.* Much

fluid between the pia mater and arachnoid, and a good deal in the ventricles. Half an ounce at the base of the brain and upper part of spine. Substance of brain healthy; membranes of medulla oblongata dark. *Spinal Canal.* No water external to the theca, which was lax and contained hardly any fluid. The substance of the cord was perhaps softer than usual, and the nerves of the cauda equina appeared red, but on examination, it was found that this arose from an almost total decay of the white nervous matter, allowing the vessels of the membranes to shine through, and not from any unusual vascularity. There were no marks of previous severe inflammation of the membranes. *Chest.* Lungs healthy, but posteriorly contained spumous fluid. There were several long adhesions between them and the costal and diaphragmatic pleura. The right lung was pushed up to the nipple by the enlarged liver. The heart, its valves, and the great vessels were healthy. There was a broad white spot on right ventricle. White coagula in right side of heart and in left auricle. The left ventricle was empty. The diaphragm healthy. *Abdomen.* Liver greatly enlarged, its substance soft and easily broken down. Spleen and pancreas small. Stomach and intestines healthy. The urinary organs were in a singular state of disease; the kidneys greatly enlarged, pale, and soft; the cellular substance around them loaded with yellow fluid, and the kidney easily separated from the surrounding parts. The ureters were enormously dilated and their coats thickened and cartilaginous: on laying them open, their inner coat was red and in some places contracted. The upper part of the right ureter took a sudden turn towards the spine, and was contracted above, so as to give it the appearance of the cyst of an abscess, from which some difficulty was experienced in passing a probe into the pelvis of the kidney. The pelvis of the kidneys could hardly be distinguished, as they branched into great tubes passing into the body of the viscus; some of these branched into others, and the glandular part seemed to have been pushed outwards, and was pale and flaccid and its parts separated from each other; and dark soft points were found in the right kidney, as if it were gangrenous, but it did not smell badly. The openings into the bladder were natural. Behind the orifices of the ureters there was much hardened cellular and fatty matter, firmly attached to the bladder and ureters, but not to the rectum. The bladder was much thickened and contracted, its mucous coat mottled, and in some places, the ridges almost black. The mucous follicles were prodigiously enlarged. The urethra and prostate were healthy, and there were no ulcers or obstruction in any part of the canals. The kidneys, upper part of the ureter, and the bladder contained a urinous pale fluid, mixed with a white puriform matter, rapidly sinking in water. All the great vessels and the thoracic duct were healthy, and the semilunar ganglions and solar plexus did not differ from their usual appearance. Some of the cutaneous nerves of the thigh were healthy.

This case is exceedingly important, as it is, perhaps, the only one on record, of the dissection of an old beriberi patient; and the remarkable changes to which the disease leads, in the advanced stages, throw much light on the pathology, and evince the danger of suffering the symptoms to become chronic. The tendency to œdema was great but easily removed, and at one time effusion took place in the abdomen, and at another probably into the chest and pericardium, of which the weight in epigastrium and tightness at præcordia were symptoms; and the adhesions to the diaphragm and spot on the heart, however common, probably indicated occasional and slight inflammations which had arisen in the course of the disease.

The lower part of the spinal cord was evidently unfit for the performance of its functions, and at length induced those changes in the urinary organs, which result from injury of this part. Whether the change in the state of the nerves arose from long continued pressure of fluid, as the laxity of the sheath seemed to indicate, or on that process which goes on in parts, which from any cause, have ceased to perform their functions, I shall not now enquire; but there is no reason to doubt, that a similar affection had existed, as in the cases I have lately met with, where there was a severe and constant pain at the same part of the spine.[28]

But if this is the part of the canal which is diseased, how are those affections of the same nature occurring in the hands &c. to be accounted for? These observations are not intended to establish more than the existence of spinal affection, but

[28] After the paper was finished, the fatal termination of a very interesting case which had been several times alluded to, afforded an opportunity of examining the state of the cord, and the concluding part of the history and dissection were communicated as an appendix. This and other important facts, which will establish the conclusions in the text, are inserted in the sequel, but the course of reasoning from the symptoms and anatomy, is preserved nearly as in the original copy, as the evidence derived from the two unconnected sources,thus add an additional value to each other. I did not designate this division of the subject by the term pathology, partly from a conviction, that this term should be applied only to the established conclusions derived from morbid anatomy, and partly to afford an opportunity for a fuller examination of the symptoms.

there is nothing more remarkable in most diseases of the spinal cavity, than the rapid way in which affections of one part of it, is propagated to another. The following short case is selected to illustrate this.

Case 3rd. W. Rodman was admitted into Bartholomew's hospital under Mr. Lawrence, March 22d, having fallen on his back in coming down stairs. He complained of pain across his loins and soon after he lost the use of his legs; he could lift the arms but he had no power of directing their motions, and suffered from tingling of his fingers and uneasiness about the chest. By cupping and moxas, sensation was restored except to the feet. Mr. L. pointed out "the curious fact," that the nerves supplying the upper extremities should be affected whose origin was above the painful part. This extension of diseased action however very often does not take place, and in one or two instances of beriberi, where the pain of the spine had extended as high as the 3rd and 4th dorsal vertebra, and was accompanied with affection of the nerves arising below, the hands did not suffer.

The nerves both of sensation and motion are usually affected, but the functions of the former partake more remarkably of the diseased actions and present the most instructive facts.

While the affection is confined to the legs, whose nerves are derived from the lowest part of the cauda equina, I believe there is generally more or less affection of both sets of nerves. The patient will be seen to totter more or less in his gait, or if he is a muscular man, he may appear to walk steadily, but he will be sensible of a weakness and *tendency* to totter, or the limbs will feel heavy, a sensation ap parently arising in some measure from diminished power, although it is not entirely thus accounted for, having been observed to extend over the body and in one instance to be confined to the loins. When the upper parts of the body partake in the disorder, the different sets of nerves are more unequally influenced; as we would expect, from the injured nerves in the first instance, being combined into bundles in which those possessed of different functions must be, for the most part, equally affected by disease; and in the latter, branching off from distinct roots from the opposite surfaces of the cord, either of which may partake in diseased action without the other.

On this subject the discoveries of Sir Charles Bell have thrown great light, and a short abstract of a very remarkable case of remittent fever, will in the present state of the enquiry be a useful confirmation.

Case 4th. A serjeant, ætat. 28, in India 8 years, after intemperance, was attacked with remittent fever and vomiting; there was pain in right side and the stools were composed of disordered bile. The mouth was easily affected, but the ptyalism was bloody and unhealthy and he continued to have irregular attacks of fever. His stomach became irritable, and he was distressed with a burning heat in the hands and feet which soon became numb; the loss of feeling extended as far as the trunk, while the power of motion was unimpaired till the hour of his death. There was strong pulsation in the jugular veins, and the pulse was often quick and weak with a disagreeable vibrating jar.

Several days before his death he had a fit, which

he compared to a "strong pressure over the body"; while it lasted he was sensible and he appeared to the attendants to faint. The irritability of the stomach with eructations and oppression, general depression, cold sweats and a fear of dying continued, after the fever and mercurial irritation had nearly left him. His urine also was frequently made in his bed and he passed mucous stools; on the 26th whilst saying how much better he felt himself, he fell into a fainting fit from which he could not be roused.

Dissection four hours after death. The convolutions of the brain much separated; some water under the arachnoid and in the ventricles, and at the base of the brain. On opening the spine from behind, a great deal of water was found to lie on the back part of the theca in the neck and loins, to which it had probably gravitated, as none was found in the part of the back which was raised above the other parts, the body having been some time lying on the face. None was found anterior to the theca. There was also a little fluid within the sheath, in the loins. The nervous matter was healthy and there was no engorgement; and it was clear that the fluid must have pressed on the posterior or sensatory roots of the nerves, which were very distinct. The lungs were entirely healthy as was the heart and its valves. The liver was large, gorged with blood, and the gall bladder full of pale bile and angular gall stones. Spleen a "putrid gore." The mucous coat of stomach slightly vascular. The right kidney large and congested. The other appearances, though interesting, do not bear on the subject we are considering, nor on the cause of death, which seems to have happened in a way very like some of the terminations of beriberi, to which it had other analogies.

The numbness affects both sides of the body but not always equally, and in the early stage, very generally extends no higher than a little below the middle of the thighs and in slighter cases not above half way up the legs, and as the disease declines, successively descends to the ancle, instep, and toes; and when the arms are affected, the skin is usually sensible over the upper two thirds or half of the forearm, but in either case the numbness seldom terminates quite abruptly. In an interesting case of an anæsthesia recorded by Dr. Yelloly in the 3d volume of the Medico-chirurgical Transactions ; in hepatitis where numbness extends down the arm, and in various other affections of the nerves of sensation, the same thing is remarked. The explanation in the majority of cases is sufficiently evident, by attention to the origin of the nerves, and to the fact, that when the functions of a nerve are impaired, by artifical pressure or disease, the extreme branches suffer first and as the obstruction increases, the larger trunks in succession ; and that on removing the pressure, the functions are restored in a reverse order. If the pressure is made on the spinal cord itself, this is greatly modified, by the origins of different classes of nerves being unequally injured.

The injury of the roots of the ischiatic nerves, formed of the anterior sacral branches will fully account for the loss of sensation of the legs, and the numerous branches of these nerves which are distributed on the soles of the feet, about the roots of the toes above, and on the calf of the leg, will explain the fact that these parts are more affected than almost any other, while the higher origin of the obturator, anterior crural and cutaneous nerves explains the common termination of numbness one-third above the knee. These nerves were of healthy appearance in case 2d, and the patient had seldom experienced any numbness of the thigh, although its muscles were nearly paralytic. In a very important case in which every symptom that has ever been noticed in beriberi, was at one time or another present, the numbness was *confined* to the lower part of the *legs*, and to the *hips*, which derive their cutaneous nerves from the sciatic or sacral plexus, formed of the last lumbar and four upper sacral nerves.

From these and other facts, there cannot be a doubt that the lower part of the spinal canal is the seat of disease. I am not possessed of sufficiently numerous and accurate observations, to follow up in the same manner, other peculiarities in the affections of the nerves of sensation, but I am convinced, that careful study of these minute but important differences, will enable any one who has sufficient opportunity, to throw much light, not only on the phenomena of beriberi, but also to unravel some of the difficulties which surround the physiology of the nervous system.[29]

There is frequently diminished sensibility over the body, when the motory nerves are little affected. I believe this often arises, not from the posterior column of the spinal marrow alone being injured, but from that general law of the nervous system, by which the more delicate function of sensation is disordered, by slighter causes than the motory ; and

[29]These facts only attracted my attention of late, and afford the most certain proof of the part of the system involved in the disease. *Original note.*

on which is founded, the favourable prognosis in palsy and also in beriberi, when sensation alone is impaired, or disordered by feelings of tingling, &c. In many examples however, the distinct nature of the two classes of symptoms is evident ; sensation may continue unimpaired when the powers of motion are entirely lost, and instances occur in which entire loss of feeling has extended to the umbilicus, the nipples, and even to the neck without palsy of the muscles of the trunk.[30]

Numbness of the lips is a common symptom in Ceylon, and is not unknown in the circars : the

[30] The following extract from the history of a case of beriberi is taken from one of Dr. Herklot's reports. It is to be regretted, that the removal of Dr. H. from the regiment, the day after the patient's admission, prevented his observing the progress of the case which terminated fatally on the 6th March. The striking similarity of the symptoms to those described in the extract from Abercrombie's work, confirm in an unexpected manner the views in the text.

" Cumboo. Recruit boy. 5th February (1823) admitted yesterday afternoon. His complaint commenced thus ; about fifteen days ago had a slight *pain of left shoulder* and left extremity, both swelled, and a few days after the right lower extremity also swelled and all became painful. Since then, the œdema of the feet is removed ; but the rest of the lower extremities and left upper extremity is at present very much swelled, and excessively painful, *no numbness, has completely lost the use of the affected limbs ;* in turning his body from one side to another requires his arm and legs to be lifted and moved by an assistant, *and in so doing experiences so much pain as to scream and cry ;* bowels rather costive, appetite good, sleeps well, tongue white and dry, pulse 140 and natural ; there are three parts slightly blistered on hip, leg, and ancle, which the father says, broke out by itself, but has the appearance of having been scalded."

MENINGITIS OE THE CORD.

" In another case, the symptoms were, at first, more obscure. There was an expression of suffering with a retention of urine, but no defined complaint, except that *the patient screamed when his lower extremities were moved, and they became paralysed without loss of feeling.* There were afterwards rigidity and partial paralysis of the arms, rigidity of the trunk, and retraction of the head ; and he died in ten days. Between the membranes of the cord there was an extensive deposition of false membrane and flocculent matter, in some places four or five lines in thickness. It was most abundant on the posterior surface of the cord, and towards its lower extremity ; and there was some softening of the substance of the cord." Abercrombie on diseases of the Brain, 2d edit. page 349.

In a somewhat similar case given in the preceding page there was *pain of the shoulder* and upper part of the chest. Coagulable lymph was effused between the cord and the membranes, and these were remarkably vascular.

lower may be alone so affected.[31] This does not take place except where the diseased action would seem to have extended to the upper part of the cord and the medulla oblongata. The insensibility of the face appears to depend, on affection of the origin of the ganglionic branch of the 5th pair, which according to the latest researches, is the medium of sensation to the face and anterior part of the scalp, and partakes in all the characters of the sensitive branches of the spinal nerves; and has been traced into the column from which they arise.[32]

[31] "It was discovered that the 5th nerve bestowed sensibility on all the "cavities and surfaces of the head and face. It was also observed, that "where the sensibility of the integuments remained after the division of the "5th nerve, it was only to the extent of surface supplied by the nerves of the "spine. Where certain fibrils of the spinal nerve extended upon the inte-"guments of the side of the jaw, they were equivalent in office to those of "the 5th Nerve." The Nervous System of the Human Body by Charles Bell, F. R. S. 1830.

[32] The numbness of the face in beriberi is occasionally confined to one spot. In case 37th of the appendix to Bell's Exposition of the Nervous System, both the 5th and 7th nerves were involved in disease at the base of the brain. The insensibility was at first confined to a spot above the eye, but extended over the side of the face as far as the vertex and external ear. The integuments of the back of the head retained their sensibility; the 10th nerve of the head being healthy. Taste was lost. The cheek was œdematous. The partial loss of sensibility of the face is well illustrated by the following extract from a case described by Messrs. Geddes and Macdonell.

"Appiah, sepoy, 41st regiment N. I., aetat. 26. Admitted 12th Septem-"ber, 1832. This man had beriberi last year. Complains of pains in his "limbs, and a smarting sensation with heaviness and numbness, no distinct "œdema but the limbs are tense. Numbness extends up to his loins and he "has a benumbed spot on his forehead. No fever. Pulse 118, full, and "round, the heart's action felt all over the chest, tongue a little white, "bowels open, appetite good, tottering gait; these symptoms of eight days "standing; there is numbness of the arms to the wrist, urine scanty and "high coloured. ℞ Ol. Croton. gtt. ij, syrup. simplic. q. s. statim. *Ves-"pere.* Tinct. digital. gtt. xxx, pulv. scillæ gr. ij, mist. camphor ℥ 1. 13th "Pulse 108, not so full. Bowels purged yesterday, legs not so tense, com-"plains of smarting at the soles of his feet. A flannel bandage to his legs, and "the draught three times a day." In December the numbness was confined to the balls of the great toes. He was in other respects quite well and was discharged to duty.

Dr. Herklots also mentions a case where the numbness was confined to the ball of the great toe. The internal saphenus nerve a branch of the anterior crural is lost at this part.

Dr. Herklots notices a sweet taste as having occurred in a beriberi patient. I attended some years ago a patient who suffered from a constant sensation as if his mouth was full of sugar. His stomach was disordered but there were marked symptoms of cerebral congestion. By the advice of Dr. Abercrombie he was bled, &c, He subsequently became amaurotic. It

I have never observed loss of muscular power in the face in beriberi; it is not uncommon in local palsies from "strokes of land wind," in which the portia dura suffers, and in one instance where the muscles of the cheek and eyelids were palsied, ophthalmy succeeded, probably from the irritation consequent on inability to close the eyelids. There will be sufficient proof adduced hereafter, that the brain seldom partakes primarily in the disease: and to this cause we may refer the general healthy state of the muscles supplied by the fifth pair of nerves and the portia dura, and indeed of all the respiratory muscles not supplied with nerves from the spinal cord itself, or involved in morbid actions in a manner we shall point out by and bye.[33] Phenomena

is probable that the 5th pair had suffered in both. See case of Professor Roux. Bell on the Nerves, appendix, page 88.

The back of the head, supplied by the 10th cerebral or 1st spinal nerve is perhaps more frequently affected than the face, but the observations on this point are few and imperfect. A case will be found in a succeeding page in which the whole head was deprived of sensation.

[33] When the morbid actions have extended to the upper part of the spinal marrow, the medulla oblongata, the nerves arising from it, and from the parts immediately adjoining are disordered in their functions. Accordingly disorder of the motor branches of the 5th, notwithstanding their higher origin than the sensitive, appear to have been the cause of a remarkable train of symptoms in the following abstract of a case, recorded at great length in Dr. Herklot's report already quoted. It was the only one of 65 cases in which there was any cerebral affection.

A sepoy, aged 48, was admitted 5th May, 1823, with symptoms which at first resembled tetanus but ended in beriberi, the upper and lower extremities were rigid and bent to one side, "the jaw was locked at times, "occasionally it unlocked and at that time, when questioned, on opening his "month to reply his jaws remained open and he could not shut his month." He could not articulate but made loud noises in crying for food, for which he had an inordinate appetite. Some delirium and fever supervened and he pointed to his head. In two days the stiffness of the lower extremities left him, but some degree of it remained in the arms, for a longer time. The jaw ceased to be locked but for some time remained open and the power of articulation was very slowly recovered.

The urine was obstructed for one day (on the 10th) and he sweated much. Ten days after, the lower extremities became nearly paralytic and he could not grasp any thing firmly. There was no numbness or pain till the 13th June, when the loins were insensible, and on the 19th slight numbness extended over the whole of the lower extremities which shook under him in attempting to walk, which he did "with the assistance of a stick to prevent his falling." The jaw was stiff and opened with difficulty. His whole body trembled exactly like that of a superannuated person, but the hands were more affected than the trunk. The progress of the case till recovery and its

of a nature exceedingly analogous and strongly confirmatory of these views, might be easily collected from the detailed cases of anæsthesia and of spinal disease in various collections; and the disease of the nerves, known under the name of "burning of the feet," and those examples where that distressing sensation extends over the entire surface, affords a novel illustration. (See case of W. K). Besides the circumstances here noticed, it must not be forgotten, that the intimate inosculations of the nerves, will often produce effects difficult to distinguish from original disordered action; and that sensations are modified by effusion into the cellular substance, by the state of the circulation, and by the sensation of internal parts being referred to the surface.

In palsy it has frequently been observed, that when the motory nerves are affected without the sensific being interfered with, sensibility is greatly increased, and Dr. Cook and others point out, the occurrence of violent pain in the affected parts; for which Dr. Good attempts to account, by supposing, that the proportion of nervous influence destined for the palsied organ, is distributed irregularly to the other parts. The theory is not

treatment was that of beriberi. The black oil and various other native remedies were used.

The distribution of the motor branches of the 5th pair to the muscles which *close* and *depress* the jaw, as represented in the 7th plate of the Nervous System by Sir Charles Bell, explains the tetanic symptoms. "Hoffman mentions a boy who after a blow on the sacrum, was seized with a violent convulsive affection nearly resembling tetanus, with loss of memory, difficult articulation and delirium." * * * * "Upon the whole, however, the truth appears to be, that though symptoms strictly tetanic do accompany various affections of the spinal cord, the disease properly to be considered as idiopathic tetanus is entirely of a different nature, and that the pathology of it is still involved in great obscurity." Abercrombie on Diseases of the Brain, 2d edit. page 412.

The motions of the tongue and of the parts supplied by the par vagum and glosso-pharyngeal have been disordered in several instances. The 1st, 2d, 3d, 4th, 6th, and 7th nerves have not been observed to be injured in beriberi.

consistent with the improved physiology, which refers motion and sensation to different sources; and in beriberi, in a man now under treatment and in several others, the paralytic muscles of the legs have been tender to the touch and the skin itself numb. In explanation of this, I am not able to offer more than a hint taken from Dr. Bostock, that the nerves of the surface have more relation, in function, to the cerebral nerves of sense than to those distributed to the muscles, and may take on dissimilar diseased actions; and to direct the attention to the minute anatomy of the cutaneous and muscular nerves, in which the explanation will in many instances be found. To this head Dr. Good refers formication and other varieties of troublesome itching, and in some cases this is probably a just view of these symptoms; but in others they are combined with numbness and are only aggravated examples of the pricking of a sleeping limb.[34]

The violent pains in the limbs are of a different

[34] I have been much struck by the imperfect views of these symptoms, given in systematic works published since Bell's discoveries were laid before the public, and regret that I had not an opportunity of perusing the original papers and the appendix of cases, before the essay was written. The following extracts will place the subject in a more correct light. Referring to the case of a patient, who suffered from numbness of the left side of the face and severe pain of the same parts, with burning sensation of the left half of the tongue, supposed to depend on tumor or abscess engaging the root of the 5th nerve, Sir Charles Bell observes—" I must remind you, that upon an injury " to a nerve any where in its course, the pain is referred to the extremity " of that nerve." * * * " And you will observe at the same time, that it is " quite consistent with this opinion, that the parts which are the seat of this " morbid pain, should still be insensible when touched: for the disturbance " in the root of the nerve which causes the false impression of pain in the " extremities of it, prevents the course of sensation being conveyed from the " surface towards the sensorium." Sir C. Bell on the Nervous System, ap- " pendix, page 27.

" A portion of the skin may be the seat of excruciating pain and yet the " surface, which to the patient's perception is the seat of that pain, will be " altogether insensible to cutting, burning, or any mode of destruction." " ' I have no feeling in all the side of the face, and it is dead; yet surely it " cannot be dead, since there is a constant pricking pain in it.' " * * * " The " disease destroyed the function of this nerve of the head, as to its property of " conveying sensation, from the exterior; and substituted that morbid im- " pression on the trunk which was referred to the tactile extremities."

Bell on the Hand, page 177.

character from this increased sensibility. Every one in this country has observed, the combination of acute pain of the shoulder, loss of power of the deltoid, and numbness of the arm in hepatitis. Acute pains of the limbs, apt to be confounded with rheumatism precede many varieties of palsy, and may be confounded with them. I witnessed a melancholy instance of this in an eminent surgeon on this establishment, in whom pains in the limbs, mostly in muscular parts, but sometimes affecting the joints, preceded for many weeksthe paralytic stroke of which he died.[35] The brain was softened, effusion had taken place, and the anterior cerebral arteries were obstructed by hardened lymph.

Any irritation in the spinal canal more certainly causes pains of the limbs, especially affecting the calves of the legs. Lisfrank found pains in the lower extremities, the only symptom of a collection of matter beneath the arachnoid, and in two interesting cases of injury of the spine, when after inflammation was subdued, arnica was useful in removing the palsy, severe pain of the lower limbs followed the restoration of the powers of motion and sensation. *(Graffe in Medico-chirurgical Review).* In strict accordance with these, are a very important class of symptoms of beriberi. Severe pains in the lower extremities often precede the disease, and are very difficult to distinguish from rheumatism; they prevail most in the early cases of an endemic, generally disappear as the other symptoms supervene, and frequently return when these are removed. These pains rarely attack the joints and never pro-

[35] This termination was predicted by a medical friend, before any other symptoms appeared. *Original note.*

duce swelling or heat, although more frequently combined with pyrexia than is usual in Indian rheumatism. The calves of the legs are their most common seat, and next to these, the muscles of the soles of the feet and of the thighs, and generally both limbs suffer, but not always in the same proportion.[36] The upper extremities are so seldom affected, that I for some time thought they never were, but the following cases will show, that they do not always escape, and that when they do suffer, there are other signs of diseased action, having extend- higher than the origin of the nerves of the leg.

Case 5th. Shaik Emaum, ætat. 30, admitted 3d September, 1826, with severe pains in calves and other parts of lower limbs, as also of the wrists and elbows. Œdema of feet; slight fever; pulse quick. Bowels costive. Purgatives, and calomel and antimony till the mouth was sore, did little good; and on the fever leaving him, it was observed that he could not move off his cot. On 23d he complained of numbness and loss of power of lower extremities. Pulse was quick and slight pyrexia still continued, but the pains had gradually subsided and left him. He used Dover's powder, antimonials, stimulating frictions, blisters to calves and knees. October 5th. No better; a blister has been applied

[36] Numerous cases illustrative of these remarks might be given. Dr. Herklots in his second half yearly report for 1822, notices the cases of two sepoys entered with rheumatism, who after suffering from spasms in the calves were found to labour under beriberi. In the second of these, the numbness extended to the forearms; in a few days fever came on in the afternoon with rapid feeble pulse. There was no headache. He had an emetic and calomel. gr. vi, and slept well. Next morning dyspnœa came on suddenly, and he died in an hour. In his first report for 1823, he mentions a sepoy named Soobay-raidoo who was, by mistake, returned as ill of rheumatism. He laboured under beriberi, and had pain of the calves and loss of sensibility of all the parts below the umbilicus. He went to his duty but soon returned with severe pain of the knees and ancles. These were not removed till calomel and antimoy were prescribed, so as slightly to affect the mouth. Common rheumatism had supervened.

to loins and has caused a foul ulcer. October 9th. Dyspnœa came on suddenly at noon yesterday. Pulse was low and quick, and *he was sensible of water moving in the chest.* He was thirsty, but had no pain. Breathing grew shorter, the extremities cold, the pulse sank, and he died at 8 P. M. It appears from the reports, that a purgative did harm, and that stimulants afforded some relief to the fatal symptoms. Dissection. A small quantity of water was found in the chest, and a few ounces in the pericardium. The heart was enlarged and flabby.

Case 6th. Abdul Cawder. Admitted 12th September with severe pains in lower limbs, especially in the calves, and slight in wrists and elbows ; slight pyrexia at night, quick pulse and troublesome cough. Touching his gums with calomel and antimony did no good. October 2d. Pains better, but legs are numb, and they and the face are œdematous, and " the stomach weak." 3d. Pains gone. 8th. Face much swollen. Feet pit very slightly, but the swelling is considerable. Abdomen numb; pulse quick; urine high coloured and clear. 12th. Pains return in knees and the stomach is irritable. 15th. Fever at night, the limbs are powerless, the belly tumefied, and all the symptoms are increased. 17th. On the night of the 16th, on which day he had a dose of jalap, dyspnœa came on, the abdomen was drawn in, there was much thirst, pulse small and quick, the breathing became gradually shorter, and he died at 3 A. M.[37]

[37] A similar case is alluded to by Mr. Paterson in his first half yearly report for 1824. " Previous to our leaving Masulipatam, only two fatal cases " happened, both of which were rheumatic." * * * " The second, notwith- " standing the chief symptoms indicated rheumatism, I am inclined to con- " sider as a case of beriberi, particularly from its sudden termination. The " lungs exhibited precisely the same appearances on dissection, as those " who died of beriberi—" (effusion of water into the air-cells of the lungs).

It is evident that this case and another which occurred at the same time, were mistaken for rheumatism, which was treated in that hospital with remarkable success, by small doses of calomel and antimony, which however in no instance seemed to exert any salutary influence in cases similar to these; and purgatives, nitrous æther, &c. were evidently unequal to the cure of so grave a malady. It is to be regretted, that the valuable cases I have obtained from the same source, are generally deficient in the account of the thoracic symptoms, and in minute anatomical details. The pains returned in this instance, while the other symptoms were aggravated, and it is to be expected that this will occasionally happen.

Many complicated cases of an intermediate nature, between beriberi and rheumatism, will be met with in districts where both prevail; and I have seen rheumatic pains of the shoulder, scapula, and other parts continue unaltered, by an attack of beriberi, and recovery from that disease.[38]

[38] Mr. Lawrence remarks (*22nd lecture, Lancet Vol. 1st,* 1829-30) that painful affections of muscular parts, ought rather to be considered as neuralgic than rheumatic; and Dr. Pearse is of opinion, that beriberi may be distinguished from chronic rheumatism, by the muscles of the calves of legs and their tendons, particularly the tendo achilles, being the chief seat of pain, and by the joints never being affected. This observation is, for the most part, sufficiently correct for practical purposes, but as is stated in the text, pains in the joints (and in some cases tenderness to pressure) not unfrequently accompany those of the muscles, and correspond in their progress with them, so as to leave no doubt of their depending on the same cause. Some time ago, I requested my friend assistant surgeon W. G. Davidson, of the 43d regiment N. I., who was about to proceed to Ellore with his regiment, to observe the minute differences in these and the other symptoms of nervous disorder ; and while the preceding sheets are in the press, he has favoured me with the perusal of a number of cases, of which the histories are given with greater accuracy than in any I have had an opportunity of seeing, and furnish an important confirmation of the statements made above. I have no doubt, that much light will be thrown on the history of the disease by his enquiries.

The painful sensations noticed in these cases are of various kinds, and all more or less evidently connected with disorder of the spinal nerves. The pains of the muscles are either heavy, shooting, or gnawing, or only amount

Burning sensations in the feet and calves of legs, have been several times complained of; and although in a few examples occurring before the peculiar disease, of which burning in the feet is the principal symptom, had quite disappeared from the troops returned from Ava, there was a doubt as to its being a symptom of beriberi, subsequent observation has shown it to arise in the course of that disease, as in other affections of the nerves of the spine; and a certain relation between it and the other symptoms has been traced. In one example it extended with numbness and disordered sensation half up the thigh, and in several instances has occu-

to a sense of soreness, and are most frequently complained of in the calves of the legs; but the thighs, the fleshy parts of the foot and the forearms are also frequently affected; and if the disease has spread upwards, the abdominal muscles may be tender and easily excited to contraction; the pains are much aggravated by pressure, by attempting to walk, or even by bending the joint.

The muscles frequently feel rigid to the patient, and occasionally they are found to be hard and to roll under the skin when touched, and in one, some permanent induration of a portion of the gastrocnemii took place; there are drawing sensations, often of a painful nature, in the hams and ancles, particularly of the tendo achilles, and the joints may be stiff. In one instance, the knees were loose and as if dislocated, the muscles of the thigh being weak and tremulous, and the ancles stiff from rigid contraction of the muscles, the toes being permanently extended, and the power of moving the feet lost. Like the numbness and other symptoms of nervous disorder, they are occasionally aggravated at particular times, generally from 8 or 10 P. M. till 3 A. M; and they sometimes leave rather suddenly for a short time, but generally return in the evenings, though with less violence; and very slight causes, as eating a full meal or lying on the back, may increase them.

The pain on pressure is sometimes so great, that the patient cannot walk from being unable to bear any weight on the soles, and in one instance he screamed out when his calves or feet were touched, and in another, the heel felt as if there were a painful ulcer rudely pressed upon. The extensors do not always escape; the instep has been very painful, and in one example where the flexors were so, and the toes extended, sensations of pricking of pins were caused by pressure along the front of the legs and thighs. The connection of the painful sensations with the paralytic symptoms is very clearly seen in all these cases, but the former frequently exist for several weeks before the latter are observed, and power is restored in other instances, without the pain being removed. Numbness of the skin is frequently present, where the painful sensations are severe; or there is tingling of the surface, occasionally moving from one part of the affected limb to another, or induced by slight pressure as from the weight of the other limb; sometimes there is painful stinging compared to biting of ants, or a smarting of the surface, or a sensation as if ants were running over it, and this is even felt as if it were between the rigid or painful muscles; or the skin of thigh which is sensible, may be so affected, while the tendons are rigid. The soles of the feet were

pied the soles of the feet and calves of the legs; and has been complained of in the flesh of the latter part, when the skin was free from it and the muscles were rigid; and in another, where there were other marked signs of spinal disease, it extended from the upper dorsal vertebræ to the sacrum, over the space supplied by the posterior spinal nerves.

More accurate observations are required, to enable us to form a judgment, as to the nature of the general painful sensations often associated with rigidity of the muscles and torpor of the limb, and of that peculiar spasmodic rigidity, shooting from the limbs to the chest and obstructing respiration. It

severely pained in a case, where there was pain at the junction of the last lumbar vertebra and sacrum, and in the hollow of the arch of each foot, a circumscribed spot of thickened skin and cellular membrane formed, in which there was occasional throbbing pain, relieved by pressure. In the same patient, there was pain of the groins and thighs; and in another, the pain shot from the groins towards a painful part of the loins, along the course of the musculo-cutaneous nerves. This symptom does not appear to be uncommon. In case 134th of Abercrombie's work, it was the result of meningitis and suppuration of the lower part of the cord; and in case 140, of ramollissement. Another observation confirming the neuralgic origin of these symptoms deserves attention. There was numbness of the hands, and pain and tenderness of the muscles of forearm and wrist, and from this, the patient traced the course of a pain along the forearm and arm to the axilla, and down the side of the chest, in the course of the thoracic branches. Pressure on the ulnar nerve caused no morbid sensation. Mr. Davidson's experience confirms the opinion, that pain may be produced in the *joints* by irritation of the spinal cord. Severe pain has been experienced in the knees and for a few inches above and below, and their connection with the spinal affection has been shown, by the two limbs being equally affected, by the peculiar and agonizing nature of the pain without any swelling and heat, and by the singular circumstance, that the pain left the part entirely devoid of sensation. Pains of the same character afterwards returned to the calves and tendons, with increase of numbness and tingling in his fingers, but the knees remained " dead like a stone." In a patient already alluded to, who had severe pain of the spine, and in whom there had been numbness of the lower half of the body, the joints of the fingers were very painful, and there was a degree of loss of power of the hand, evinced by the pen slipping unconsciously out of the fingers. The pains left the fingers, but remained for some time fixed in the thumb, which more frequently suffers in spinal disease than any other part of the upper extremities. See Bell on the Nervous System, appendix, p. 160.

The sensations of heaviness appear to be peculiar, and to depend on affection of the nerves of sensation, although instances occur in which the numbness is removed, leaving the loss of power and sense of weight in the part unalleviated. It occasionally is felt, as if it were in the rigid tendons, or may occupy the soles, while the calves are painful, or after declining over the rest of the limb, may continue over the tense bodies of the gastrocnemii. It is felt when at rest, but is increased on moving; even here a relation is perceived

appears to be common in Ceylon, and occupies a place in Good's definition, but neither Drs. Wight or Herklots have noticed it in their description of the disease in the circars. The following case will show, that it is not unknown in these districts. My attention was first directed to it, by the perusal of this and other cases which occurred to Mr. Price, when Zillah surgeon at Chicacole.

Case 7th. Mahomed Saib, admitted 4th July 1827.

13th July, 1827. Is very fat; has been in hospital sometime with all the symptoms of chronic rheumatism, in addition to which, he complained of a numbness in his legs. He now appears to have beriberi; his legs and thighs have become stiff and

between it and the other symptoms of the same class, the numbness and heaviness in the legs coming on together, and both may be felt only on walking and be preceded by a feeling of ants running on the surface. In one case there was a sense of numbness all over the body on awaking from sleep, but at no other time; constant heaviness over the body (especially in the œdematous legs) was at the same time complained of, and as it declined, the insensibility of the surface on awaking, was no longer experienced. Its course was in this case singular, being at first, like the numbness, extended over the body; it left the legs with the exception of the calves, then the thighs, and last of all the face, and again returned for a short time to the left arm. The numbness in a few singular cases, follows the same course; extending at first over the lower extremities and arms, and gradually subsiding from below upwards, so that it may remain only from the umbilicus to the knees and from the shoulders to the middle of the forearms. Exactly similar phenomena are described by Dr. Abercrombie, as symptomatic of affection of particular parts of the spinal marrow, and in some of them, the general affection of the cord spread from one part, and remained in that secondarily affected after the original morbid state had been removed. In one of Mr. Davidson's cases, the numbness was confined to the knees and ancles; and in a woman in whom partial loss of power, spasmodic affection, sense of burning, and severe pain in the soles on pressure, succeeded severe labour in which the sacro-sciatic junction was loosened, there was a feeling of deadness of the patella as if it were covered with clay. A similar fact is recorded in a case of anæsthesia in the Medico-chirurgical Transactions, and may be considered as of an allied nature with the pain and tenderness of the patella in a beriberi patient. Attention to the minute anatomy of the nerves explains some of these anomalies, but many, as Dr. Abercrombie remarks, still remain inexplicable.

Mr. Davidson has remarked, that the disease always declines in the right extremities before the left. If this is a general fact, its explanation may be found in the remark of Sir C. Bell, that the superiority of the right hand over the left extends to the constitution, and "that disease attacks the left extremities more frequently than the right" (Bell on the Hand), and favours the supposition, that the cause of the symptoms is in many instances, nothing more than weakness of the nervous power.

locomotion is impeded. Pulse small and weak; urine of a red colour.

Habeat ter die haust. ex pulv. zingiberis gr. xl, spt. ammon. aromat. ʒi, aquæ ℥ iss. Liniment. ol. terebinthin.

Gives a wrong account of his symptoms, being afraid of blisters.

15th. Yesterday he was very ill, and this morning was extremely so; spasmodic rigidity of the lower limbs much increased, shooting to the chest, and obstructing the respiration and the voice; no pulse. He has no pain of the body. Died at 7 A. M.

The same symptoms occur in tetanus, to works on which I may refer the reader, for the explanation attempted.[39]

The general temperature of the body has appeared to several observers to be lower than natural. I have found it generally about 96° or 97°. When

[39] The allied nature of the cause of beriberi to that of the forms of tetanic affection referred to by Dr. Abercrombie, as arising from spinal disease (note 83) is illustrated by the following abstract of a case of beriberi, which occurred to me 6 years ago. I was at that time ignorant of the occurrence of such symptoms, and erroneously considered the complication accidental.

Dauniah, sepoy. Was admitted on the evening of the 10th December, complaining of great stiffness of the limbs and slight numbness. Occasional spasms of the whole body, brought on by any slight exertion or surprise. Jaws are at times very stiff and opened with difficulty. Swallowing any thing excites spasms. Was in hospital 8 days before with a spasmodic affection, which was removed in two days by a purgative. Pulse very small and feeble. He had a dose of colomel and a purgative. On the 13th when rising to go to stool he says he fell, and the right shoulder was dislocated. It was thought, that this was caused by the morbid action of the muscles of the shoulder. Had 20 leeches to the shoulder. On the 14th the pulse was very weak, and he had a drachm of tincture of opium with some diluted brandy; and 15 drops of the ol. nigrum three times a day were prescribed. On the night of the 19th, had difficulty of breathing and spasms which were relieved by frictions of volatile liniment. Had taken two grains of opium which he said prevented rest. Pulse was still feeble. The brandy was repeated and the oil continued. On the 23d had still spasmodic affection of limbs but the mouth could be freely opened. He could not take a full inspiration on account of a pain in the region of the heart (over which he lays his hand), which came on the preceding night. Action of heart diffused. Felt a sort of sudden catch or hardness two inches below the nipple. The pulse continued small, and the respirations 22 in a minute. A blister was applied to the painful part, and calomel and opium prescribed. The remainder of the history has been lost, but the patient recovered and is now alive.

there was fever, it has risen to 101°. In confirmed palsy, where the muscles are extenuated and the skin dry and withered, the limb is a very little colder than the body; but diminished temperature is most remarkable in more recent examples, where it is accompanied with a profuse transpiration.

Extract from case of James Hicks, Indo-briton, April 24th, for some time ill of beriberi. "Limbs cold, moist, and numb; œdema of back and legs, partial loss of power of lower extremities, tendons in hams sometimes contracted and legs are extended with difficulty, spasms of calves; urine pale, depositing earthy phosphates. 26th Heat of feet nearly restored; numbness much the same. 27th. Feet mostly warm, when they sweat they get cold. May 4th Less numbness, and cannot bear the heat of sand, in which he has been walking at noon for some days; coldness of toes and heels only, cold sweat of forehead. 19th. Legs to-day cold and covered with sweats. Vespere. Skin very hot all day. Pulse 100. Thermometer in axilla and palms of hands 101°; between soles of feet, which like the rest of the benumbed parts do not feel hot 77°, and above the knees a little higher. Temperature of the air 89. Barometer 30°. 20th. Fever left with sweating. Temperature of axilla and hands 98°, feet 91°, and says they are not so cold as before. Temperature of the atmosphere 86°. Barometer 29° 58′ Hardness of the flesh over the lower part of calves, and a cold sweat covers the part. Internal feeling of heat in right leg Says the veins are now getting a colour from the blood, and that before, they were empty." After this, while the temperature of the air varied from 89° to 93° (Barometer 29° 48′), the feet were of the same temperature as the air and the hands 97°, but when that of the air fell to 83° and it was loaded with sensible moisture, the feet were at 87° and the hands at 94°. The numbness was not complete, and slight œdema extended apparently, into the interstices of the muscles. In the progress of the case, burning sensations in the feet and calves of legs came on, but the surgeon into whose care he passed, did not ascertain the temperature. The arterial action did not seem to have been weakened in the cold parts, but the colour of the blood in the veins, as far as could be judged from that of the vessels, was not of the usual dark hue.

In a native woman, in whom numbness extended up to the middle of the thighs and one third above the wrist, the hands were smooth, covered with sweat, and felt cold like the moistened body of a corpse. May 25th. Temperature of air 89° (barometer 29 55′), in axilla 97°, in hands 94° and in feet, which felt *less* cold, 95°. The temperature did not diminish in proportion to the decrease of numbness, but there was an evident connection between them. It will be observed, that although the limb had the power of generating a certain quantity of heat sufficient to keep it above a temperature of 83°, it was not capable of raising it above the surrounding medium, when that was between 87° and 92°. The moist state of the atmosphere may be thought to account for this, by diminishing the evaporation, and Good ascribes the cold in similar cases, to the evaporation of the morbid halitus, which the application of hot bodies to the relaxed and debilitated limb throw out. The same explanation suggested itself, while these cases were under observation, but the temperature was not different when the limbs were closely wrapped in woollen, or when the thermometer was held between the soles of feet or hands and free evaporation carefully prevented; and in one case (an European) where the skin of the feet was soft and bathed in perspiration and the veins of a fine blue, the temperature was natural. The remarkable change in the colour of the veins, seems strongly to support the opinion, of the evolution of heat from changes in the blood, taking place in the capillary vessels, influenced by the nerves. To ascertain the last part of the proposition, and whether nervous influence and galvanism were analogous to each other in influencing these changes, galvanism was applied, but the imperfection of the instrument prevented a proper trial, and the patient passed from under my care before it could be remedied.[40]

The only analogous phenomena, I am acquainted with, are those observed in cholera, where the skin is sometimes colder during life than after death, and *partial* rise of temperature over the trunk is fre-

[40] The change of temperature bearing no exact relation to the state of sensation or powers of motion would suggest, that the nerves connected with the generation of heat and changes in the blood, are from a different, though intimately connected source. *Original note.* In one of Mr. Davidson's cases the feet felt cold at night, the power of regulating the temperature being lost, and this Dr. Abercrombie considers to be the ordinary, if not the only influence of a paralytic state of the limb on the temperature. With this opinion the above facts are at variance. The sensation of cold is sometimes unconnected with the temperature of the limb, and dependent on affection of the nerves of sensation, as in the sergeant, whose case is alluded to in the following extract. "Sense of excessive coldness occurred in the limbs of seve-" ral patients, but never reached (with one exception) above the knees or " wrists; in two of these instances, the coldness was experienced at night and " heat in the day; but in one case it was the reverse, the patient complain-" ed of his feet and legs feeling warm and heavy during the nights, and cold " and light during the day. In two or more instances the patients felt as if " their legs, up to their knees, were all day and night immersed in ice cold " water. The above exception alludes to our serjeant major who used to " be, for a couple of hours for several nights successively, subject to a sense " of coldness throughout his whole body, immediately after the use of any " liniment; the coldness begun at his feet and rapidly spread over his whole " frame." *Dr. Herklots' report for the 2d half of* 1823.

quently a fatal symptom.[41] The constant occurrence of cold sweats in these circumstances is not yet ascertained, and the lowest forms of collapse, according to my experience, are without them. A careful enquiry into this subject would be of great physiological and practical use.

In an abstract, by Dr. Wight, of a valuable report by Dr. Herklots on 65 cases which occurred at Chicacole in 18 months, there are some singular facts connected with the subject we have been discussing. Sixty had more or less paralysis, and in the other five, it appeared to have been prevented by the early use of remedies; in one, almost the whole body was affected, and in some, only a finger or toe; 57 had numbness of the feet or hands; in a few, a spot only on different parts of the body was affected, and in others, the head and breast were the only places not benumbed; 48 had pain or soreness; 40 œdema; 33 spasms; 11 had the gait of the sheep; 12 tottering in walking; 24 had sense of weight of "limbs or thorax" as if they were increased or had a weight attached.[42] There was a sense of

[41] Mr. Brodie has remarked, that increased heat of the body follows certain injuries of the spine.

[42] It is unfortunate that these symptoms are thus grouped both by Drs. Wight and Herklots, which renders their observations as to the nature of the symptom of no value, and accounts for opinions the reverse of each other, both professing to be drawn from experience; the one, stating "the sense of weight" to be easily removed; the other, very difficult. Sense of weight in the limbs is seldom obstinate; that in the thorax always. Dr. Herklots seldom found the thorax or pulse much affected at Chicacole, which he ascribes to the disease differing, at that station from others; but I believe this was in consequence of the early application of the sepoys, to one they must have placed so much confidence in, from his intimate knowledge of their language and opinions. No where does the chest suffer more than at Chicacole. *Original note.*

The following extract from Dr. Herklots' original report will show, that he referred to the peculiar feeling of heaviness in the limbs, although he elsewhere seems to confound the sense of weight in the chest with it. The account of Dr. Herklots' observations in the text, is taken from an essay by Dr. Wight, drawn up for the Madras Medical Society, principally from the reports of Dr. H. and Mr. W. Geddes. "Sense of weight in the legs has oc-"curred both about the beginning and towards the termination of the dis-

coldness in the extremities in 5; of biting of ants in 3; in 10, sense of tingling, which in one was only felt on standing, and then extended upwards from the soles where it commenced; and in 4, of the feet being covered with clay. In three patients there were copious sweats, of whom one had them general, another over the benumbed feet and a third, in whom the numbness occurred throughout the body and extremities in patches here and there, every where except on the benumbed parts.[43] Various disorders of the chylopoietic viscera were com-

" ease; in the latter case, when all signs of œdema, numbness and spasm " had been removed, a sense of weight and weaknes in the limbs remained " for a long time after. In several cases the sensation was compared to that " of dragging along a log of wood fastened to the legs; in one case, the sense " of weight was confined to the knees; in a second, to the scrobiculus cordis, " and in two others (both of whose abdominal parietes were affected with " numbness), to the abdomen."

[43] This curious fact is not inconsistent with the opinion, that the exhalent vessels are influenced by the state of the nerves distributed to the part; on the contrary, it shows that a relation exists between them, although it is in different cases of an opposite kind. It is important to trace the exact similarity, of even the apparently anomalous symptoms occurring in the disease we are considering, and in the most carefully studied and unequivocal cases of spinal disease. At page 364 of Abercrombie's work, there is the case of a gentleman who, in October 1827, began to be affected with pain in the lower part of the back, stretching round the abdomen and shooting into the groins. In a short time, this was succeeded by numbness and coldness of his feet, which gradually extended upwards with diminished power of motion. Benefit was derived from frequent cupping and blistering, but he soon began to be affected with spasms of the muscles of the back, sometimes resembling opisthotonos, and of the abdomen, with a very uneasy sensation of tightness across that cavity, and at times, across the lower part of the thorax. He had violent hiccup for several days. The pain of spine and the numbness extended upwards, and at length reached nearly the upper part of the dorsal region, " but there never was *complete* loss of sensation of the affected limbs; he " had only complained of it occasionally at *particular spots* and of a general " feeling of numbness and coldness." " After this he became liable to feve- " rish attacks at night, terminating in the morning by very profuse perspira- " tion, but this was *strictly confined to the parts which were not palsied*, and " there *never was the smallest moisture on the lower extremities.* He had also, " in the upper extremities, a frequent feeling of intense heat, while the " *lower continued cold* and benumbed." In July 1828, the head partook in the disease and he died comatose. The whole cord was of a pale rose colour and in every part entirely diffluent, and the ramollissement extended into the crura and adjoining part of the brain. In one of Dr. Herklots' former reports, there is a case in which severe pain and profuse sweating of the feet, occurred at the same time; and Mr. Wright had a patient under his care, who recovered from an attack of beriberi, but returned to hospital complaining *only* of numbness of the feet, which were continually covered with a cold clammy perspiration, whilst the skin of the rest of the body was *perfectly dry.*

mon. The general accuracy of this statement, as far as it goes, is confirmed by my experience. Whether the numbness, pains, &c. were present in any of the 5 instances where palsy of the muscles did not occur, the report does not notice; I have little doubt they did. Coldness seems to have occurred when there was no sweating, but without minute details no inference can safely be drawn.

On the morbid affections of the muscles additional observation is required, and from the little progress which has yet been made, in illustrating the causes of the varied forms of irregular and impaired muscular power in the genera chorea and tetanus of Cullen, synclonus of Good, and in arachnitis of the French, there is reason to fear, that much of the enquiry will receive but little illustration from anatomy.

Palsy appears to be the most constantly present of all the muscular symptoms, generally coming on slowly but now and then very rapidly, the knees being suddenly so weakened, that the patient on awaking from sleep has been unable to rise without assistance; in the majority of recent cases spasmodic rigidity is also present, and in a few, the flexor muscles were permanently contracted. The recti muscles of the abdomen, in one instance, felt hard and contracted, the patient comparing them to sticks. The cramps are most distressing in the calves of legs and soles of feet, and in one example, the muscles of the back were thrown into such rigid contraction as to give the appearance of opisthotonos.[44]

[44] The following additional observations are too valuable in themselves, to require any apology for the length of this note. Dr. Herklots describes the

lating gargles, and spread along the arch of the palate to the uvula. He had evening fever. The gums were again made sore and he went to his duty the end of February, but the arm was still painful, stiff and swollen. On the 20th March he was readmitted, with severe pain of the inner side of the left knee joint extending to the thigh, and of the elbow and right shoulder. Leeches gave temporary relief, and blisters increased the pain and irritation. The pains extended to the arms, chest, right thigh and fingers, and were increased at night and by thunder storms; his appetite was bad and his tongue white. Various remedies as wine of colchicum, turpentine, guaiac and bark were used with little benefit, and in May his mouth was again slightly affected by blue pill, tartrate of antimony and opium. In August a grain of calomel and opium were given but griped him, and the stools were green. In September, a swelling of the second joint of the third finger of right hand, which had been sometime soft, ulcerated, and left a deep white indolent sore with undermined edges. In December he was emaciated, his general health bad and he suffered from occasional evening irritative paroxysms. On the 12th January he was sent to the coast where he arrived on the 12th March; the pains unrelieved, the elbow swollen, the joint motionless, the right knee was stiff and painful, his nights sleepless and he was much wasted. He improved a little at first, but in April an abscess formed behind the knee which never healed, although it put on a healing appearance, and the right tibia became painful; he used anodynes, sarsaparilla, quinine, &c. On the 24th April vomited in the night; this was relieved by an emetic, but recurred occasionally and proved the first symptom of the fatal disease about to follow;

the bowels were yet regular. The tongue was red and perfectly clean. In May took muriate of mercury in decoction of bark. 14th June. Sore on knee painful, and the painful and swelled part of left elbow above the inner condyle ulcerated, an abscess has formed at the top of the right shoulder, and loose bone was taken from the sore on the finger. July 12th. Purging set in; stools at first dark and watery. 20th. Stomach irritable. August 3rd. Ulcers sloughy. 23d. Right foot swollen and the other knee and hand partook of the diseased actions. 28th. Stools frequent, copious, liquid, light coloured and passed without straining. Pains about the umbilicus increased on pressure and vomiting. Pulse quick and feeble. Urine high. September 1st. Stools scanty, watery *and white*, vomits thick clotted greenish matter. Purging was relieved by opium, chalk, and Dover's powder. 15th. Vomiting, and frequent scanty stools at night; they are occasionally greenish and mixed with mucus. Died exhausted on the 26th September. In a good many instances ulceration of the skin is not, as in the above example, a local disease depending on that of the subjacent parts, but is caused by the constitutional disorder. The ulceration is commonly slow, indolent, superficial, the edges thick and white, and heals at one side or in the centre and extends at the opposite margin or all round the edges. The upper and lower extremities are equally liable, and sometimes the ulcers form over the trunk. In two cases they took on a phagedenic appearance, destroying the muscles, laying open the veins of the inner side of the arm, and killing the patient by repeated hæmorrhage. The following case I saw after the ulcers had healed, and was favoured with a notice of his former history by the surgeon under whom the disease commenced, and by whom he was sent to the coast. The careful enquiries that gentleman* has long been making, into the constitutions in which Indian diseases most prevail and into the succession of these to one another, is a guarantee of the correctness of the opinion he gives, as to the absence of the ordinary causes to which we would be inclined to ascribe the disease.

Case 27th. A very corpulent man of florid habit but without mental energy was subject during 1828 to rheumatism: the end of 1829 the tendency to unhealthy ulceration commenced over the lower extremities, chest and arms; there were also nodular swellings on the bones, irregular febrile exacerbations and tendency to looseness. In January 1832 he was sent to the coast where he arrived in March. Fulness, pain and hardness with tumid belly came on during the journey; the legs were œdematous; the wrist swollen and the pains severe from 7 P. M. till midnight; severe pain shooting through the diaphragm. Ease after eating hot things. Tongue scarlet red, and moist. He was temporarily relieved by blisters, baths and Dover's powder, but they weakened him: the urine was red and scanty and abdominal fluctuation was distinct. Cold sweats towards morning. Bowels costive and stools dark. Liver projects beyond the edge of the ribs. April 11th. Severe pain in the lower part of thorax worse at night,, pulse 120, very soft; vomiting, urine muddy, pale or yellow with occasional copious white deposit. 26th. Stools frequent, of various colours, watery, pale, or composed of mucus tinged with blood, or green with clusters of white subtance embedded in transparent mucus. Vomiting. Four ounces of blood were drawn, which coa-

* Surgeon W. Geddes.

gulated firmly and had little serum. He died the end of May. *Dissection.* The brain was healthy, as were the contents of the spinal canal, which contained only a very little fluid such as is often found in chronic disease. Heart small, pale and flaccid. Lungs healthy. Mucous membrane of the œsophagus dark and that of intestines thin, with dark tints and slight excoriation. Great engorgement near the cæcum. Colon livid, with marks of old ulcers. Liver enormously enlarged and all its fissures very deep, the substance having increased without encroaching on them. The great fissure was almost a complete canal into which the finger could be pressed during life, and gave the feel of a collection of fluid, through which the aorta could be felt to pulsate. On the surface of the organ there were some nine or ten deep scarlike irregular fissures, from some of which fibrous processes penetrated into the substance of the liver; but that they were not real scars appeared from some natural hepatic substance being found close to some of them, from large healthy vessels passing through them, and from others not penetrating the substance of the viscus, which was seen to be *healthy immediately below them.* The structure of the liver was altered: it was partly changed into a pale white gristly substance, in which minute orange red spots were seen with a magnifier, or numerous white waved lines separated small portions of the natural hepatic matter. The convexity of the organ felt soft like wet sand, but contained no matter; the lower and back part tore like rotten leather. It appeared to me from the examination of this liver, that the marks usually considered as the scars of old abscesses are formed, by the irregular enlargement of the organ caused by its shape, the position of large vessels, and the change of old or deposit of new parts less susceptible of distension. Inflammation may cause this, and the change has also appeared to act as an excitement of the vessels of the peritoneum, thickening it over the depression. Since the notes of this case and the conclusions suggested by it and others were recorded, I have had the pleasure of finding, that Dr. Bright has noticed the appearance and cause of the marks in nearly the same words. The white substance is probably *cholesterine* found in these livers by Dr. Bostock, and the orange deposit was perhaps of the same nature as that found by him in the bile, which was deficient of its usual ingredients. It appears that in chronic disease of this kind adhesions are rarely formed, and the liver protrudes downwards instead of towards the thorax as in acute cases. The kidneys were dark and gorged, and part of the right embedded in the enlarged liver. The coats of the urinary passages were pretty natural. The urine had deposited much white matters. A case hardly differing in any respect from the above was under treatment at the same time; he had laboured under rheumatism, got sores over the body, which had not healed at the inner part of the left arm, his pulse was frequent, feeble and irritable, there was a red patch without fur on the tongue and a red streak in its centre, the urine was pale, copious, generally with white deposit, not coagulable by heat and of sp. gr. of 1012. Some effusion took place in the abdomen, the liver became painful and greatly enlarged, and the pains in the arms and legs were severe. He had profuse sweats at night, and diaphoretics were injurious. He was several times bled, and the blood was buffy and cupped with much serum, apparently from the rheumatic diathesis, rather than the slow hepatic inflammation; accordingly, the evacuations gave no relief, but his health did not seem to be injured by them, although they caused increased paleness of the countenance, and probably did ultimate injury. The stools were at first pale and of natural consistence and frequency; ultimately he was purged, and stools were slimy with traces of blood, there was tenderness about the umbilicus and in right iliac region, enlargement in epigastrium, swelled glands in the neck; and swellings of the bones under the scars of the old sores began to form, when he was sent to another station. I have little doubt that he died soon after.

Abscesses seen rarely to form, notwithstanding the extensive disease of the liver, but in one man who had long suffered from rheumatism of the joints, puffy abdomen, and occasional purging of pale yeasty stools; after recovery consequent on residence on the coast, the liver took on subacute inflammation and ended in extensive suppuration. It was, however, probably a distinct affection, although no doubt the previous disease predisposed to unhealthy action.

Obstruction and chronic enlargement of the liver and disease of the hollow abdominal viscera, are well known to follow long continued gout, and Broussais has asserted it to be a gastro-enterite with a developement "of irritation in the joints;" an assertion which may be reversed, and applied with more justice to many forms of Indian rheumatism. If the conjunction of the external and internal disease had been accidental, it is not probable that so many remarkable cases corresponding in their principal features should have been seen by one individual,[16] in a comparatively

[16] I proposed giving some cases of natives with similar terminations, but the paper is already too long. *Original note.*

short period; and the numerous instances in which the health was broken by long continued rheumatism, in which symptoms evidently of the same nature though in a less degree occured, confirmed the evidence of a pathological connection. It does not seem to be confined to any particular district, although comparatively rare in stations, where simple rheumatism is little prevalent and mild. The very accurate and careful observer who communicated the early history of the last two cases, in allusion to the ulceration succeeding rheumatism observes, "that there is a class of diseases connected with a peculiar cachectic state of the body in this country, which have not as yet been sufficiently pointed out;" which so far confirms my remarks on the subject, by shewing that there has been little attention paid to it. Nor will it appear improbable, that in a climate in which the original affection differs so widely from that of Europe; in which the known complications especially that of pericarditis is so seldom present, and then in a different form; and where the liver and abdominal mucous membrane are so prone to disease, that they shouldbe liable to take on secondary morbid actions. Some remarkable cases have occurred, in which a still greater variety of tissues have in succession been altered in structure or disordered in function, but the details are too voluminous to be introduced at present. A slight notice of two will conclude the subject. A man subject to rheumatism got pain in the cardiac region, tenderness between the ribs to pressure and some other symptoms, which were thought to be caused by chronic pericarditis. He then suffered from cough, viscid expectoration, irritable stomach, rejection of some small dark clots of blood either from the chest or from the œsophagus, on food passing through which there was pain and obstruction.[17] After some months the affection of the heart was aggravated, and a swelling formed in the groin which pulsated violently and had so much the appearance of an aneurism, that it was only distinguished from that disease, by feeling the artery on strong pressure, to be for an inch as if included in a hard cylinder painful to the touch, and probably formed by inflammation of the sheath of the vessel. The loins, right hip, and thigh became violently painful and the latter permanently flexed, a very hard circumscribed moveable swelling which did not appear to be connected with the colon and over which there was tenderness, was detected above Poupart's ligament; on the pains being alleviated, oppression at the chest recurred, bowel complaint, and discharge and violent pain of the ear succeeded, and with aggravation of the original symptoms have completely broken his constitution.[18]

The following is more instructive, as showing the tendency to sudden metastasis of diseased actions, in some respects analogous to those we have been con-

[17] In a man of the name of Connors who was long subject to rheumatism, difficulty in swallowing and afterwards loss of power of the right arm occured. Symptoms like those of palsy may arise from and be mistaken for rheumatism, but a mistake of an opposite description is more common. *Original note.*

[18] This patient died on the 2nd May 1833, soon after the paper was transmitted to the Board, having derived no benefit from blisters and moxas to the loins and hips, extract of conium and Dover's powder, iodine, and whatever other means seemed to afford a hope of alleviating his sufferings. The moxas to the hip caused troublesome ulcers, and sores formed over the sacrum. The body was examined 4½ hours after death.

Spine. Fatty matter external to the sheath, from 6th to 11th dorsal vertebræ posteriorly, and a slight deposit of lymph opposite to the 5th lumbar vertebra. Within the lumbar vertebræ there was a quantity of bloody fluid, of which a good deal was also found within the sheath, round the cauda equina. *Head.* Some congestion of the vessels of the brain and red points on cutting into its substance, with slight effusion below the arachnoid and in the ventricles. Considerable vascularity at the base of the cerebrum and cerebellum. *Thorax.* Numerous strong adhesions of the lungs to the pleura costalis, particularly at the upper parts; many minute tubercles in their substance, a few of which contained pus. The pericardium contained a good deal of fluid, but neither it or the heart were diseased. The valves were healthy. A loose cellular substance hung from the root of the aorta, apparent-

with the severe pain experienced in some cases, in the situation of the cul de sac formed by the junction of the membranes; it may safely be proposed, as a probable inference, that the sheath of the cord partakes principally in the disorder, and that through the continuity of the arachnoid, the morbid action is communicated to the proper membrane of the spinal marrow and nerves.

A careful study of the symptoms, and of the general anatomy of the parts, will not often greatly mislead the practical observer; and an hypothesis derived from evidence of this kind, whether it is confirmed or modified by future observation, by directing enquiry and preventing our being presented with vague statements of morbid appearances such as have, as yet, only been laid before the public in this disease, gives a value to individual facts which they would not otherwise possess. That above given will, I believe, be rendered more probable by some of the complications we shall have presently to consider; and the morbid appearances in the succeeding cases, corresponding as they do with these enquiries, are invested with an importance they would not otherwise possess.

Irritation of the vertebral column communicated to the cord, is attended with some symptoms resembling beriberi, but there is much less paralytic affection, and the spinous processes are tender to pressure; this has not occurred when there was pain in the spine in beriberi, which confirms the opinion that the membranes are the parts affected. By a reference to Bichat's work already quoted, the sheath of the cord will be found to be a compound membrane, partaking of the qualities of the fibro serous structures, and readily taking on similar diseased actions as others of the same class, or of the simple ones of which it is formed. One remarkable exception to this exists, in the fibro serous structure of the joints, which do not sympathise with others of the same class, in dropsical affections ; a fact, perhaps analogous to the diminished secretion of the joints, which appears to cause that peculiar cracking sound in the knees, occasionally heard in beriberi, and which, as it continues long in patients otherwise thought to be cured, affords, when minutely watched, some useful indications.

The following case, I consider to be of great importance in relation to the preceding observations, and therefore offer no apology for extracting from the hospital journal, as much of the history as is necessary to the understanding of the morbid appearances.

Case 10th. November 25th, 1832. W. K., an European soldier, in India 5 years. Admitted last night complaining of pain and great tenderness at pit of stomach, where there are occasional palpitations ; action of the heart was extremely strong in the cardiac and epigastric regions. He was bled to 16 oz. which were natural, and he experienced great relief; the pulsation nearly ceased and he felt much lighter. Pulse on admission was 108, firm and sharp, now 100 ; epigastrium tender, action of heart heard over the left side of chest, and can be felt jarring against the hand, a little above the nipple and in epigastrium. Lungs are freely traversed, unless for some way round the cardiac region. Dyspnœa on exertion only. Is easiest in the recumbent posture and on the right side. Urine acid, red, clear, scanty, and made with pain, but never obstructed. Pain and tenderness in the region of the bladder, œdema on admission as high as the pelvis,—now confined to the shins. He had severe internal pain, without tenderness, of the sacro-lumbar region for many months, followed by change in the urine. The affection of the chest has been coming on for two months. For four days there has been a feeling of sleeping and numbness of thighs and legs with soreness of the flesh, especially of the *left leg*. He does not totter in his walk. Had eight grains of calomel last night. Rept. v. s. ad ℥xvj. Pulv. jalap. comp. ʒj. 26th. Much relief from bleeding, only two stools; was cupped over the back but blood not obtained, and had no relief. Twelve leeches were applied to the stomach which is much better, and there is now no pulsation or tenderness in epigastrium. Says there was swelling there, but it has disappeared. Pulse 84, soft; tongue white and furred. Calomel. gr. v, et post horam pulv. jalap. comp. ʒj. 27th. Well purged. Back and pubic region no better. Breast and stomach easy. Pulse 80, firm and regular. Œdema and numbness gone.[46] 29th. Pain shoots from the painful part of the

[46] This part of the case was introduced into the body of the essay, in illustration of the fact, that general bleeding, when most beneficial in relieving the thoracic symptoms and general excitement, has little influence over the local affection of the spine, and that it is consequently necessary to employ local depletion and counter-irritation. The following remarks were added to this report. "The remainder of the case does not bear on the subject "before us, it will therefore be sufficient to state that leeches to hypogastrium relieved the tenderness there, and that the pain of the back was much "lessened by repeated leeching and cupping, but that blisters were afterwards more efficacious and removed the pain, after which the affection of "the limbs slowly left him under the use of frictions, &c. On the 28th November, phosphatic deposits first showed themselves alternating with highly "acid urine, often holding phosphate of lime in solution. At one time the "alkaline state of the urine with phosphatic deposit seemed to be confirmed, but in the progress of apparent recovery, it again became clear and "acid, and the only apparent morbid condition of any of the functions which "could be detected, was the excess of acid in the urine, holding much phos-

spine (about sacro-lumbar junction) in the course of the ureters to the kidney. There is again some pain in epigastrium.* December 2d. Leeches have greatly relieved the back, and he can now turn from side to side without much pain; urine the same; bowels open. Cont. treeak farook. Hirudines x dorso. 3d. Pain of back further relieved, no abdominal uneasiness; after making water has an inclination to make more and cannot; it is high coloured, acid, and without deposit, but on standing 24 hours, deposits a white light sediment. Bowels three times opened. Fowl diet. 4th. Soreness of the *flesh to the touch and numbness of the back of left leg* all night, which is now better. Feels easier, the pain of back being now slight. Urine one pound, and of very red colour with very little sediment; no scalding but pain for a minute after voiding it. Tongue white and loaded; appetite rather better; two stools. 5th. Improves. Back of left leg still "without life," and sore to the touch. Urine 23 oz., very red with little sediment. No pain now extends along the ureters and has much less in the back, but loins feel weak. Emplast. vesicator. parti dolenti h. s.—Liniment. saponis. 7th. Blister appears to have removed the pain of back, but there is a degree of deadness and numbness of both legs below the knees, and of tingling in the toes. Temperature natural. Strong pressure above the pubis,

"phate of lime in solution." Before the paper was forwarded to the Medical Board, however, the case terminated fatally and the remainder of the history was sent as an appendix, as noticed in the following foot note. "The termination of this highly important case will be found in the appendix with a "full detail of the morbid appearances, which throw much light on the history of the disease, and forcibly impress the necessity of local remedies to "the spine."

* A few extracts from the voluminous reports from this date till the 5th March, are all that can be introduced.

and in back where the kidneys are situated pains him, although he does not suffer at other times. Urine ℔iss, paler and slightly ammoniacal perhaps, without sediment and passed easily. Pulse 84, a little sharp. Bowels open, stools brown. Omitt. treeak farook. Habeat pulv. jalap. comp. ʒj. Frictions with ol. terebinth. 8th. Physic operated well in the night, stools of a deep green colour. No pain in back. Legs the same. Pulse 72, small. Urine ℔iss, clear, and of a deep red colour, stains his linen yellow. Rept. pil. treeak. Cont. liniment. Extra bread ℥viij: milk lbij. 9th. Legs less numb. Urine passed easily but it continues red. Cont. medicament. One measure of gin. 10th. Blister not healed. Less numbness and he feels the feet warm; before, they were cold to his sensations but on touching them they felt warm. Urine still red and acid, and now deposits on being neutralised by lime water, a pink precipitate. Bowels lax. On the 12th the pain returned in the lower part of the back and across the region of the kidneys; the former was of a dull character and constant as at first. Tenderness to pressure over the kidneys in the upper and anterior part of lumbar regions, and to each side of the upper lumbar vertebræ. Leeches to the region of the kidneys, and a blister to the lower lumbar vertebræ removed the pain, and the numbness descended to the instep. 17th. Pain in back *on standing and turning in bed, none on pressure.* Numbness rather increased and extends up the inner side of calf of left leg. Feet feel cold. Pulse in leg the same as in the wrist; cold sweats especially of back of hands, and he occasionally brings up several ounces of clear fluid from the stomach. 23d. Only a little numbness of left ancle. January 2d. No change. Phosphatic diathesis strongly marked. Countenance pale and depressed. Flatulent, and has fetid eructations. Pulse 60, feeble, and feels as if the coats of the artery were thick. Stools like blue clay. An issue is inserted on each side of the last lumbar vertebra and over the seat of each kidney. 8th. Pain extends from lower issue to *left* groin and root of penis. Soreness of the flesh of back of *left* leg, below the skin. On 16th, pain seemed to come from the upper issue to bladder and to both groins, with soreness of the skin. On 22d, sediment disappeared but urine was loaded with phosphates in solution in free phosphoric acid, and on 23d, they were again deposited from slightly alkaline urine. February 9th. Professed himself well, and urine appeared natural although acid, and there was some tenderness of the kidneys and bladder.

From March 5th the relapse of the acute symptoms which proved fatal may be dated, and the reports are copied at length from the hospital journals.

March 5th, vespere. The urine on the 3d was quite clear and without deposit, spec. gravity 1032, acid, and on adding ammonia giving a free deposit; yesterday it was again alkaline with deposit, spec. gravity 1034. Now complains of a sensation of burning heat on each side of spine, from upper dorsal vertebræ to the sacrum, and confesses to have had it for three weeks. Epigastrium tender to pressure, and is painful on full inspiration. Tongue covered with the same thick fur as before, and edges are a little red. Pulse 60, small. Urine passes off in a feeble stream. Emplast. vesicator. dorso. 6th. Urine high coloured and clear, with deposit. 9th. Blister applied on the 6th, and rose well. Heat has nearly left the back since the 7th. 14th. Heat was removed, but has returned again in the back. Urine not alkaline but deposits the phosphates. Great tenderness to strong pressure below the ribs. Rept. emplast. vesicator. dorso. 21st. Urine has been getting scanty and clear for some days, is powerfully acid but still precipitates lime on adding ammonia, but in smaller quantity, and the spec. gravity did not on the 19th, exceed 1025. Face has been puffy, and yesterday I observed œdema of the legs and the whole skin seemed to partake slightly in it. Pulse was 100 after walking for some time and its stroke a little hard: the impulse of the heart was also strong, and slight shortness of breath was excited. The sound on percussion is natural, as well as the respiratory murmur. When at rest in recumbent and sitting posture pulse is 72 and small, and the stroke of the heart clear and rather vibrating, but not stronger than in health. Urine last night 8 oz. Œdema in the morning mostly along the tibia. No heat in back. Some tenderness in epigastrium and hypogastrium, and there is much less pain in the loins and the sense of weakness is diminished. Appeared to gain flesh before the present attack. Tongue with thin white fur and reddish edges. Twenty eight respirations in a minute. Much thirst for four days. Urine does not come freely and when it does, flows in a feeble stream. Had a purgative yesterday morning, and two doses of forty drops of tinct. digitalis and half an ounce of cream of tartar in the evening. Habeat supertart. potass. ℥ss in die. Tinct. digital. gtt. xxx ter die. Hirudin. xvj præcord. 22d. Rather less œdema, only sixteen ounces of water in 24 hours

Relief at stomach, from leeches ; pain in bladder on making water. Pulse 68, small. Bowels open. 23d. Sickness and weight at stomach, and some drowsiness. Urine only 12 ounces ; sweats. Pulse 64. No stool. Spoon diet and a pudding. Omitt. tinct. digital. Cont. potass. supertart. Habt. pulv. jalap. comp. ℈ij. 24th. Physic operated ; much nausea and some vomiting yesterday, and had a drachm of aromatic spirit of ammonia and twenty five drops of laudanum. Urine only 8 ounces. Œdema gone. Pulse 74 ; skin moist. Cont. supertart. potass. 25th. Vomits the cream of tartar. Epigastrium tender and there are occasional strong pulsations at the lower part when the heart is quiet, and even now the abdominal aorta beats hard ; pulse 64 small. Bowels costive ; swelling gone. Urine 8 oz. only, and high coloured. Omitt. supertart. potassæ. Recipe-Acet. potass. ℥ij, spt. æther. nitrici ʒiss, aquæ ℔iss. Fiat solutio. ℥iij quater die. 27th. Urine increased to near a pound. Had a blister on the stomach on the 25th, which has relieved the nausea and load he complained of. Last night was taken with severe pains of the limbs, especially of the thighs and forearms which are tender to pressure. Pulse 92, small, and slightly sharp. Skin moist but feels a little warm. Action of heart rather strong. Face puffy, no œdema. Cont.—Hirudines x regioni cordis. 28th. Was feverish yesterday evening and there was strong pulsation in the epigastrium, neck, and cardiac region. He felt a great heat over the body and was much relieved by a purgative injection, the bowels being slow. Pulse 80, small. Face and neck a little puffy. Urine still scanty. Pain in bladder in the morning before he makes water. Cont. medicament. 29th. Action of heart increased (not diffused) and rapid, especially in the night, and after taking his gin and water. Pulse 96 small and a little sharp. Tenderness in each iliac region. Urine not at all increased, and bowels costive. Now confesses to having pain of an aching kind, at last lumbar vertebra, increased by moving, and has had it since the commencement of this relapse. Omitt. med. Habt. pil. treeak bis die. Enema purgans. Cup over the spine to 6 oz. 30th. Four ounces of blood obtained with relief to the back. Was feverish in the evening and pulse was 108; it is now 86. Respiration short on exertion, but natural when at rest. Urine very deep coloured and only 8 oz. Cont. treeak. Six leeches to each groin. Vespere. Emplast. vesicator. dorso. 31st. Feverish in the night but has less beating at the heart, much easier at epigastrium. Pulse 92 with an occasional intermission. Cont. treeak. Omit the gin. Vesp. Œdema of legs and thighs, notwithstanding he is constantly in bed. Bowels costive. Habt. h. s. pulv. scillæ gr. iij, calomel. gr. i. Enema purgans. April 1st. Pain in back easier, but still complains of tenderness in groins. No better. Little complaint of bladder, but very tender over the kidneys from which pain shoots occasionally. Thinks the pain in groin is sometimes increased by that in back, but is not certain. Respiration free while at rest, and chest sounds well and lungs are well traversed. Sound of right side of heart rather loud, impulse not diminished, and that of one cavity is not stronger than the others (more than natural); no morbid sound nor is the impulse too extensive. Pulse 96, small, and a little sharp. Urine 7 ounces of a deep green. Three stools, reddish. Abdomen full. Pulv. jalap. comp. ʒj. Cont. treeak et pilul. h. s.

2d. Œdema along the back, and the abdomen is generally tender and considerably swollen, with obscure fluctuation. Four reddish stools. A white fur on tongue. Pulse 96 with some sharpness. Occasional nausea and vomited part of the jalap, retains the treeak. Great thirst. Perspires. Urine 6 ounces, and spec. gravity 1031.; coagulates slightly, and deposits a quantity of white sediment on adding ammonia. V. S. ad ℥xxvj. Cont. treeak. Hirudines xx abdomini. Habt. ter die calomel. gr. j, pulv. scillæ gr. ij in pilul. Nitric acid drink. Vespere. Bore the bleeding well and wished more to be taken, blood natural, perhaps too much serum and the coagulum is soft. Has felt weak all day, and has made no water. One frothy stool. Breathes heavily but is not sensible of it. Sweats. Pulse 104, a little sharp but weak. Abdomen greatly relieved by the leeches. Cont. medicament. Habt. h. s. tinct. opii ʒss, spt. æther. nitric. ʒj, magnesiæ ʒss, aquæ menthæ ℥ij. 3d. Slept a little. Urine increased, but is of a dark greenish red colour. Starts from sleep. Still some tenderness in abdomen. Œdema the same. Pulse 100 rather sharp. No uneasiness from beating at the heart, in the night. Cont. medicament. Hirudines xvj abdomini. 4th. Had no stool yesterday and took two drops of croton oil, which caused much pain till they operated, and have left the abdomen tender. Five dirty coloured stools. Urine a little increased. Pulse 104, small, and a little sharp. Less abdominal tumefaction. Little pain now in the back. Complains of a "weak stomach" and there is pulsation in epigastriun. Cont.

medicament. Hirudines viij epigastrio. Vespere. Leeches could not be procured ; worse. Face more tumid, abdominal fluctuation, and much tenderness, especially over the kidneys. Breathing oppressed but lungs are traversed, and chest sounds well unless a little dulness to the right of sternum at 5th and 6th ribs. Impulse of right side of heart very great, sound not diminished. The epigastrium heaves at every impulse : no sound indicating local disease. Hirudines xij regioni renis. Omit. treeak. Cont. alia. Habt. tinct. digital. ʒss, spt. æther. nitric. ℈j stat. et h. s: 5th. Relief from leeches to pain about the lumbar vertebræ, to which they were applied. He says the draughts greatly reduced the pulsation about the heart. Cannot sleep any time without starting. Pulse 112, slightly irregular. Action of heart less violent but is still strong, especially in epigastrium and is communicated over the liver ; sound rather dull to right of sternum but the lung is well traversed, a jarring pulsation communicated all over it. Gums tender. Urine about 8 ounces. One stool. Pulsation of carotids very strong. Great œdema along the spine, especially of right side, on which he lies. Pain in back easier. Sweats much. Omitt. pilul. Rept. haust. ter die. Ten leeches to the region of the kidney. Tea 2 pints. 6th. Some sleep. Is better. Urine now ℥ x. No pain of back above or below ; less tenderness. Pulse 108. A yellow fur on tongue, edges red. Cont. haust. Cream of tartar drink. 7th. Worse. Urine 6 oz., less dark. No pain but abdomen is tender and more swollen. Respiration hurried. Œdema all over him, face puffy. Urgent thirst. Pulse 108, slightly irregular and sharp. One stool. Cont. medicament.

℞ Ol. croton. gtt. ij, calomel. gr. iij, ol. menth. pip. gtt. iij. Fiat pilul. statim sumenda. Rept. hirudines xij regioni renis. Vespere. There is less tenderness, but the œdema and oppression is increased and pressure in epigastrium pains him. Breathes heavily. Only one stool. Pulse 102, easily compressed, but with some hardness. In great distress. Cannot drink cream of tartar. One pint additional tea. Rept. pilul. h. s. Rept. tinct. digital. sine spt. æther. nitric. 8th. Vomited greenish fluid after the pills, which griped him very severely; several stools, pale, not watery. Had much dyspnœa in the night, but says he is now much easier. Urine only 6 oz. Respiration heavy, 32 in a minute, lungs well traversed; action of heart less violent, but refers the uneasiness which shortens his breathing to the apex of the heart, which when it acts violently brings on dyspnœa. Much tenderness over the whole abdomen especially in epigastrium, where there is pulsation. Sweats over the face and head only, while before the relapse he perspired freely. Face puffed and gives the appearance of a double chin, great œdema of the back, and on lying on one side it does not leave the other. Urine made easily. Thinks he was better after the last bleeding. V. S. ad ℥x. Hirudines x epigastrio. ℞ Tinct. digital. min. xv, tinct. scillæ ʒj, spt. æther. nitric. ʒss. M. quater die sumend. ℞ Calomel. gr. j, pulv. scillæ gr. ij. Fiat pil. ter die sumend. To have 3 pints extra tea to which 2 ounces of sugar and 3 pints of water are to be added. Fotus. Vespere. Face got pale when ten ounces were taken which were cupped and buffy; thinks the bleeding relieved the breathing, and there is less tenderness of abdomen, but feels very weak. Pulse 108, very small and feeble. Heart beats strongly. Wishes for a warm bath. The whole body feels heavy. Temperature of skin 98° Cont. medicament. A warm bath of 96°. 9th. No sleep. Complains of feeling of heat all over him, and felt the bath too warm. Skin cool and moist. Impulse of heart strong. Pulse a little sharp and small. Urine scarcely 6 ounces. Dry yellow fur on tongue. No stool. Cont. medicament. V. S ad ℥vj. Enema purgans ex muriat. sodæ ℥j, infus. sennæ ℥xij. Vesp. Bore the bleeding well which was carried to ten ounces, blood a little buffy. Has been restless and very low all day, complaining greatly of burning heat all over him, and of great distress at the lower part of cardiac region Has made no urine to-day. Breathes heavily and sighs deeply and loudly. Lungs loudly traversed, chest sounds well, heart's action obscurely tumultuous, impulse less strong and not diffused. Pulse 96, very small. Hands clammy and cold, skin cool. Abdomen more swollen. Pupils large, but contract. Expression glassy and anxious, a cold moisture on the face. Could not take his medicine. It gives him too much inconvenience to turn off his back, but obscure œgophonism perceived as far back as can be reached. Gin two measures in punch. Habt. h. s. tinct. opii min. lxx. 10 P. M. Rather worse. Habt. hora xii, tinct. opii min. lxxx, æther. sulphuric. ʒj. 10th. Made no water. A restless night but says he was considerably relieved by the draughts, although he did not sleep. Respiration very laborious but easiest in the recumbent posture. Oppression at heart less and its action is more moderate. Has been again worse for an hour, and hands and feet have got cold, especially the former. Face less tumid. Tongue brown and dry. Pulse 72, so feeble as to be felt with difficulty, and seems to be influenced in its frequency by the frequent (34) very deep respirations. Had two measures of gin. ℞ Tinct. opii min. lxxx, spt. æther. nitric., æther. sulph., āā, ʒss, aquæ ℥ij stat. Warm frictions to the back, hands, and feet to be diligently employed. Gin, two measures in punch. Enema. Sunk gradually and died at 9 A. M.

Body examined at 11.

The body appeared fat from infiltration of the cellular substance with serum, there was also a good deal of fat over the abdomen. The serum in the neck was much redder than below, and almost bloody. The lips were livid.

The spine was opened from behind, and did not appear to contain any fluid except what passed from without on opening it, and some slight infiltration of the cellular substance. There was no fluid external to the theca anteriorly, and the contents of the canal at first view, from the 2d dorsal to the 4th lumbar vertebra, appeared healthy. At the 4th lumbar vertebra, to the *left side* posteriorly, there was a small mass of reddish coagulated lymph. This increased towards the sacrum, the cavity of which was nearly filled with a thick mass of firm lymph, evidently organised, of a reddish colour, with some fine vessels and longitudinal and transverse fibres. Towards the coccyx it passed into the fatty substance. It was not confined to the posterior surface, but passed between the bone and sheath anteriorly, and some way along the sacral nerves, especially those of the *left side.* It was more firmly adherent to the lining of the canal than to the sheath of the nerves, which in several places appeared healthy below the limph: in some others the lining of the canal came away with it; and anteriorly the bone seemed softened, but this was very doubtful. The membranes and nerves did not appear otherwise diseased. Of these appearances the drawing gives a sufficiently accurate representation. Pursuing the dissection upwards from the second dorsal vertebra to the *attachment of the sheath* to the occiput anteriorly, a red mass like a coagulum of blood of considerable thickness and well defined was found, which was probably the cellular membrane injected with a bloody fluid. It was confined to the anterior surface of the cord. On opening the theca, no fluid, congestion of the vessels, or disease of the arachnoid or of the proper membrane or substance of the cord could be detected. The nerves supplying the lower extremities, and some of the abdominal twigs, without the spine, were healthy.

Head. Much bloody serum escapes from the scalp; a very little fluid between the arachnoid and pia mater; convolutions well marked and the substance of the brain is firm and healthy, a very little water in lateral, none in 3d, and a little in 4th ventricle. No fluid at the base of the brain, and the cerebellum is healthy.

Thorax. Upwards of two pounds of fluid in the cavities of the pleura; the lungs healthy, pale, crepitous and without œdema. The larynx and bronchi also healthy. One old adhesion of right lung. Œdema of the cellular substance of the mediastinum and pericardium. Pericardium large and lax, but free from disease and contained only two ounces of fluid, entirely coagulated by heat (but not firmly).

which that of pleura was not. Heart enlarged; several irregular white membranous spots on the right ventricle, the largest of which is easily torn off from a fatty layer of considerable thickness which covers the heart anteriorly: other small spots are easily rubbed off from the red substance of the ventricle beneath, and appear to be recently effused lymph. The right auricle is much enlarged and distended with a coagulum, partly white. The ventricle is enlarged, its substance scarcely thickened, pale, easily torn but otherwise of natural appearance. It is full of a firm white coagulum, passing into the vessels. The left auricle small, and as well as the ventricle contains coagulated blood; all the valves are healthy. The left ventricle slightly enlarged and its substance firm. The great vessels are every where healthy.

Abdomen. A very little water in the abdomen, and it forms into jelly immediately on being put into a glass. The peritoneum healthy; the intestines large and full of fluid. Strong white fur on tongue, and a dark spot internally in the œsophagus where it passes behind the pericardium. Mucous membrane of stomach reddish from minute star-like dots. It is not thickened nor are the vessels congested. Duodenum and jejunum healthy, but there are some dark flocculi in them and the stomach. Upper part of the ileum contained a dark adhesive mucous substance, and on its being wiped off the mucous coat is seen of a fine red colour. The mucous membrane is then pretty healthy almost to the colon, and contains yellow matters. The colon is not thickened, but its whole mucous membrane is pulpy and very red, and this increases towards the sigmoid flexure and descends into the rectum. The contents of the lower part of ileum and of the colon are greenish, and none of the dark matters are mixed with them. (See dissection of a pauper in a subsequent page). Liver healthy, dark bile in gall bladder. Spleen and pancreas natural. Left kidney externally pale, of natural size, firm in its structure: white and red lines well marked. Where the tubular portions end in the calices they are rather red; a clear fluid may be pressed out of them. The right kidney more easily torn, very red, and a white puriform matter may be squeezed from its tubular part. Ureters rather thickened, especially the left. Bladder contains a good deal of clear urine; is small, and with the exception of some thickening of the muscular coat, is healthy. Urethra not diseased. The vessels of the kidney healthy, as are the nerves of the solar plexus to this and the other viscera.

Remarks. The great importance of this dissection, will be evident to any person who has attended to the reasoning, founded on a minute attention to the symptoms, and the known structure and phenomena of the diseases of the parts, supposed to be involved. These leave no doubt of the lower part of the spinal canal being diseased, and the peculiar symptoms and manner in which the disease extended or was limited, induced me to propose as a subject for enquiry, whether it was not an affection of the membranes of the cord; and in this individual, the disease is found to occupy the *situation*, inferred from the symptoms and from the dissection of case second; and is found without the theca, where the propagation, limitation, and transfer of morbid action, as previously described, is more satisfactorily accounted for, than if it had been in any other part of the canal.[47] The lymph effused on the *left side* of the cord, accounts for the greater suffering of the left leg and foot, and demonstrates the relation of the whole morbid appearances to the symptoms. The comparatively healthy state of the urinary organs, after so long a period of diseased action, and the partial recovery from such severe disease of the spine, will encourage us to persevere steadily in the use of every means of cure; and the nature of the spinal affection, enforces the necessity of remedies to the part, and the propriety of long continued rest in all *severe* cases. It is not necessary to point out, how completely the thoracic and abdominal symptoms, and morbid appearances, correspond with the other observations in this paper, which were made before this case had terminated.

(The appearances above described are not likely

[47] The absence of tenderness of the spine, led me at one time, to overlook the probability of disease existing between the bone and theca; a case however has occurred, in which there was some degree of tenderness of the spine with symptoms not very dissimilar to the above, and great tendency to relapse; and in one of Mr Davidson's patients, there was a severe pain in the middle of the lumbar region, felt deep in the part, as if the bones were broken, and much increased on any sudden motion; pressure also aggravated it, and caused it to be felt in the 7 or 8 superior vertebræ, which were also tender to pressure. This we might expect to find occasionally, in disease of the sheath. In another of Mr. Davidson's cases, the pain in the spine was felt only at night; as in a patient of Olivier's, in whom there was severe pain from 10 P. M. till 3 A. M., at length shooting into the legs, with muscular rigidity and spasms. Pus and false membrane were found between the membranes of the cord, and the matter had found its way out between two of the lumbar vertebræ. It will be observed that the pain was felt, in this example, at the same time as that in the limbs, has occasionally been most troublesome in beriberi. See note 38, page 79.

An accurate coloured sketch of the morbid appearances, was made on the spot by Lieut. Ryves of the Madras European regiment, which has been engraved by Mr. Gantz, of Madras, and will I believe be thought creditable to that artist.

Reference to the drawing.

A. The cord.

B. Sacrum.

C. Coagulable lymph on the posterior surface of the theca, at the 4th dorsal vertebra.

D. The same in the sacrum, which should have been represented somewhat thicker.

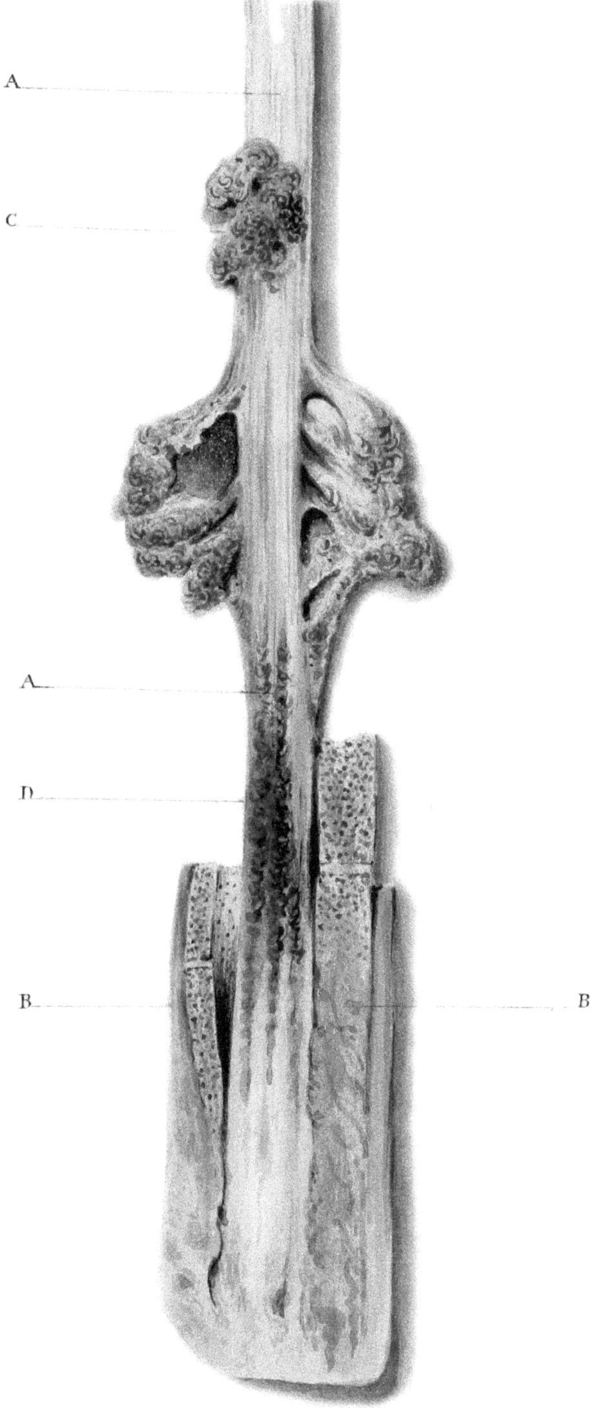
A
C
A
D
B
B

to be often met with, as the symptoms of local affection in the spine are seldom so well marked, and such decided proofs of inflammation are only occasionally produced, even where it has existed with considerable violence. It will rarely happen, that the inflammation does not extend to the other tissues, and render it difficult to trace the precise nature, seat, and progress of the affection; which can only be done, when distinct proofs of inflammatory action are left, and the local distribution of these well marked, and in strict relation to the defined and characteristic symptoms of irritation of the particular part of the cord affected. It is this, that gives the preceding case so much importance, both in referrence to the observations previously made, and to the following case communicated by Mr. B. W. Wright of the 8th regiment Native Infantry.

Case 11. "Mootoo-Roydoo, camp follower. Has resided in the lines, and states that he accompanied the regiment on its march from Hyderabad.

10th August, 1833. Admitted with the usual symptoms of beriberi: œdema and weakness of the lower extremities, when he attempts to walk the legs appear incapable of supporting the weight of the body, pulse 86 small, skin dry. Is of a weakly habit, and states that he has been unable to walk for several days. Habt. calomel. gr. x., pulv. scillæ gr. ij, mane et vespere. Infrict. liniment. ammoniæ cruribus. 11th. Passed a restless night; there is less œdema of the lower extremities, has slight difficulty of breathing, and complains of numbness in the fingers. Pulse 90, rather weak. Bowels have been freely opened, evacuations dark coloured. Cont. medicament. Habt. stat. mist. camphor. ss, tinct. opii.

min. x. 13th. The dyspnœa increased gradually during the day; there was nausea, restlessness, and anxiety about the præcordia. The medicines were continued, as ordered the day before; last night the breathing became very laborious; there was throbbing, palpitation of the heart, with irregular action of the diaphragm, and the pulse at the extremities was weak and intermittent. A blister was applied to the chest, and the draught of camphor mixture and laudanum was repeated. The dyspnœa however continued to increase, and he expired at noon.

Dissection. There was slight serous effusion between the dura and pia mater, without signs of diseased brain. On examining the spinal marrow, there were redness and vascularity of its investing membranes along their whole extent; and slight effusion of *reddish coloured serum* with general vascularity of the substance of the cord, in the lumbar region. The lungs were found turgid with dark coloured blood. There were four ounces of effusion into the pericardium, and its internal layer appeared red and inflamed, with turgidity of its vessels; thus it appeared as if the patient had been finally carried off by pulmonary apoplexy, connected with disease of the heart."

There is much ambiguity attending the inferences to be derived, from serous effusion between the dura mater and the inner membrane of the cord, on account of the free communication which this space has, with the cavity of the cranium; but Abercrombie has remarked, that this is removed when the fluid in the spine is bloody, while the effusion under the arachnoid of the brain is colourless, as was the case in this patient. The following remarks by Mr.

Wright will therefore, I believe, be considered just: they were communicated, along with other valuable observations, in the course of a correspondence which I had been induced to solicit, by anxiety to have the opinion of one, who had observed the disease so carefully, on the views I had been led to adopt. It was long after the paper was written, that I enjoyed the advantage of his communications; and the facts therefore are more important, as confirmations of what was there advanced. Mr. Wright observes, that —" The symptoms of beriberi seem to me to justify an inference, that the disease takes its orgin in the lower part of the spine, at the lumbar region, where the great nerves of the lower extremities are given off. I have observed vascularity and effusion on examining the spine, chiefly in the lumbar region, and the symptoms of beriberi point out the frequent occurrence of some local irritation there, unconnected with encephalic disease: thus we frequently find a patient labouring for months, under the loss of the powers of progressive motion, whilst the functions of the brain, and all the natural functions are undisturbed; and the local application of a blister over the loins, is at times attended with relief. In the more aggravated forms of the disease, the disturbance of the natural functions soon becomes general; but it will always be observable, that the disease was ushered in by paralysis and œdema of the lower extremities, and that there were symptoms of some local irritation in the lumbar region; thus in the case of Mootoo-Roydoo it seems to me, that there was at first, disease of the lower part of the spine, there being paralysis of the lower extremities without functional disturbance; shortly, however, the disease became more extended, and it appeared as if the spine were more generally affected; there was excessive dyspnœa, irregular action of the diaphragm,[48] probably from affection of the phrenic nerves, and this was followed by symptoms of general thoracic disease, palpitation, and general anxiety."

In two other instances, Mr. Wright found slight serous effusion in the spine. A few cases occurred to him in which there were signs of phrenitic inflammation, but the ordinary consequences of cerebral palsy, such as impaired intellect or memory, were never observed; and the only morbid appearances in the brain, consisted in engorgement and slight serous effusion, which, as he found them, he considers to be uncertain signs of morbid action. In one of the cases in which the spine was opened, there was slight vascularity of the pia mater, but no effusion or trace of any morbid condition of the brain. The membranes of the cord were unusually vascular, and there was slight serous effusion, but sufficient, in Mr. Wright's opinion, to be the source of disease. The patient had been ill several weeks before he was seen; the lower limbs were then œdematous and unable to support him, the joints were relaxed, there was hurried respiration, and a small, quick, and irregular

[48] The most marked case of disease from serous effusion in the spine, that occurred to Dr. Abercrombie (page 374), had similar symptoms; a child after being feverish and oppressed for two days, got convulsions followed by coma. " During the fits and for some time after them, there were violent " and irregular action of the heart, and a peculiar spasmodic action of the dia- " phragm." Only very slight vascularity and effusion were found in the skull. Between the membranes of the cord there was much bloody serum; and a copious deposition of colourless gelatinous fluid betwixt the canal of the vertebræ and the dura mater of the cord, which was most abundant in the cervical and upper part of the dorsal regions, where the cord was softer and more easily torn than natural. " When the effusion is contained in the cavity, " formed betwixt the dura mater and the canal of the vertebræ, there can " be no doubt of its connection with the disease of the spinal canal."

pulse, with an anxious expression. There was also swelling and fluctuation in the abdomen. In a few hours violent dyspnœa came on, the pulse became imperceptible, and he died.)

There are no appearances in the dead body so deceptive, as simple congestion in the spinal canal, and I have seldom found it wanting where the circulation had been obstructed, either from disease of the heart, lungs, or brain; I do not therefore place much confidence, in the inferences drawn by Mr. Hamilton from the appearances observed in a single case, accompanied as they are, by a wild, dangerous, and indiscriminating application to practice.[49] It has

[49] I have not been able to procure Mr. Hamilton's paper, but various reviews give lengthened extracts, and the treatment he recommends is, I fear, by their means, becoming popular. *Original note.* I have since had an opportunity of perusing the paper itself, and from the similarity of the symptoms to those occurring in the case of ootoo-Roydoo, am inclined to think, that it confirms in some degree the opinions suggested by the preceding cases; the congestion however was more remarkable in the lungs and liver than in the spine, *and this state of these organs, was considered to be the principal cause of the obstructed circulation and of the symptoms which characterise beriberi*, not only in the individual examined, but *in all others.* The state of the heart and the effusion into the pleura, more especially, if the blood were fluid as is common in fatal cases of beriberi, sufficiently account for the turgid state of the lungs, liver, mesentery, brain, and perhaps of the spine. In the appendix, a more remarkable state of the spinal canal is described, associated with similar pectoral symptoms, but without any affection of the nerves of sensation and motion. The following remark is also in great part erroneous. "The numbness, spasms, and loss of power in the limbs, which take "place in this disease, I consider as principally, if not entirely, dependent "upon congestion of blood found to exist in the internal parts, and more "particularly in the brain," (why then are the upper extremities so seldom affected) "and along the course of the spinal cord." Edinburgh Medico-chirurgical Transactions, vol. 2, page 22. The case, notwithstanding the erroneous inferences founded on it, is valuable, and as the work in which it is published is seldom met with in this country, it is here introduced. "The "symptoms were as follows: great debility, with difficulty of respiration, "a sense of weight and oppression at the lower end of the sternum, and an "almost paralytic state of the thighs and legs; which soon after the com-"mencement of the attack became œdematous, as did also the face and in-"deed the greater part of the body, with a general sense of coldness over "the surface; pulse 120, small, feeble and intermitting. All these symp-"toms went on increasing until the death of the patient, which took place "within forty eight hours from the time that I first visited him. A short "time previous to his death, he was seized with a violent fit of vomiting, "spasms of the abdominal muscles, and increased dyspnœa, which carried "him off." * * * "Sectio cadaveris. Upon removing the skull cap, I "found upwards of an ounce of serum effused between the pia mater and "tunica arachnoidea, and in two or three different places there appeared "dark red coloured patches, one of which was exceedingly vascular, and ex-

been already remarked, that there is reason to believe, from the effects of certain remedies to be hereafter noticed, that in many cases of beriberi, the disorder of the nerves is probably only functional; and even when we must suppose, that alterations in the state of the parts have taken place, we must be prepared to find, as in other forms of palsy, that the alterations elude our search. Sometimes it may depend on diminished energy of the circulation in the spine. This seems to have been the case in a gentleman, who had numbness of the lower limbs extending to the abdomen, and of the upper as high as the wrist, with diminished muscular power and feeling of unsteadiness in walking. Evacuations and spare diet were hurtful. After two months he determined to try the effect of violent exercise, and walked six miles as hard as he was able, in a warm evening. He returned tired and heated. Next day he had severe pains in the calves of his legs, but his other complaints were much diminished and in a few days disappeared. (Abercrombie, p. 423).

"tended into the substance of the brain, to the depth of, from a quarter to "half an inch. There was likewise found considerable effusion in all the ven-"tricles except the fourth. In the base of the cranium, upon the brain be-"ing removed, there appeared upwards of four ounces of fluid tinged with "blood."

"The lungs were very much loaded with dark coloured blood, and in both "cavities of the thorax there was found extensive effusion. The heart was "of a healthy appearance ; nor did the pericardium seem to contain a much "greater quantity of fluid than usual ; both on its external surface, however, "and internally, there existed very evident marks of inflammation. The "diaphragm, particularly toward the right side, appeared considerably in-"flamed. The stomach was of a healthy appearance, and contained about "six ounces of a dark brown liquid."

"The liver was very evidently larger than natural, and appeared even "still more loaded than the lungs. On cutting through its substance, the "blood, from different points, trickled out in a continued stream, and in-"deed all, even the most minute vessels, seemed completely gorged ; as were "also those of the mesentery and pancreas. In several places on the surface "of the intestines, there appeared a sort of efflorescence ; but upon the "whole they presented nothing remarkable. On examining the spinal mar-"row the same evident marks of congestion were found to exist, more par-"ticularly in the dorsal region. From three to four pounds of fluid were "found in the cavity of the abdomen ; and in the cellular texture, almost "all over the body, there was very extensive effusion. No other deviation "from the healthy appearance of the parts was found."

(In the following singular case of paraplegia which occurred to Mr. Simm at Nellore, the excitement of a paroxysm of fever seemed to restore the healthy state of the circulation in the cord, which could scarcely have taken place, had the preceding inflammation induced any organic change.

Case 12th. " The case of local paralysis was " originally one of rheumatism. The patient com- " plained of a severe pain in the small of his back, " which prevented him from walking or even stand- " ing upright, without difficulty. The pain was " much worse in the night than in the day time. " He had this complaint on him for fifteen days be- " fore he applied for assistance. His skin was cool, " his pulse slow and feeble, his bowels regular, and " his tongue furred of a white colour. He was ad- " mitted into hospital on the 27th February. Twenty " leeches were applied to his loins, some calomel and " compound powder of ipecacuan were given to him " at night, and a dose of salts the next morning. On " the 28th, the pain in his loins still continued but its " severity was greatly diminished. On the 1st March, " the pain returned with its former violence. Leech- " es were again applied to his loins, and afterwards " a blister. On the 7th, he was entirely free from " pain in his loins. On the 8th, the patient per- " ceived that his lower extremities were completely " paralysed, and that he had no feeling in his legs. " On attempting to stand, he found that he was un- " able to do so without support, and that he could " not guide the motions of his legs. Blisters were " now applied to his legs, and the carbonate of iron " was prescribed for him. These remedies appear- " ed to render him no service, for on the 14th he

" was much the same as on the 8th March. On the " 15th, he was attacked with what subsequently " proved to be a quotidian fever. It lasted but for " four days. Each paroxysm of fever, however, was " of decided advantage to him. The first restored " some degree of sensibility to the legs, and each " succeeding paroxysm increased it. From this pe- " riod, there was a very slow but gradual recovery " of the lower extremities from their paralysed state. " On the 9th April, the patient was a second time " attacked with a quotidian fever. He derived " nearly as much advantage from this second attack " as he did from the first. He is now sufficiently " recovered to be able to join his corps."[50])

The spasms are of two kinds: the first, which are of a tonic character, have already been noticed. The others, differ in nothing from those spasmodic affections common to all diseases, where the supply of nervous energy is interrupted; and are like them, most distressing at night, when the whole nervous system is weakened. In a few fatal examples, " spasms of all the body" are noticed in the reports, and an experienced friend considers, the cause of death in many cases to be a transference of these to the internal parts. In some cases the patient is ob-

[50] A very important case of chronic inflammation of the intestinal mucous membrane, in a native who had laboured under beriberi a number of years before, has been communicated by Mr. W. G. Davidson, by whom a very careful examination of the body was made. In addition to the abdominal tenderness, nausea, constant thirst, red aphthous tongue, and ultimately dysenteric purging, there were œdema of the limbs and smarting sensations in the feet. Since the attack of the disease supposed to have been beriberi, he had a degree of numbness of the lower and outer part of right thigh, and occasionally, for a few hours at a time, sensations of ants running over him. Nearly half an ounce of serum escaped from near the cauda equina on opening the spine, and a number of large apparently congested vessels were seen on the membranes, but no decided morbid appearance could be detected. The cord felt firm when held betwixt the fingers, but on cutting it across in the upper part of the back, a part like thick curdled milk oozed from it, but it did not appear to be diseased.

liged to adopt a running pace, as in many other examples of nervous debility, wherein, a great and rapid motion is more easily performed than a slow one requiring direction. The toes and forepart of the feet usually first strike the ground, as in "shaking palsy." The motions are often performed freely when the power of regulating them is impaired, hence a staggering takes place when the muscular power is little diminished, or the fingers, though not palsied, have a tendency to move irregularly over each other. When the power of motion remains but feeling is blunted, the regulation of the muscles becomes difficult and imperfect; thus, a woman who could lift a considerable weight was constantly letting things fall out of her hands,and the dragging of the feet, in many cases, seemed principally to depend on the patient not being *directly* sensible of his touching the ground, and unwilling to leave the support which the "sensation of action" enabled him to judge of.[51]

The power of deglutition is in a few instances destroyed a little before death, and in those I have met with, the base of the brain seemed to have been affected. A more important symptom is spasm of the larynx, which appears to be one cause of sudden death. In the following interesting case, the slow pulse and singular hemiplegic tendency indicated by the distribution of the œdema, render it probable, that the brain was oppressed and the recurrent nerves directly affected. In other instances, we shall see, that they probably suffer indirectly through irritation of the extremities of the 8th pair.

[51] These phenomena as they occur in common palsy have been admirably illustrated by Sir C. Bell, and his remarks apply to these observations, which were made before I had an opportunity of perusing either of his late treatises,in which the subject is discussed; the facts may,therefore, be received with more confidence, as having been described solely from nature.

Case 13th. "Ramaswamy, sepoy, aged 38. Admitted 8th April, 1828, with beriberi. Has been ill one month with this disease. Is not able to walk, has a swelling of the whole body ; at present no weight or oppression at the præcordia, respiration free, complains of great numbness of the lower limbs. Pulse 70 and weak. Took a strong purgative yesterday. Habt. ol. nigri m.xv bis die. 10th. No better, the general œdema as yesterday ; pulse small and weak. Cont. ol. nigrum. 12th. If any thing, the general œdema is less. 13th. As yesterday; the chief seat of œdema is on the back of the hands and on the forearms. Pulse slow. Cont. ol. nigrum. 15th. No better, the general swelling of the whole body continues, respiration not oppressed. Cont. ol. nigrum, et habt. cras mane pulv. purgans. 17th. The œdema of the hands and arms has considerably diminished, had four stools from the purgative. Cont. ol. nigrum. 19th. The œdema has returned to the hands and arms, and it is now as much as ever. Cont. ol. nigrum. 21st. No better. Cont. ol. nigrum. Habt. cras mane pulv. purgans. 24th. The œdema suddenly leaves one hand and returns to it, but the swelling of the lower limbs remains stationary ; had several stools from the purgative. Omitt.ol. nigrum. 26th. The œdema of the left leg is subsiding. Nil. 29th. Is exactly in the same state as he was on his admission. Habt. pulv. purgans. Rept. ol. nigri m.xv bis die. 2d May. Had several stools from the purgative, the œdema of the right hand and of the upper part of the left leg is diminished. Cont. ol. nigrum. 4th. Last evening he was taken suddenly worse, not being able to speak, but his speech has now returned as well as ever ; complains frequently of much thirst. Pulse weak and slow ; the œdema of the left half of the body has much diminished, but that of the right half has rather increased, particularly about the neck, shoulder and arms ; respiration free and bowels open. Cont. ol. nigrum. 6th. Was again taken suddenly speechless last night at 7 o'clock, and died 3 hours afterwards. He expired very easy."

Had the loss of voice depended on effusion of fluid in the chest, it could not have been suddenly and completely restored.

In a young sepoy of the extra regiment, the left side of the body was palsied, the mouth drawn to the right side, and speech impeded. It came on in the night along with symptoms of beriberi. He was relieved, but not cured. A case of hemiplegia in a beriberi patient in Tulpius, is referred to in Good's nosology.

Having taken as extensive a view of the more easily understood and essential symptoms of beriberi, as my engagements will permit, I shall endeavour to throw some light on various and singular phenomena which frequently occur in this disease, and constitute its chief claim to a distinct place in a nosological system ; but as none of them are universally present, and as they occur at no particular stage of the disease, they cannot be looked on as essential to it. Those rules of philosophy which are so important in physical enquiries, although logically true, must not be applied practically, in enquiries into diseased actions ; the causes of which are usually very complicated, and the effect of disease of one part on others, can never be positively predicted, however intimate and well ascertained the connection may be. This want of correspondence of effects to apparent causes, probably depends on our ignorance of their intimate nature and attendant circumstances; and is in no part of the economy so observable as in the nervous system, in which, the most extensive diseases of the brain and its productions are found to have caused little inconvenience during life, and the most fatal diseases are produced by causes that elude our scrutiny; and this is perhaps still more remarkably the case, where irritation of one part of the nervous system is communicated to another.

The affections of distant organs produced by spinal irritation, have been recently illustrated by several practical physicians of eminence, and a few of their observations may be usefully introduced in this place. They are, generally, pains of limbs, palpitation of the heart, irritation of the bladder, throat, and stomach. When the lumbar nerves are affected, there is abdominal tension, the chylopoietic viscera and bladder principally suffer, and various hypochondriac symptoms precede the paraplegia; when the lower dorsal vertebræ are diseased, there is a tightness, weight, or feeling of oppression at length amounting to pain in the epigastrium, various affections of the breathing, and a tightness in the course of the diaphragm; and in a case of inflammation of the spinal marrow at the head of the back, Olivier found the pericardium inflamed, and the skin yellow; when the upper dorsal and lower cervical vertebræ are affected, there are various thoracic symptoms, pricking, numbness, sense of cold in the arms, stiffness of the elbows, cramps, spasms of the muscles, weakness of the limbs, and the fingers are insensible to the objects they contain. As Wilson Philip remarks, the important "tendencies of these depend on the direct influence "of the nervous on the sanguiferous system, on the "fact, that continued nervous irritation always tends "to produce inflammatory action." We are not prepared, however, to trace the effects of the disease of the spinal canal in inducing the affections of the viscera, until we have stated some facts regarding the morbid changes in the urinary organs, which appear to have an important influence in their production.

As the subject has not been heretofore attended to and is of considerable difficulty, I shall state at full length all the facts I have observed, and call attention to those points, which my opportunities have not enabled me to examine or establish. The investigation will certainly reward any person, who has the opportunity of prosecuting it.

In almost every recent case, I have seen or read a history of, the urine has been scanty, of a deep red colour and pellucid. In some instances it is suppressed but more generally, even in the worst cases, it is secreted in small quantity, and as is observed by Sir H. Halford, it is remarkable how little of this evacuation is sufficient for the purposes of life, although not of health; two ounces in twenty four hours have been all that were voided or could be obtained by the catheter, when the constitution exhibited none of the effects which follow a total suppression; but rapidly increasing dropsy of the cellular membrane and of the cavities was induced. I have not been able to ascertain positively, whether this change in the urine precedes or follows the symptoms of disease in the cavity of the spine. The two usually exist together when the patient is seen, and he seldom can give any information. The probability is, that the kidneys suffer secondarily. An intelligent man, who had long suffered from severe pain at the sacro-lumbar junction, before the functions of the nerves of the extremities were disordered, informed me, that the urine did not become red and scanty for some time after the commencement of the complaint. In a few cases, the urine did not appear to be altered in any remarkable degree throughout the disease, and in rapid cures, effected by medicines which principally act on the nervous system, the urine speedily regains its healthy appearance; while the benefit derived from diuretics seldom extends beyond increasing its quantity, and the removal of the effusions into the cellular structures, leaving the paralytic symptoms but little changed, and the tendency to relapse very great. In protracted cases also, the urine is of a very different quality, and one which is known to follow injury of the lower part of the spinal cord.

Some urine sent me by a medical friend, was stated to have been voided in small quantity in the morning, by a sepoy beginning to recover from a severe attack of beriberi, attended with symptoms of inflammation of the thoracic viscera which induced him, though averse to the measure in general, to bleed freely and with relief. The blood was buffy. The urine was perfectly clear, of a deep red colour,[52] with a very slight appearance of opaque matter, only observed on close examination, and almost or entirely free from smell. Its specific gravity was only 1013. and it did not exhibit any coagulation by

[52] "When the urine contains a free acid, it is commonly more transparent than usual, and of a bright copper color." Prout's Enquiry, p. 129.

heat or acetic acid ; on adding a solution of corrosive sublimate, it became slightly opalescent, and after standing sometime a precipitate was obtained, but it was dissolved on adding a little diluted nitric acid, and therefore was not albumen, but some of the salts of the urine decomposed by the muriate. To obtain the comparative weight of the urea, one thousand grains were evaporated to a syrupy consistence, which on cooling did not become solid but remained a gummy adhesive mass ; this residuum was dissolved in alcohol and filtered, and again evaporated, but sufficient care was not taken in this delicate part of the process, and the heat being too high it boiled and part was lost, so that the exact quantity could not be correctly ascertained. Thirty hours would be required for this part of the process. Another specimen could not be procured at this time, but the deficiency of urea in urine not coagulable by heat was sufficiently demonstrated. My servant had suffered from slight beriberi in March, and in October had a return of the complaint, but in its mildest form ; the only symptoms being slight œdema and numbness, with sense of stiffness below the knees, and a very little oppression at præcordia, and palpitation at pit of stomach on ascending stairs. The pulse was small, soft, and a little frequent. He had taken the treeak farook for three days, which had nearly removed the symptoms. The urine had the red colour of the urine of beriberi but to a less degree than before, and was powerfully acid. Its spec. gravity was 1025. 5 and it did not coagulate by heat. It did not-contain bile, as muriatic acid caused no green tinge. Nitric acid, carefully added to it in a watch glass so as to remain at the bottom, produced no change in several hours, proving according to Professor Turner a deficiency of urea. By evaporating the mixture to less than half in the sun, the fine laminated crystallized mass indicative of urea was formed.

To find the quantity of urea and salts, it was attempted to evaporate 2000 grains in a low vapour bath heat, but the process was exceedingly tedious, and after two days close attention it was neglected for a short time and boiled, but this did not decompose it, as would have happened had it contained the usual proportion of the animal matter, and no alteration in colour or smell took place. After this, it was exposed to the sun in a shallow vessel for two days and was not yet evaporated or offensive, and continued to exhibit acid properties.[53] Two days after, another specimen was procured. The recovery had made great progress, and the urine had increased from about a pound and a half to upwards of two. Its spec. gravity had also increased two grains, being now 1027.5. A distant march prevented further examination. In every example of the disease I have since met with, the exact agreement of the urine with these observations was ascertained, but in a camp afflicted with cholera, it was impossible to arrive at greater accuracy.

In comparing these facts with the recent admirable researches of Drs. Bright, Christison, and Gregory, on dropsy depending on disease of the kidneys, they will be found to throw much light on the disease under consideration, and to suggest some

[53] The quality of resisting evaporation of the acid urine is very remarkable, and probably depends on the presence of phosphoric acid. *Original note.*

reflections on the conclusions of these eminent physicians. The deficiency of urea was in their cases united with albuminous urine, and Dr. Bright appears to consider the latter, the most important part of the morbid state; but Dr. Christison (*Edinb. Medical and Surgical Journal, No.* 101, *page* 283) has shown, that the fundamental change is a diminution in the proportion and quantity of urea, a conclusion however founded on only a few observations, but singularly confirmed by the deficiency of urea in this disease, being in no instance coincident with coagulable urine.[54] From the great variety of ways in which the urine may be diseased, low specific gravity will not, in all cases, be found to indicate deficiency of urea; a necessary caution in examining complaints of a different nature, from those regarding which the rule was first stated, in which the salts were also deficient. The reverse is the case here, as to two saline bodies at least; and the lightness of colour of the urine must not be at all trusted to, as is done by Dr. Christison in his remarks on Campbell's case, although he notices red urine as occasionally existing in the height of the complaint.[55] The most remarkable effects of the altered secretion, was a strong tendency to inflammation of a masked character in the serous membranes, especially of the chest and pericardium, (*Edinb. Medical Journal No. 96*), and to serous effusion into these structures

[54] Since this was written, a slight appearance of coagulated matter was observed in two cases, in one of which abdominal and cardiac inflammation existed, and the blood was buffy. *Original note.*

[55] Professor Berzelius and Dr. Prout have shown, that urea is destitute of colour, that of the urine depending on other substances generally accompanying it. (Dr. Henry on Urinary Calculi, Medico-Chirurgical Transactions vol. x, page 133). When there is an excess of urea the urine is commonly, but not always, of a pale colour. Prout, page 10.

and the cellular membrane. Indeed to this cause, many cases commonly called inflammatory dropsy arising suddenly in debilitated subjects, on exposure to cold and wet, are to be referred; and Dr. Bright remarks that, there is a strong tendency of disease in the kidney, liver, and heart to succeed each other, an observation which applies with great truth to beriberi.

The liver is very often disordered in its functions and sometimes altered in its structure, a circumstance we might expect from the intimate connection of these two glands, the one being seldom diseased without remarkable changes in the functions of the other. Rose and Henry differ from Dr. Prout in stating, that urea is deficient in acute hepatitis, and Dr. Graves of Dublin has advanced an opinion, on the authority of two cases, that pale urine of a low specific gravity and slightly coagulable, indicating deficient urea, is rather a symptom of chronic hepatitis than of affection of the kidney. As might be expected from a pathologist of his eminence, the observation is not unfounded, but he has been led into error by reasoning on two cases only, and therefore I may venture to point out facts, which will modify his assertion. In an example of acute liver becoming chronic, there was copious hæmorrhage evidently into the right colon, and the urine after some days was of spec. gravity 1017., very red, with a slight darkish deposit; a copious white precipitate was formed on boiling and by adding solution of corrosive sublimate. Here it was evidently an admixture of a portion of the blood, a tendency to the extravasation of which was induced by hepatic obstruction, that rendered the urine coagulable.[56] In a man (Bruce) long in a dangerous state from chronic hepatitis, the urine was copious, pale, spec. gravity 1008.5 and not at all coagulable : in another, during chronic liver two months after a severe attack, spec. gravity 1018., slightly coagulable. In a case of dropsy from diseased liver and colon, the former of which was enlarged, hardened, with much white structure surrounding red parts, the urine was red, turbid, with a slowly subsiding white deposit, but the urine was not coagulable and had a spec. gravity of about 1015. In a man long subject to rheumatism and whose liver was greatly enlarged, it was pale, copious, spec. gravity 1011.5 and not at all coagulable. In a lad (G. Smith) long ill of chronic liver, consequent to a severe and acute attack, the urine varied much, sometimes being

[56] The mixture of blood or serum with the urine, is probably not an uncommon effect of obstructed circulation in the liver and spleen, and as the same cause gives rise to dropsy, the indications founded on the coagulability of that secretion must be received with caution. Soon after the observation noticed in the text was made, a man who had long laboured under physconia, died dropsical. Before his death he had frequent attacks of hæmatemesis, and passed much grumous blood by stool. There were numerous fibrous white flocculi in the urine, and when boiled, and when acetic acid was added, a considerable quantity of coagulated matter was deposited : there had been an interval of two days without any hæmorrhage. The urine was occasionally muddy, or deposited a white sediment, when the fluid was not coagulable by heat, or it was copious and limpid and passed rapidly into putrefaction. There was no trace of inflammation of the membranes, which were remarkably bloodless ; the liver was converted into a mass of white hard tubercles of different sizes, and the spleen was enlarged and firm, but it had diminished in size some months previous to his last illness. Several pints of clear fluid were found in the abdomen, and some dark coagula in the stomach, but the source of the hæmorrhage could not be detected. The peritoneum over the kidneys had numerous red vessels : the glands were pale and in other respects healthy externally ; internally the same paleness existed, the striated appearance was not altered, and on tearing them, the sensation and surface of torn leather were perceived. In the right kidney, near the middle of its cortical substance, there was an oval perfectly smooth cavity, lined with serous membrane and surrounded by a red fleshy cyst about a line thick, which separated from the substance of the organ, to which, except in its firmness and the direction of its fibres, it bore a great resemblance ;—the ureters and bladder were thin and pale, and the latter full of limped urine. Fourcroy asserts that blood is sometimes passed with the urine, from a deviation of another sanguineous evacuation, as the hæmorrhoidal discharge. System of Chemistry, vol. x, page 253. See also Dr. Well's paper on the presence of the red matter and serum of the blood in the urine, in the Transactions of a Society for the improvement of medical and chirurgical knowledge. Vol. 3, page 194.

scanty, at others copious ; at the time the other observations were made, its spec. gravity was 1024., with a slight precipitate from muriate of mercury and heat. He was subject (since the hepatic affection had become chronic), to remarkable hysteric fits, attended with copious flow of pale urine with distension of stomach, and consequent disordered action of the heart. The urine of healthy or otherwise diseased persons, at the time the experiments were made (thermometer above 90°), was usually 1027. to 1030. In acute liver it is generally 1030. It will be seen from these cases, on what a great variety of causes the coagulability and colour of the urine may depend. The low specific gravity is always present, but in no direct relation to the nature of the symptoms. The two lowest were from patients very long ill ; and when the intimate relation between these glands is considered, and that acute diseases of the liver have so remarkable an effect on the secretion of the kidney, we shall not be inclined, in the face of the observations of Bright and Gregory (*Edinb. Journal No.* 109, *page* 320), to adopt the conclusions of Dr. Graves.[57] In beriberi the urine is always altered, the liver frequently not at all disordered, and I think I have observed a peculiar alteration to occur in its secretion when the phosphates were deposited, a change in which the state of the liver can have no influence.[58]

[57] The importance of these remarks in themselves, and the bearing they have on several phenomena of beriberi, will excuse their insertion in what may appear an improper place. *Original note.*

[58] Dr. Prout has traced the deposition of the various forms of lithic acid deposits, to chronic disease of the liver. (Pages 124, 125, and 136). Brande, however, ascribes the occurence of phosphatic deposit to hepatic derangement, (Quarterly Journal of Science, vol. 6, page 201), but he does not appear to have attended to the order in which the urinary and liver symptoms occurred ; however, as all forms of urinary derangement tend to produce the phosphatic diathesis, the uric acid will probably gradually give place to the mixed phosphates.

Returning from this digression several other similarities deserve to be noticed, as dysuria, frequent micturition, and partial suppression of urine, tenderness across the upper part of abdomen, obstinate vomiting, and a very great tendency to relapse. Effusion on the brain occurs more frequently than, according to my experience, is the case in beriberi. During the examination of the urine of the servant mentioned above, it was observed, that it possessed powerful acid properties which could not have been from uric acid, as it neither was precipitated by cold nor acids. Lime water was added, and a copious precipitate of phosphate of lime fell to the bottom. A thousand grains of that voided on the second occasion, when its spec. gravity had increased to 1027.5, and its quantity and appearance had become more natural, was examined six hours after it was passed, by which time healthy urine would have lost its slight acidity. It acted powerfully on litmus paper. Pure lime water was cautiously added, stopping short of complete neutralization, and a precipitate of a white colour was formed, which, after repeated washings,was dried and had then something of a brown colour, and weighed 13 grains. It was again well washed, boiled in rain water, and dried in a strong sand heat, after which it weighed 11 grains, giving by the table of equivalents 5.5 grains of phosphoric acid ; the precipitate from another portion having been previously ascertained to be phosphate of lime, by solution in weak nitric acid and precipitation by pure ammonia, and a copious precipitate was afforded by the acetate of lead added to the nitric acid solution. After neutralization, a further addition of lime water caused a precipitate of the phosphate of lime, from the decomposition of the natural phosphates of the urine. The more accurate method of examining the immense precipitate, caused by the addition of a salt of lead, has yet been unfortunately prevented by the causes above mentioned.[59] When the free acid was almost neutralized, the colour of the precipitate changed to a most beautiful pink; purpuric acid appearing to be developed, by the lime water precipitating its colored salt, after precipitation of the free phosphoric acid, which can be conceived only to take place, as a free acid of less affinity. I have been much gratified by the approbation of that eminent chemist James Prinsep Esq. F. R. S. and Secretary to the Asiatic Society, to this view of what he considers to be a very curious fact. The deep red of the urine is not diminished by the separation of these substances, and is destroyed by nitric acid and boiling, and is altered by sulphuric acid.[60] The urine kept for two weeks retained its acidity and red colour, and its smell; though disagreeable, was not urinous or ammoniacal.

Berzelius has stated that acidity in urine is caused by the uric and lactic acids, and appears to think that phosphoric acid, from its powerful affinity for the alkaline and earthly bases, must always be neu-

[59] The behaviour of the precipitate with muriate of magnesia and ammonia, also proved the acid to be the phosphoric. *Original note.* The examination of the precipitate formed by acetate of lead was commenced, and had not circumstances prevented its completion, would have obviated the objection to which the observations in the text are liable, from the phosphate of lime in the urine being held in solution by its existing in the state of a supersalt, and being precipitated by the removal of the excess of acid. Many facts showed, that the powerful and *permanent* acid state of the urine in these cases, was of a different kind from that of health.

[60] Purpuric acid is of a yellowish colour and acquires its purple hue on entering into combination with ammonia, according to Prout pages 13 and 17. It is evident that the colour of the urine did not depend on this acid, as he supposes frequently to be the case, but on some other principle.

tralized (*Medico-chirurgical Transactions*); but its existence here cannot be doubted, and there is no proof that the alkalies are in sufficient quantity to neutralize the whole acid. Various chemists have also found much free phosphoric acid, although in none so great a proportion as above stated. The whole quantity, *free and combined*, in the extensive series of experiments of Scudamore being seldom 2, often below 1, and in one instance only out of 40, nearly 4. So great an increase of phosphoric acid, must have an important influence on the healthy state of the functions, and on the remarkable changes which take place in the secretion in chronic cases; but until we know "something of the laws according to which chemical affinities are altered in the living body, we cannot expect that the chemical examination of dead animal matter will give much assistance to pathology." (*Alison's Physiology, page* 53.) However this may be, organic chemistry, by detecting peculiar changes in the secretions, in which the senses alone will often deceive us, affords valuable aid in forming a correct diagnosis. Since I observed the state of the urine here described, I have had much gratification in ascertaining, in several obscure cases, the nature of the disease by so simple a test as the use of litmus paper and lime water. The first instance was in a woman, who was supposed to be suffering from the effects of a severe labour, and subsequent fatigue and exposure. It was difficult to obtain an accurate history of the early symptoms, but having seen that the urine had the appearance of that of beriberi, I examined it and found it powerfully acid, and that it afforded the white and pink precipitates above described, and also corresponded in other points. More accurate information was now obtained ; it was found that the affection of the limbs, of which she had nearly lost the use, preceded the labour, at a station where beriberi prevails, and the whole history and especially the fatal termination could not be mistaken. It was cause of deep regret that this was not tried sooner, as the disease is tractable in its early stages, but, as in this example, often difficult to recognize by the general symptoms. Should this be borne out by enlarged experience, as from the unexpected confirmations I have met with I believe it will, I shall consider myself well repaid, for any trouble I have taken in drawing up this essay.

When the disease continues for a considerable time without being relieved, or the patient experiences frequent relapses, the urine is remarkably altered in its characters, and does not differ from that of a patient with ordinary paraplegia, or injury of the lower part of the spine. It is then copious, sometimes as much as 80 or 90 oz. in twenty four hours ; generally pale in colour, although sometimes reddish, of a spec. gravity from 1020. to 1025., uncoagulable by heat, and exhaling a strong ammoniacal odour without fetor. The whole vessel is sometimes covered with a thick froth, from the spontaneous separation of the ammonia, and thick fumes of muriate of ammonia are formed on bringing muriatic acid near it. On adding any acid to the fluid, a very strong effervescence is caused by the separation of the carbonic acid. In the bottom of the vessel, a plentiful white heavy precipitate is always found, of an earthy feel and weight. The deposit dissolved very rapidly without effervescence in much diluted nitric acid, and was precipitated again by the addition of pure ammonia. The nitric acid solution afforded a very copious precipitate on the addition of acetate of lead, further proving the acid to be the phosphoric. It appeared interesting to ascertain whether magnesia existed in the sediments, as it was probable, that the triple phosphate of magnesia and ammonia was mixed with the phosphate of lime; but various processes laid down in the latest works were pursued by myself, and by Mr. Smith of the Engineers, whose enquiries into the composition of the lime stones and cements of this country, had rendered him practically familiar with the various methods recommended for the separation of lime and magnesia, without being able to detect the presence of the last mentioned earth. The specimens were obtained from the urine of two patients long ill of beriberi, and in which the phosphatic deposit had existed for a considerable time. When the disease is further advanced, or the irritation in the bladder greater, the earthy matter is mixed with a lighter substance, which gives it a glutinous appearance and feel; when half dried, it adheres in cakes of a dark colour and peculiar smell, and is less completely dissolved in much diluted acid, some mucous flocculi remaining on the filtering paper. The portion dissolved was filtered, and the precipitate afforded by pure ammonia was equal to that dissolved. Oxalate of ammonia, when care was taken that there was no free acid, afforded, after some time, a free precipitate.

Remarkable symptoms attend these changes in the state of the urine: there is distressing sense of weakness in the loins, and pain in the region of the kidneys ; on pressure being attempted over their situation in the loins, the patient shrinks, as he does, occasionally, when it is made through the abdomen, in front. At times, a sharp shooting pain darts along the ureter to the bladder or groins, and these symptoms may be mistaken for disease of the vertebræ, if the examination is not careful. In a patient in whom the change from the acid to the alkaline state of the urine was about to take place, this pain and tenderness of the kidney, was observed previous to the earthy deposition. In one case the ureters themselves could be distinctly felt thickened and tender, through the abdominal muscles, during life. There is great tenderness in the hypogastrium, increased on pressure, and often severe on awaking in the morning, or if the urine is not voided immediately there is a call, although a pint is sometimes made at a time. When the disease has made much progress, there is a fulness and sense of weight above the pubis, and the bladder can be felt thickened, and may be grasped between the fingers and thumb, and the patient complains of a hard body, like a bladder, rolling about in the pelvis on his moving in bed.

The urine is usually more or less turbid when voided, but sometimes it becomes more so and the deposit increases after it has stood for some time, probably from the extrication of ammonia ; the addition of which, to the urine of a patient in whom it had changed two days before from alkaline to acid, threw down the phosphate of lime, as did slow decomposition in the same urine ; but *none* was afforded by this means, when the phosphatic disposition had not yet been exhibited, or in the same person some days afterwards; and (as Dr. Prout has remarked), if lime is in excess, acid urine may deposit the phosphate. I have also occasionally observed the urine very alkaline without deposit.[61] The urine was in one instance very thick at the end of micturition; in another the first voided was most turbid. It is seldom retained, or voided in a small stream, but strangury and pain along the urethra, and after passing it, usually occur: in one it seemed to have a tendency to come away in an interrupted manner, as if there were a want of correspondence in the muscles of the urethra and bladder; a phenomena noticed by Dr. Alison in an interesting case of caries of the third dorsal vertebra causing paraplegia and alkaline urine; (*Lecture on Peter Elder's case. Lancet vol.* 1 *for* 1829-30 p. 627). The patient has usually complained of coldness of the extremities, flatulence, costiveness at times, seldom of diarrhœa, and the stools are often dark or clay-coloured; the patient is languid and uneasy, and the only European I have seen in this state, had a peculiar sallow leucophlegmatic countenance. The pulse is soft and often slow. These are all symptoms of the phosphatic diathesis, and although I have not found nausea a frequent symptom, the stomach is easily irritated and becomes tender, with a red tongue or fiery edges. In two cases, a thick adhesive mucus was passed with the stools several times; and in one patient, they sometimes presented a curious greyish brown appearance, like a mixture of fine sand and mucilage. This was unfortunately

[61] It has been justly observed, that the essential part of the morbid alteration in the urine, is the excessive secretion of the earthy matter.

not examined, but had probably a relation to the urinary secretions, and was perhaps of a similar composition to the ammoniaco-magnesian phosphate, passed in circumstances not very dissimilar, by two of Dr. Scudamore's patients, (see his treatise on the gout, page 87). In a pensioned sergeant much given to drinking, who died of supervening dysentery, besides ulceration and sloughing of the colon, the spleen was found studded externally with calcareous tubercles; the lungs were healthy, with the exception of some adhesions, and a few superficial insulated tubercles of the same character.

As might be expected, in organs so much disordered, the secretion of urine is not uniformly copious, but is occasionally greatly diminished; and the consequence has been, anasarca unattended by inflammatory symptoms, and not difficult to remove;[62] or as in case second, a febrile action is set up which proves fatal. On comparing that case with the symptoms here described, the whole series of morbid actions are explained, as far as they depend on the sensible alterations in the structure of the parts. The opposite states of the secretion alternating with each other, would appear to prove, that the actions of the kidneys do not depend altogether, as supposed by Ruysch and by the latest writers, on their intimate structure, but that they are as much under the influence of vital causes as the more complicated glands.

[62] Dr. Prout observes that the form of diuresis, occurring in the phosphatic diathesis, "is not *constant*, but takes place at certain times only, either spon- "taneously or from the slightest exciting causes." Page 179. He objects strongly to the use of mercury, and to salts containing a vegetable acid, as Seidlitz powders, and Rochelle salts, and considers that "all remedies that act as diuretics should, in general, be shunned." Of the justness of this opinion, in ordinary circumstances, I entertain no doubt; but when dropsy is making rapid progress, we must not refrain from the cautious use of diuretic medicines, which fortunately, act powerfully and rapidly in this state of the constitution.

However that may be, the nature of the changes ultimately induced in the kidneys and bladder, must render the hopes of cure very slight; and powerfully impress the necessity of an early adoption of the most effectual means of curing the affection of the nervous system, and of preventing relapses; and should make us averse to the cautious plans, recommended by the latest and best authors on palsy, of waiting till all chance of excitement is over, before having recourse to such peculiar stimulants as are useful in diseases of the nerves. Of nine histories of cases of this description which I have before me, five never shewed any sign of recovery, one got well, two were lost sight of, and a patient now under treatment, who was watched at its earliest approach, and in whom the affection of the spine and limbs appear to be entirely removed, yet continues in a precarious state, although the urine has at length become in appearance natural, and the thickened bladder, although painful on filling, is no longer felt above the pubis, and pain in the kidneys has entirely left him.[63] Paraplegia is generally fatal,

[63] The change was deceptive, the urine was found to be acid, and to hold the lime dissolved in sufficient quantity to raise its specific gravity as high as 1034. at a temperature of 90°. It got more and more scanty; anasarca, pain in spine, increased action of heart, abdominal tenderness and effusion came on, under which he will probably soon sink. He was not discharged as he desired, merely from the discovery of the lime held in solution in the urine, and his life has been thus prolonged and perhaps may yet be saved. *Original note.* He soon after died. See case 10. Minute attention was paid to the state of the urine only a few months before the paper was written, and various circumstances concurred to bring under observation, principally, confirmed cases of beriberi in which the phosphatic deposit had existed for sometime; the prognosis is therefore probably not so bad as it would appear to be, from the result of the cases alluded to in the text. Injuries of the spine are followed by a morbid state of the urine, so soon after they are received, that we may expect to find the same changes in many recent cases of beriberi, in which a favourable termination may be expected. The following remarks of Prout in reference to the phosphatic diathesis appear to give a correct view of this subject. "The prognosis in this form of disease will depend entirely on its cause, and the length of time it has existed. In general it may be considered as unfavourable; particularly if the cause be some injury of the spine." Page 182. Although all the other forms of urinary

and that form of beriberi which affects old drunkards and most resembles it, also, sooner or later ends fatally, in a great degree, I am convinced, through this distressing secondary complaint.

Notwithstanding the excellent researches of Dr. Prout and Mr. Brande into these peculiar changes, a diligent search into recent works, and cases in medical periodicals, even of the latest date, have afforded little information of a satisfactory kind, and the cases in which they occur appear to be very generally misunderstood. Dr. Elliotson, from some of his remarks, appears to have directed his attention with success to the subject; but I have unfortunately been unable to procure his lecture on paraplegia published in the Lancet, vol. 1st, 1829-30, to which he refers, which would probably render it unnecessary to enter into further discussion of the observations I have had an opportunity of making. Should our views be found to coincide, it will be extremely gratifying to me.[64]

Two very important cases of apoplexy of the spinal cord are given in the *Edinb. Medical and Surgical Journal, Nos.* 104 *and* 108, from the Nouv. Bibl. Med. November 1829, and the "Archives Generales de Medecine" January 1831, in which the appearances in the kidney and bladder exactly cor-

derangement "converge towards the formidable state of disease we have "been considering, which may therefore be viewed as the last and worst "state of things; yet if the original cause of irritation can be mitigated or "removed, a healthy state of the urine may be again reproduced, and the "patient will thus recover. But on the other hand, if this cause be of such "a nature that it cannot be mitigated or removed; or if the disease be once "fairly established, be permitted to proceed unchecked, or be combated by "inefficient or irrelevant treatment, the patient will be doomed to much "misery and his recovery will be exceedingly doubtful." Page 201.

[64] The information I expected to find, is not contained in the paper, which is in other respects very valuable, and should be studied by every one who has to treat beriberi.

responded to those in case second, and although they are considered as complications only, and the kidney described as riddled with purulent cavities, a comparison with the apoearances there mentioned and with various cases of paraplegia on record will show, that these were probably only dilatations of the natural openings, and the secretion in great part, mucus and earthy phosphates.

Case 14th. A man after suffering from pain of spine, lost the use of one limb and sensation of the other, also power of the bladder and rectum ; the palsied limb was œdematous ; sensibility gradually diminished as high as the nipple. Pulse and skin natural. On the 22d day, urine was loaded with purulent matter ; respiration became difficult, apparently from paraplegia extending upwards. The dissection shewed blood effused in the spinal canal and whole of marrow. Kidneys were riddled with purulent cavities.

The second case occurred to Breschet. Case 15th. A young man was seized with a feeling of coldness, especially of the back and loins, followed by pain in the region of the kidneys and afterwards retention of urine, constipation, and weakness of the right leg of which he gradually lost the power, and sensation of left side as high as the nipple. Pulse natural, tongue white, urine *clear and red :* on the 7th day had fever and vomiting, incon tinence followed, right kidney became more painful and very tender. On 12th day was worse, and the catheter brought away fetid urine loaded with pus : on the 26th day, chest and upper extremities began to suffer from palsy : on the 38th he died with dyspnœa and exhaustion. The cord at the lower dorsal vertebræ was loaded with blood, membranes red; kidneys twice their natural size, the pelvis and ureters of each dilated, the mucous membrane red and covered with lymph and ulcerations. Urine in kidneys purulent; pus in mamillary protuberances and substance of the kidneys. Renal veins contained no pus. Bladder thickened, urinary membranes red with black patches, ulcerations, and softening. (*See case second, page* 63.)

The puriform appearance of the discharge passed with the urine, is exactly what is found in the strongly ammoniacal excretion, in injury of the lumbar vertebræ; and in the second instance, the kidney was affected sometime *before retention* came on, as has been observed to be the case in beriberi; it cannot then be supposed, that obstruction to the urine through the passages, induced the remarkable organic disease; and in case second, the left kidney was disorganised to the same extent as the right, although no obstruction existed in its ducts; and the extraordinary enlargement of the mucous follicles of the bladder could not be accounted for in that way, the urethra being perfectly healthy in every part. Dr. Alison in his physiology published 1831, pages 146-149, remarks, that the inordinate action of the bladder and consequent incontinence of urine in affections of the spine, may be regarded as an example of increased vital power from physical "irritation of nervous matter, and the inflammatory condition and increased and altered secretion of this organ, may be regarded as examples of dependence of nutrition and secretion on the same causes." There is an approximation to the true theory in this passage, but the author having adopted an opinion, that the influence of the nerves on secretion, is confined to those parts most influenced by sensation, both in the work referred to and in his clinical lectures, supports (no direct facts are adduced) the opinion, that the kidney is diseased in consequence of the extension of irritation from the bladder. To me, the bladder has appeared to suffer in part from the irritating secretion, and also from a similar irritation to that affecting the kidneys, probably communicated along the numerous branches from the anterior sacral and lumbar nerves distributed to the pelvis, and that the diseased action of the kidney preceded, or was in no way commensurate to, the disordered functions of the bladder. That the kidney is previously affected appears, from the pain early experienced in its site, and by the facts above noticed, regarding the occasional excess of lime and acid in the urine, and the effect of ammonia, either naturally produced or added to it, in causing the phosphatic deposit *only* when the change in its qualities had first taken place. The nearly total absence of mucus in the deposit in the early stage, also shows that the secretion of the bladder is not, as supposed by Alison, first increased or altered; and the products of its decomposition, are evidently very different from the almost pure carbonate of ammonia extricated from the urine, even immediately on its being passed.[65] (*See clinical lecture on Peter Elder's case.*) The same fact also appeared to be a satisfactory refutation of an opinion of Sir C. Scuda-

[65] The change of the urine from alkaline to acid the same day, and the latter not containing mucus in unusual quantity, is an additional argument against this opinion. It would be important to ascertain the relative proportions of urea in the ammoniacal, healthy, and acid urine, and in that of persons labouring under hepatitis. I tried to do so, but the results do not deserve to be recorded. *Original note.*

more, that the white deposit is prevented from crystallizing, by the admixture of mucus. I have the satisfaction to find in several works of authority, that the phosphate of lime is seldom any thing but pulverulent, the crystallized phosphate being the ammoniaco-magnesian compound. The absence of magnesia, clearly ascertained by experiments conducted with care, will therefore account for the phosphate seldom being crystallized. The phosphate of lime calculus rarely occurs, and is supposed by Brande to be formed only in the bladder, "as the phosphates do not separate till the urine is at rest," an opinion which can only be received, in so far as the deposit arises from the slow extrication of ammonia. In case second it lay in the pelvis of the kidney, and in all, it is formed too quickly to be the result of the decomposition of any animal product. In one case of beriberi imperfectly recorded, several calculi were found in the kidney, and described as "bone imbedded in it," but the similarity of the external aspect of the two substances (*see Baillie's plates of morbid anatomy, page* 147), and these bodies being found in the situation of calculi, where bone can hardly be formed, render it probable that in this instance, the phosphate was deposited in concentric layers in the pelvis of the kidney.[66] The mixed phosphates have been found, in one case, to compose the sediment from the urine of a beriberi patient, which was kindly examined for me by Mr. Prinsep. It is remarkable that this occurred, when this morbid state of the urine first showed itself, and was as yet not confirmed or con-

[66] Nephritic calculi composed of the phosphates are very rare, and are only found in severe and obstinate cases of the phosphatic diathesis. Prout, p. 211.

stant; the same series of actions appearing to exist in this disease as are described by Prout, who found the fusible sediments to be deposited in the early stages and milder cases of the phosphatic diathesis, and that, as the symptoms became more decided and severe, the proportion of phosphate of lime to the ammoniaco-magnesian phosphate gradually increased. The sediment, in the instance referred to, was very fusible, which was not the case with the deposits previously examined. It is probable that magnesia existed in some of the others, as it is difficult to separate it, when in small quantity, from lime, and the only specimens which were examined with care, were from very obstinate cases, in which the triple phosphate may be supposed to have gradually disappeared. Dr. Scudamore states, that white sediment is seen only after the urine is cold, an evident error, it being deposited, whenever the excess of acid necessary to the solution of the earthy phosphates is neutralized, should they be present, which it would appear from the analysis of Berzelius is not usually the case, to any extent at least. Prout has remarked, that as the lithic and phosphatic diatheses often alternate, it is probable they are in some way connected; a remark more applicable to the acid and alkaline states of some examples of this sequela of beriberi. Thus, the urine suddenly loses its alkaline qualities, the sediment is diminished or the urine is limpid, and on examination is found to be acid as in the early stage of the disease, holding the lime in solution, and is consequently of high specific gravity. I have found it 1034. at a temperature of 86° and 90°. Ammonia separated the lime, and led to a correct diagnosis, that the disease still existed ; the patient was detained in hospital, the deposit returned, and he confessed to a return of pain in the spine which he had concealed. From the tendency of urea to pass into carbonate of ammonia by spontaneous decomposition, it is generally supposed that the ammoniacal quality of the urine is produced in this manner, but without more definite observations on this point, it appeared to me more probable, and consistent with the fact that urea never runs into such rapid decomposition in health, that the change is effected by the organs themselves, either by an imperfect union of the elements of urea or by some other mode ; but as, (Mr. Lawrence has observed), the causes of the formation of calculi although diligently studied, are not at all understood, it is probable that mere chemical observations will be found defective.

There is another point however, on which these cases throw some light. In a case in which the deposition of the phosphates was about to commence, the urine was very acid, but did not show any pink deposit on neutralization with lime water. Next day there was a spontaneous deposition of very white phosphates from the acid urine, and after filtration the precipitation continued, as decomposition went on and set free more of the earthy salt. In a few days the deposit ceased, the urine was again acid, and on adding lime water, the pink deposit formed when the acid was about being neutralized, as in the other cases ;[67] and a few days after a co-

[67] I am quite unable to account for the change of colour in the phosphate of lime, in the following observation of Mr. Smith's, which he conjectures may be in some way connected, with the formation of the pink precipitates produced by the neutralization of the phosphoric acid, in our previous experiments. Speaking of Dr. Prout's theory of the formation of purpuric acid, he remarks in a letter dated 2d April, 1833. " I have myself observed that

pious *spontaneous* deposition of the phosphates, of the fine pink colour produced in the preceding experiments, was observed, and on examining the urine it was discovered to have no acid or alkaline properties ; thus, leaving no doubt of the connection of the observations, establishing the fact of the mixture of the deposits, and throwing some light on the way this takes place.[68]

heat appears to have a similar action on the phosphate of lime, as Dr. Prout supposes the nitric acid to have on the lithic acid. Some phosphate of lime prepared by dissolving calcined bones in nitric acid and precipitating with ammonia, was *well washed* and calcined in a furnace, and I remarked, on taking it out, that it had a very decided pink colour, which was permanent Probably the fact is explained by the recent researches into the modifications of phosphoric acid.

[68] The pink deposits are considered to be purpurate of ammonia or soda, but this is perhaps not the case in beriberi. The spontaneous deposit only happened once, and was principally composed of the mixed phosphates and probably purpurate of lime. *Original note.* The remark of Prout, that the pink sediments are principally found in patients labouring under dropsical affections, and where there exists some chronic visceral affection or irritative fever, applies to the individual here referred to (case 10th) ; and to three patients whose cases have been communicated by Mr. Davidson. In the first (Mahomed Khassim ætat. 39) who had been long ill, there were œdema, partial palsy, and muscular rigidity and pains of the upper and lower extremities, pain shooting along the spine, debility, irritative fever, and slight disorder of the heart. The urine was alternately acid, and alkaline with deposit, which was dissolved by acids with effervescence filling the vessel with white fumes. The deposit in October varied in appearance from a greyish pink to purple. The urine from which the purplish sediment was deposited, was of a deep colour and did *not affect litmus paper.* In the progress of the case,a clayey pale yellow gritty deposit subsided from pale ammoniacal urine. In a few months he nearly recovered from all the symptoms. The second patient (Meer Kumroodeen ætat. 40) had muscular pains but no palsy, the principal symptoms having been dyspnœa on any exertion, tense swellings of the greater part of the body, rapid rather strong pulse, anxiety, burning sensations of the skin and abdomen, and yeasty evacuations. The urine was at first slightly acid and not coagulable by heat, but deposited a pinkish flaky mucous like matter only partially dissolved by nitric acid,with effervescence probably from the presence of carbonate of ammonia. In a few days, the urine was high coloured and for sometime afforded alternately a buff, pink, or brick dust deposit. Subcarbonate of potass and lime caused the extrication of ammonia. The urine when the deposit was pink coloured had, in this case, weak acid properties, litmus paper dipped in it *becoming red when dry.* In a few days the deposit became whitish, the pale urine leaving a chalky mark on the floor. Notwithstanding the urgent nature of the symptoms the patient recovered. In the third case (Shaik Emaum),which like the first was of long standing, the pink deposit occurred in connection with œdema, nearly total loss of power of the lower and partial palsy of the upper limbs, evening fever, and cardiac affection.

The following additional facts are gathered from the cases which occurred to Mr. Davidson, to whom I am under great obligations for his kidness in communicating the minute and accurate histories contained in his journal. In the cases above noticed and in others, buff, greyish, or brick dust deposits were occasionally observed to subside from high coloured urine. In several

There is a question of great practical importance connected with this subject, on which I would venture to give an opinion, founded on my own observations and the examination of published cases. Berzelius in the Medico-chirurgical Transactions, vol. VIII, notices a case, where the deposition of the phosphates was followed by paraplegia, and he and others considered the altered action of the kidney, as the cause of the frequent occurrence of loss of power of the lower part of the body, and of the universal prevalence of symptoms of affection of the nervous system. In examining a great many cases, in which the urine was alkaline and deposited white

instances a portion of carbonate of ammonia was present, causing the effervescence on the addition of acids; and the acid character of the fluid was always feeble, affecting litmus paper only after drying, as if from the presence of lithate of ammonia. The addition of subcarbonate of potass, chalk, or lime, caused the extrication of ammonia, and in such cases, part of the deposit was insoluble in diluted nitric acid. This form of deposit occasionally alternated with white soluble sediments from alkaline urine, and in one (Syed Nubbee) after an alternation of this kind, the urine became whey-like and ammoniacal, and deposited white sand and flakes. In this and other protracted cases, the deposit was latterly copious, like butter, sinking slowly to the bottom of the vessel, half of which it filled, and much acid was required to neutralize the ammonia and dissolve the sediment. That decomposition of the urine after being voided, did not cause the precipitation appeared, from the white marks left on the ground. The urine which afforded the coloured deposits occasionally acquired strong acid properties and became clear, and in a patient in whom there was severe pain at the sacrum, the urine was decidedly acid, or alkaline with phosphatic deposit, several times in the course of the disease.

The region of the bladder was frequently tender and micturition painful when the urine was alkaline, and in one patient in whom there was severe defined pain in the lumbar vertebræ, the hypogastrium was painful on pressure and micturition, although only a slight tendency to morbid alteration of the urine was remarked. The scalding in making water ceased, in one case, on the appearance of the buff coloured deposit. It may be proper to mention, that a yellow sediment took place on one occasion from yellow urine.

These observations sufficiently prove, that in this disease as in the ordinary phosphatic diathesis, the amorphous sediments, composed principally of lithate of ammonia, are occasionally the first indications of a tendency to the phosphates; and that the transition takes place by the deposit becoming paler, (sometimes crystalline), from the substitution of the triple phosphate for the lithate of ammonia, and ultimately the secretion of phosphate of lime. See Prout's Enquiry, p. 108 and 170. However, while this last stage of the disease has not yet taken place or is only observed at intervals, we may expect a favourable termination, if the original source of the mischief can be removed. It is difficult to say how far the acid state of the urine occurring in the first days of the disease, influences the subsequent changes, but that it is an important part of the chain of morbid action is very evident.

sediment, it appeared that the patient had frequently received an injury of the loins, and that the appearances on dissection resembled the inflammation and thickening of the bladder and diseased kidney, found in the bodies of men who died in the London hospitals from injured lumbar vertebræ, and in several, the ascertained effects of injury of the spine could be traced, notwithstanding they had been overlooked by the medical attendants. The probability, then appeared to be, that in all cases, the phosphatic diathesis arises from affection of the spinal cord. To this it will be objected, that the phosphates are frequently deposited before the limbs become paralytic ; but it is so common for disease of the spine to exist a long time, before it is indicated by its usual symptoms, that this can have little weight, when opposed to the established connection of phosphatic deposition with spinal injury : accordingly, in a case of beriberi several times alluded to (page 98), severe pain arising from disease within the spinal canal was suffered, at the last lumbar vertebra, for many months before any paralytic affection was observed, and before the urine deposited the phosphates.[69]

The following abstract of a case is still more im-

[69] Various distressing sensations in the limbs and even palsy, are said by Prout to be caused, in some instances, by the thickened bladder pressing on the nerves. Page 253. I doubt whether this effect could be so produced. At page 180 he makes the important observation, that the white amorphous sediments have, in a large proportion of cases been distinctly traced to some injury of the back, in which the patient has received a violent general concussion of the spine. He adds in a note, that he never had an opportunity of inspecting a body after death, and that it is " a very old observation, that in-" juries of the back produce *alkaline* urine ; yet what is surprising, no one " seems to have thought of applying the remark to the present form of dis-" ease." The same effect had been observed in jaded worn out horses and dogs of the sporting kinds, in whom the deposition of the phosphate, probably, arose from some injury of the back.

portant, notwithstanding some deficiency in the narration.

Case 16th. A sepoy, ætat. 20, suffered in March from febrile exacerbations in the afternoon, his urine was at first high coloured, but soon became loaded with white deposit, and there was scalding and irritation in passing it. This was mistaken for gonorrhœa, but it was afterwards discovered that the sediment was passed after the urine. He was weak, emaciated, and suffered from pains in the lower limbs. He was sent to Masulipatam for change of air. These pains had so much the character of those preceding beriberi, that I was very anxious to discover what became of him, and with some trouble I obtained the remainder of his history. He returned from Masulipatam to Ellore without benefit from the change, and was admitted November 4th, complaining of numbness, weight, and pain of the lower extremities which were œdematous; weight and oppression in chest increased on any exertion ; short dry cough, and dyspnœa not increased in the recumbent posture ; body, arms, and face, were œdematous and the latter bloated and of a glassy appearance; eyes yellow, bowels slow and irregular. Pulse languid and irregular, tongue fiery red, moist, and clean ; urine was stated by the patient to be scanty, and is unfortunately not again noticed. Jalap prescribed in the morning and colocynth at night. 6th. Well purged, less œdema, more dyspnœa. The treeak farook prescribed. 8th. Œdema and dyspnœa less. 10th. No dyspnœa, œdema nearly gone. 12th. Œdema, dyspnœa, and numbness all gone. 14th. Omit. medicament. 18th. Weak. Infus. cheyrettæ. 27th. Discharged cured.

There cannot be a doubt from the character of the pains, that spinal affection had existed at the commencement, and the change in the character of the urine, and the subsequent symptoms, are similar to those which I have observed in other examples. The rapid cure by the treeak is very striking.

Case 17th. The following singular case is an exact counterpart of one of paraplegia communicated by Dr. Hutchinson to Dr. Cook (*vol. 2d, page* 43 *of his treatise on nervous d·seases*), and referred to by Good, vol. 4th, page 672, edition of 1829. A man named Venkiah was admitted into the hospital at Ellore in March, having previously had some afternoon fever ; he was much emaciated, very weak in his loins, "dull and heavy," and never moved off his cot. Bowels regular, urine free and deposited a thick white sediment. His gums were made sore without advantage and he was sent to the coast for change of air, and returned without improvement towards the end of May. He had irregular fever at intervals of a week or more, face sallow, edges of tongue red ; belly puffy and large, bowels rather loose, urine deposited much white sediment ; very weak. He was again injudiciously salivated, and took quinine. The end of June a large abscess was opened at the top of right thigh. His future progress I could not learn. It is probable that there was a lumbar abscess, but whether it arose from irritation of the kidney, or was itself the cause of affection of the limbs and kidney, it is impossible to determine from the imperfect record of the case. The occurrence of two such examples in one month, renders it probable that the symptom will be found very common, when attention is directed to it.[70] The practical conclusion from these remarks is, that the treatment should be directed to remove the spinal affection, and that remedies which have not this effect, however beneficial in alleviating particular symptoms, can never cure the secondary disease.

Of the Dropsical Symptoms.

An attentive examination of numerous cases has shown, whenever attention has been paid to the accession and progress of the œdema, that it bore a certain relation to the symptoms of affection of the nerves, and also to the state of the urinary secretion; with only such occasional exceptions and anomalies as we find in every other action, dependant in any way on morbid states of the nervous system. It is sometimes absent altogether, and very frequently soon leaves the patient, and then the secretion of urine is often either natural, or in the progress of the disease has become too copious; but in a few examples there is no œdema detected, when the urine is high coloured and scanty, as Dr. Bright has also

[70] Mr. Davidson's cases establish the fact that these deposits are of very frequent occurrence at Ellore. Most of these cases were protracted, and several of the patients had been ill for considerable periods, or had been treated for fever or rheumatism when on detachment, prior to admission into the regimental hospital. Acute symptoms were rarely present. Messrs. Geddes and Macdonell also notice the frequent occurrence of a " white ammoniacal sediment in the urine." The 41st regiment was much exposed to fatigue and fever during the harassing service in the hills, and the forms of disease prevailing were such as to indicate an atonic, or even a cachectic state of the system, and this Mr. Macdonell informs me, was strongly marked in those labouring under beriberi. Mr. M. therefore considers the use of the lancet and mercury as almost inadmissible. These statements and my own observations accord with the opinion of Dr. Prout, that "in general when acids are " formed in excess by the kidneys, the urine is commonly small in quantity " and high coloured and the disease" (may be) " inflammatory; when neut- " ral or alkaline substances, the urine on the contrary is generally pale co- " loured and larger in quantity and the diseases are those of irritation and " debility." Page 35. " In alkaline conditions of secretion the effects of " mercury are very doubtful; and when carried to any extent they seldom " fail of increasing the irritation, not only by rendering the urine more al- " kaline, but probably by their pernicious effects on the constitution." Page 271.

remarked, in the affection of the kidney he has so well described.

In its simplest and most usual form, it is confined to the lower extremities, often only affecting the parts over the tibia or about the ancles, where all the actions are weak ; it has also been observed to be confined to the calves of the legs and feet, when the nerves of these parts only were affected, either with pain, numbness, or irregular contractions ; or extending to the middle of the leg or thigh according as the numbness has extended more or less, and it is not unfrequently seen to rise up the limb, as the nerves lose their power higher and higher.[71] When the parietes of the abdomen partake of the palsy, the skin over them is commonly thick, and if the affection is chronic, will remain so for weeks, often with puffy abdomen and obscure fluctuation. When it is acute and the urine much diminished, its progress upwards is exceedingly rapid, and frequently ascends higher than there is any marked numbness, and as it rises up the chest, water is too frequently effused into the cellular structure of the lungs and rapidly destroys the patient ; of which the following is an instructive example.

[71] Dr. Herklots remarks that the œdema pursues the same course as the numbness, though with much less regularity. " It seldom proceeds higher " than the wrists, before the thighs are affected with it, and if it advances " further it ascends regularly ; first affecting the abdomen, then the thorax " and upper extremities, and lastly the head ; and in going off it observes " much the same order, only reversing the course." *Second half yearly report of* 1823. Messrs. Geddes and Macdonell ascribe the numbness, which they have accurately described as being occasionally of a partial description, affecting only the calves of the legs, hips, &c. and the affection of the gastrocnemii, to the distension of the cellular membrane by the effused fluids, and to some depravity of the fluids circulating in the limbs. The remark confirms the fact of the œdema and nervous disorder being in some way connected ; but that the numbness does not arise from the distension is apparent from the fact, that the removal of the œdema is often effected without the numbness being lessened, and that it is not unfrequently even greatly increased, when the dropsy has yielded to appropriate remedies.

Case 18th. An Indo-British woman had weakness and œdema of lower extremities, loss of appetite and strength, for two months; on the 1st November she had lost the power of her limbs as high as the pelvis, which were also œdematous. Pulse was quick, small, and irregular; and the stomach was irritable. On the 3rd, œdema was observed along the spines of the lumbar and sacral vertebræ, debility increased, and her breathing was said to be occasionally laborious, but I did not observe it to be much affected. Jalap was given on the 3d, and she commenced to take the treeak; on the 4th she passed no urine, on the 5th a very little in the morning, and took nitrous æther, squills, and a purgative. On the 6th urine continued obstructed, but stools were easily procured; there was severe pain at junction of the sacrum and lumbar vertebræ,* in the left lumbar region, and in the groins which were tender; œdema had also extended over the abdomen and some way up the chest. The bladder was not distended; and the catheter brought away only 3oz. of clear very red urine: the urethra and vagina were tender.[72] In the afternoon her breathing became laborious, she could not lie down, the pulse was rapid and feeble, and the extremities cold. Pulse was gradually lost, the breast heaved, and there was no rattle. The chest sounded well, and the lungs at the upper part were well traversed, but lower down

* See dissections of cases 2nd, 10th, and 11th.

[72] The urine drawn off by the catheter had the appearance previously described. A slight deposit was left in the vessel in which it was boiled, and the milkiness caused by the muriate of mercury was not entirely removed by nitric acid. It contained much acid, which appeared to be the phosphoric acid, in other respects the experiments corresponded with those above noticed. *Original note.* Mr. Ridley states that the urinary bladder is frequently inflamed and collapsed and its coats thickened.

the murmur was obscure, and there was a slight sound as if there were fluid in the cells; the inspirations were exceedingly full, but when the chest was enlarged about two-thirds the murmur entirely ceased, and the parietes were evidently enlarged without any corresponding increase of the space occupied by the lungs. She appeared sensible till a short time before death, when stupor came on and her jaws were locked, probably from the circulation of venous blood in the brain. I was not permitted to examine the body, but the thoracic affection could not be mistaken. I have copied from the note book the stethoscopic indications as recorded at the time, that they may be compared with Laennec, or the following extract from Martinet's Elements of Pathology. "In œdema of the lung the respiration is "laborious, the respiratory murmur is scarcely per-"ceptible although the thorax is largely expanded, "there is a slight rale, lung is found gorged with "colourless serosity and collapses only on being "freed from the fluid. It is crepitant." The cause of this appearance is said to be diseased heart or protracted fever; which will account for the lung being universally affected, while in the woman, the œdema had not yet ascended much above the nipple.[73] The pain in left loin seems to have arisen from the kidney,[74] which appears to have been con-

[73] The cause of œdema of the lung here referred to, does not appear to have been heretofore noticed. *Original note.*

[74] In the report for the 1st half year of 1822, Mr. Desormeaux, then garrison and zillah surgeon of Chicacole, gives a short history of a case of beriberi in a prisoner, in whom the kidneys were found considerably enlarged. The symptoms were anasarca with a sense of smarting, feeble pulse, dry skin, cough and expectoration. The urine was not observed to be morbid. Dyspnœa came on the 14th day of the disease and the 6th of treatment, and he expired in a few minutes. Much yellow fluid was found in the abdomen, and nine ounces in the pericardium. The lungs were shrunk and there were a few tubercles in their substance. The heart was very fat; the liver large

gested and the bladder inflamed in one of Ridley's cases, which terminated fatally from the same cause, modified by the disease of the heart; the cells of the lungs having been found gorged with reddish fluid and the heart much enlarged. (*Dublin Hospital Reports, vol.* 2.) The pleura and diaphragm had been inflamed; and in the following case, which occurred to me at Chicacole, the substance of the lung had also suffered from inflammation.

Case 19th. Beemanah, sepoy, ætat. 21. January 19th, vesp. 1827. Complains of œdematous swelling of the extremities. The right foot is much swollen round the scar of an old ulcer. Face puffy. Limbs have in a great degree lost sensation and he walks with difficulty. A burning sensation in calves and ancles, a feverish paroxysm in the forenoon, skin now cool, no dyspnœa. Pulse 96, small, but hard and firm, tongue coated and yellow at the root; says his urine is made freely. Has had the complaint for two days as now described, but the symptoms have been coming on gradually for a month. Has taken jalap and has been purged. V. S. ad ℥xij; postea habeat calomel. gr. x. 23d. He was relieved by the bleeding after which the pulse was small and quick, and has been purged by antimonial solution and salts; has also taken 20 drops of tincture of digitalis three times a day, and a grain of calomel and two of squills, and rubbed in camphorated mercurial ointment. Urine clear; pulse is now soft; œdema diminished. Pains in limbs. Skin dry and hot, and

and pale, but on being cut much blood flowed from it. The intestines and spleen were sound, but the omentum and mesenteric glands are stated to have been slightly inflamed. A protracted case will be found in a subsequent page, in which the left kidney was firm, enlarged, and very vascular; the right small, firm, and blanched.

constantly feels feverish, had a paroxysm on the night of the 20th coming on in the afternoon ; does not sleep ; mouth tender. Omitt. tinct. digital. et unguent. hydrag. Cont. pilul. et solut antimon. tartar. cum tinct. opii. 24th. Slight difficulty in taking a full inspiration and pain below the sternum. Pulse 86 small, skin cool, mouth sore, swellings subsiding. Emplast. vesicator. sterno. Omitt. pil. et mist. Rept. tinct. digital. gtt. xx ter die. 25th. Blister rose well, breathing free, burning and spasmodic sensations in calves of legs. 27th. Complains only of soreness of mouth and pains in the scar of the old sore ; respiration free, pulse full, eyes tinged yellow. Omitt. medicament. 28th. Does not sleep, constant slight feverish feel, no appetite. Pulse small and weak, tongue coated, bowels regular ; mouth complained of. 29th. About 10 P. M. had short cough and dyspnœa. Was found dead this morning at 5. Countenance tranquil.

The body was examined at 11 A. M. On cutting the cartilages of the ribs, a quantity of serum ran out on both sides, there was still a considerable quantity in the cavity of the pleura, and about two ounces in the pericardium. The right lung was of a dark blue colour, heavy, and hard like liver ; on cutting into its substance some fluid and air bubbles passed out. The left lung was less gorged, but its cells were loaded with clear fluid. Crepitus was not entirely lost. The heart was healthy and contained no coagulum. The liver was considerably enlarged and the hollow viscera were healthy. The state of the kidney not observed. This dissection, although hurried by the impatience of his friends, is important in proving that effusion into the cells is apt to supervene on inflammation, and in demonstrating the nature of that peculiar kind of dyspnœa so often fatal in beriberi ; and the necessity of the stethoscope as a means of diagnosis.

When the anasarca does not rise high, œdema of the lung is apt to occur whenever the hands are numb or swollen, the face puffy, or the heart diseased ; and often supervenes very suddenly and unexpectedly when the patient is thought convalescent. In such circumstances he can never be thought out of danger.

The following two cases and one hereafter given, leave little to be desired on this part of the subject. They were recorded ten years ago by a gentleman of deserved reputation, and were communicated after this paper was ready for transmission.

Case 20th. November 15th. Brondah Naik, ætat. 25. Complains of rigidity of the legs which are slightly œdematous. Tongue furred, urine scanty and high coloured, pulse 90, regular. Has had a number of dark watery stools from a dose of croton, and swelling is a little reduced. Small doses of calomel and squills, and cream of tartar are prescribed. 19th. Swelling rather less. Pulse 96. 20th. Worse. Pulse 116. V. S. ad ℥xvj. Omitt. calomel. Habt. supertart. potass. ℥ss die. 21st. Pulse 120 ; but swelling much reduced. 22d. Feels much easier. General sense of stiffness of limbs gone, but the pulse continues very frequent although weaker. V.S. ad ℥xx, Pulv. jalap. comp. ʒss. 23d. Only nine ounces of blood obtained, which were firm but not buffy. Ten stools. Feels better. 24th. Œdema and rigidity gone, pulse 96, appetite, two stools from senna. Cont. supertart. potass. 28th. Is affected to-day with dyspnœa, cough, and great debility. Cont. medicament. 29th. Dyspnœa and cough increased, face swollen, and complains of distension of the stomach and abdomen, and vomited his medicine this morning. Pulse 120, scarcely perceptible. Cont. potass. supertart. cum spt. æther. nitric. Emplast. vesicator. magn. pectori. Died at 9 P. M.

Sectio cadaveris. Pericardium contained much fluid, and water was also contained in the chest and abdomen, lungs dark coloured and filled with *serum like a sponge.*[75] The heart pale and flaccid. Liver somewhat enlarged, its anterior edge rather irregular. Gall bladder tinged with bile. The mesentery in some places unusually vascular, but excepting the lungs no part exhibited any great morbid change. The blood was dark coloured and quite fluid.

Case 21st. A man who was admitted November 8th complaining of œdema of feet, had impaired appetite, intermitting pulse,and on the 10th, pains and stiffness of legs. On 13th, swellings were removed by purgatives, but the pains in the legs continued and the pulse was very frequent and the skin warm. 19th. Stiffness of legs the same, and there is a little œdema. Pulse 112, hard. To omit cream of tartar, and antimony and calomel, and to take "nitrat. potass. ℨss, acid. acetic. ℥ij ex aqua." 20th. Swelling no better, pulse 116. V. S. ad ℥xviij. 21st. Same. Pulse 116. Rept. V. S. ad ℥xx. Habt. pulv. jalap. comp. ℨj. 22d. Blood not buffy. Thinks himself rather easier and not so much oppressed in the up-

[75] In the Cyclopædia of Medicine (published 1832), it is said that we know nothing of the immediate cause of death when there is little or no dropsical effusion; but Mr. Scott *guesses*, that it is from œdema of the lung. I was pleased to find my conclusions from practice confirmed by the theory of the intelligent writer, but must protest against ascribing it to inflammation, to its being the only cause of the deaths alluded to, and still more to bleeding as a remedy. *Original note.*

per part of the body ; swelling of legs and feet is much reduced. Urine still scanty and high coloured. Pulse 108, less full. Complains to-day of slight dyspnœa; seven stools. Cont. mist. 23d. Swellings and dyspnœa nearly gone, pulse 108. 24th. Slight cough, no dyspnœa, pulse 108 pretty strong. 26th. Had slight fever yesterday at 5 P. M. Swelling entirely gone, stiffness remains, pulse 100, smaller. 27th. Slight dyspnœa and cough ; pulse 90 regular, skin cool. To take nitrous æther, tincture of croton, and arrack. 28th. Got rapidly worse and died at 9 P. M.

Sectio cadaveris. A considerable quantity of water in the pericardium, both cavities of the pleura, and a little in the abdomen. Lungs dark coloured and gorged *with a serous fluid.* Heart much softened in its texture. Liver and spleen healthy. There was a stricture at the pylorus, on opening which a small quantity of pus was observed.

Blood was quite fluid and dark coloured.

It is a subject of satisfaction to me to find the examination of the records of the hospital for ten years, in which these cases occurred, confirm the views here advanced, and that the cases can be introduced in illustration of them, without a change even in the expression, except it be a more confident tone in regard to some of the inferences drawn from a study of the symptoms, when confirmed by additional cases and dissections.[76] The only defici-

[76] I am indebted to my friend Geo. Thompson Esq., zillah surgeon at Masulipatam, for the use of the valuable records of his hospital, in which these cases are recorded. They were unaccompanied by any observations from the gentleman who made the dissections ; the following extract in reference to them, from the 2d half yearly report for 1822 by Mr. Stevenson (now staff surgeon at Jaulnah) in the records of the Medical Board, supplies this deficiency, and shows that the importance of the morbid appearance referred to, had been correctly appreciated. "Considering the disease only to be a pe-
"culiar species of anasarca, it was treated in the usual mode by drastic
"purges, diuretics, and tonics, but nothing was effected by these means but

ency in these and other cases from the same source are, a want of minuteness in the account of the paralytic and thoracic symptoms, and of the circumstances of the fatal termination.

" temporary relief. Tincture of digitalis to the extent of 180 drops daily had " not the slightest effect on the pulse, nor did any abatement of the œdema " take place on this plan. The treatment by mercury was equally unsuccess- " ful. Having been foiled in every attempt at a cure for this formidable dis- " ease, recourse was had to endeavour to discover the cause of the disease " from dissection; accordingly the body of every fatal case was inspected, " and the following were the morbid appearances that were most conspicu- " ous, viz. the liquor pericardii in great quantity; the heart remarkably pale " and flaccid. The posterior part of the lungs very dark coloured, dense, " and their whole substance gorged with water. In both cavities of the tho- " rax and in the abdomen considerable serous effusion, but most invariably " in the former. In one case, water was contained in the lateral ventricles " of the brain. The mesenteric vessels generally turgid with blood. The " intestines also remarkably vascular. In every case the blood was in a state " of perfect fluidity and of a very dark colour. In consequence of the great " frequency of the pulse and hot dry skin in some cases, with the appearance " of increased vascular action exhibited on dissection, an opposite plan of " cure was immediately adopted, viz. by blood-letting and cooling purga- " tives; however, in the cases wherein this was tried, other plans of treat- " ment were had recourse to 8 or 10 days previous to its being employed, so " that no certain inference can be drawn from its want of success in these " cases. Its effects were certainly very striking in alleviating the symptoms " and removing the œdema, but as in these, it is probable effusion into the " lungs had taken place, little good could be expected from it at that ad- " vanced stage. However, in some cases of beriberi in the 15th regiment " N. I., Mr. Paterson has informed me of the successful result of several " cases treated by early venesection, which would warrant a countinuance of " that practice." Mr. Paterson who assisted Mr. Stevenson at the examination of some of the bodies has the following remarks. " The leading symp- " toms of this disease were, a considerable increase to the motion of the " blood, the pulse being seldom less frequent than 110 strokes to the minute, " small, and in general, weak; the skin rather hotter and drier than in a " healthy state; and a deficiency of feeling in the lower extremities, which " were always œdematous and pitted on pressure. The œdema constantly " began in the lower extremities, gradually extending itself upwards through " the interstitial substance, with a particular determination of water to the " organs of respiration, which was in one case sudden and fatal." * * * * " There appears to me to be three terminations to this disease. The first, " death by an effusion of water into the air-cells of the lungs. The second, a " speedy restoration to health by the means of medicine; and the third, de- " bility either connected with or without paralysis of the lower extremities, " from which patients are a length of time in recovering. There is now one " patient in hospital, whose functions appear in every respect quite natural, " except this weakness and paralytic affection of the lower extremities. " When walking he makes use of his limbs as if he had no power or command " over them. Can this affection be owing to water pressing on the spinal " marrow, where the nerves of the inferior extremities originate? or to some " morbid change induced by the disease? I can perceive no plausible reason " for designating this disease by the name of beriberi. It appears to me to " be true anasarca with a determination of water to the lungs greater " than commonly happens." *Second half yearly report for* 1822. Notwithstanding this opinion, Mr. Paterson in the succeeding report has the following observation, regarding two of those cases which remained under treat-

When œdema of the lung has made much progress, as it sometimes does before the patient is first seen, he sits on the ground leaning forward on his knees, his chest in violent motion, he is gasping for breath, the alæ nasi widely opened at every inspiration ; his skin is cold, often clammy, his pulse rapid and small, his extremities cold, urine scanty, tongue dry, thirst urgent, the face is puffy, the hands are usually numb and œdematous, and there are generally other signs of the spine being affected high in the back.[77] From these symptoms the patient sel-

ment. "Two of the anasarcous or beriberi patients have been extremely "slow in their recovery. All the functions of the body appear natural ex-"cept the action of the muscles of the inferior extremities, which are attend-"ed by a deficiency of feeling or numbness. The loss of power seems parti-"cularly attached to the extensor muscles ; one patient could draw up his "legs, but could not again extend them without aid. In walking the exten-"sor muscles seem unwilling to obey, and exert themselves in stepping out "as if with the greatest force." *First half yearly report for* 1823. Mr. Stevenson however states, that although most of the patients felt some degree of torpor and rigidity of the limbs, many of them even after the appearance of the œdema, declared that they had no other complaint.

[77] While these sheets are in the press, the 10th volume of the Medical Commentaries (1786) has been sent me by Mr. Hay, 2d member of the Medical Board. The account by Mr. W. Dick of the dropsies which prevailed during the rainy months of 1782 and 1783, in the Bengal Artillery employed in the Carnatic, is an admirable description of the more severe forms of beriberi, probably complicated and aggravated by the other complaints which arose, from the men being allowed to sink into indolence and to lie on the damp floors during the rainy season, after nine months of fatigue and exposure in the field. During the first year, the dropsical symptoms were rarely attended with affection of the chest ; in the second there was less swelling ; they complained first of an unusual languor, weakness, stiffness, and pains of the joints, hardness in the muscles of the thighs and legs, and some swelling of the ancles at night ; loss of appetite, costiveness, and scarcity of urine together with irregular heats succeeded, after which the symptoms became more decided and the patient applied for relief. The following description of the symptoms of œdema of the lungs and notes of a dissection in illustration of it, are very valuable.

"In some the symptoms of oppression were slight, and no danger appre-"hended till a day or two before death, when the swelling of the legs disap-"peared suddenly ; the difficulty of breathing, tension, and swelling of the "epigastric region, thirst, and vomiting, as suddenly came on, and hurried "the patient out of the world when he least dreaded it. From the symp-"toms, the seat of the water was easily known. * * * When the water oc-"cupied the cellular substance of the lungs, the symptoms of oppression were "more sudden" (than when it was in the cavity of the pleura) ; "the least "motion threatened suffocation ; the pain and weight complained of were "exactly felt under the sternum ; the ghastly look, anxiety, and restlessness, "were greater ; the pulse was quicker, and weaker ; the cough more trou-"blesome, and often attended with a considerable expectoration of a frothy

dom recovers. He is sensible till near the close, and gradually becomes comatose, often in proportion to the imperfect performance of respiration. When the disease was chronic, the œdema of the lung as indicated by the stethoscope, has remained stationary in the inferior lobes for a long time, and exhibited no tendency to spread above the nipple, to which the numbness and external intumescence was limited.

When the hands and arms partake of the paralytic affection, they are usually more or less anasarcous, and as in the legs, the œdema ascends gradually as the disease increases. The shoulders, forearms, or backs of the hands are also involved, sometimes in no relation to the deprivation of nervous power; and in certain rare cases the œdema is yet evidently influenced by this cause, as in Ramasawmy, page 124, in whom it affected the opposite sides of the body in different degrees analogous to hemiplegia; or in others, where one hand and the opposite foot swell suddenly, or the œdema subsides unexpectedly in one and increases in the other, as

"white fluid, resembling the scum of new milk, and which, in some cases, "was poured into the bronchia in such quantities as suffocated the patient. "When there was a necessity for lying down, it made no difference whether "he lay on his back or his sides; but, for the most part, he could only "breathe in a sitting posture."

J. Briggs had anasarca in November 1782, and in April 1783 relapsed. His face was pale, there was slight œdema of the ancles, dyspnœa on walking or attempting to lie down, bowels costive, thirst, urine high coloured and scanty. Mr. Dick concluded from these symptoms that he had water in the chest, and from the quickness and smallness of the pulse and cough, that the water was in the substance of the lungs. Next day the œdema increased, and he was not relieved by copious expectoration of a white fluid. He was restless in the night, and could not lie down, the oppression increased and he felt a pain and load of an immense weight under the sternum; he turned more restless, his pulse could hardly be felt; his thirst increased, a vomiting and hiccup came on, both of which continued for 12 hours when he expired. "The abdominal viscera were sound; but when I raised the sternum, the "lungs bursted out over the ribs, and appeared so large, that I could hardly "think the whole thorax sufficient to contain one lobe of them. On pressing "them, a torrent of the white frothy fluid gushed out at the mouth; and, on "cutting, a quantity of air and water bubbled out, and then they collapsed. "There was no water any where else. I opened two blackmen afterwards, "who died of the same complaint. The appearances were nearly the same."

in some cases of palsy the functions of one set of nerves are lost on one side and retained or recovered in the other. The œdema in some cases extended in a remarkable manner along the whole spine; more commonly the lumbar and sacral regions are only affected, and in one example, on turning from the back the fluid seemed to spread over the body, but neither in that patient nor in the others, could the position of the patient fully account, for the appearance of the swelling only where the posterior spinal branches were ramified. The throat is more frequently swollen in Ceylon than in the circars, but it occasionally occurs; and although not a fatal symptom as has been supposed, is one of danger, in as much, as it shows that the disease has extended high in the spine, or that the thoracic viscera have been involved in it. There is reason to suppose that it is influenced not only by the cervical nerves, but also by the recurrents, and that fascia, which has been demonstrated by Dr. Goodman of New York, to extend to the throat from the pericardium; and the size of the swelling, by the looseness of the cellular substance of the part.

From this general view it is evident, that the œdema in a great measure depends on the state of the nerves of the part, but a remarkable exception to this exists in the face, which is frequently swollen without any indication of impaired action of its nerves.

In a few examples indeed, this occurs where the whole of the cellular substance is loaded with fluid, as in the case of Tallent before referred to (*Dublin Hospital Reports*), and in a patient of mine where the scalp was also swollen,[78] and in others the ganglionic branches of the 5th pair of nerves were evidently disordered, but these are of rather rare occurrence. To explain this important and very alarming symptom, the records of my own practice and of several hospitals were examined, and the conclusion was forced on me, that the face was œdematous when the heart or its envelopes were diseased, especially if water were effused into the pericardium. The general fact of the face being swollen in pectoral disease is sufficiently familiar, and in several instances of beriberi, a puffy face has been one of the attendants on œdema of the lung, on pneumonia, and on the more rare complication of bronchitis, but in these there was rather a puffiness of the face than œdematous swelling, (see case 16); although there is little doubt, that, as many of the affections of the lungs and heart influence the circulation in the same way, if the former are sufficiently severe and the patient survive long enough, the same effect will be produced on the face. With these exceptions, which are more rare than would be expected, I have found, that whenever the medical attendant was in the habit of paying any attention to the state of the heart, and often from incidental circumstances casually noticed, when he entirely neglected to observe its condition, that the heart has always been impeded or irregular in its functions when the face was œdematous; and also that as the morbid condition of this organ was removed, increased, or diminished, the œdema of the face fluctuated accordingly, and now and then, without the urine being

[78] In these the effusion is often the direct result of obstructed secretion of the urine. *Original note.*

scanty. It is highly important to be aware, that the swelling of the face is sometimes the first symptom of affection of the chest, and that where it is present, even in a slight degree, there is the greatest risk of sudden death from thoracic disease; of which non-professional men who have seen much of the complaint, under European treatment, are fully aware, and conclude the patient's recovery to be hopeless. As this opinion was not first adopted, and proofs then searched for, but arose from a very extensive and laborious research, and is encumbered with some exceptions, the limits of which I am not prepared to state, I hope, that should these pages ever be laid before the public, they will not be impugned on any but an extended series of observations. Most of my own cases and those of others were recorded at distant periods, without any particular object, but the mere routine of hospital duty, with no distinct views of the nature of the disease or its symptoms, and in ignorance of the more accurate methods of diagnosis now in use, which render it difficult to find individual examples, which are at once short and satisfactory; however, many of the cases introduced for other purposes, will establish the view here advanced. Since the above was written, I have met with a striking confirmation of it, in an account of a case in England, where the face was œdematous, and there were certain indications of water in the pericardium; and in some dissections recorded for other purposes, in various medical journals, a correspondence existed such as I have described. I was also much gratified by meeting with the following sentence in a recent work. "Œdema of the face has "also been adduced as indicating dropsy of the

" pericardium." After these pages were corrected for transmission, the records alluded to at page 164 were procured, and from them, the following valuable cases are selected, which will leave no doubt as to the correctness of this highly important observation.

Case 22d. Kiser Naik was admitted November 2d, with œdema of the feet, languor and debility, slimy greenish stools, pulse 120; in a few days it is observed, that he has nearly lost the use of his legs. Takes purgatives, calomel and antimony, digitalis, and æther. On 13th complains of vertigo; pulse frequent and urine scanty. 16th. Swelling of the feet pit deeply; complains of cough, no pain of chest; dark stools, from jalap. Calomel, pills containing squills and camphor, cream of tartar, and 30 drops of tincture of digitalis four times a day, precribed. 17th. Vertigo gone; pulse 108, very small, less cough, swelling the same. Legs nearly powerless. To have a drachm of ol. terebinth. twice a day. 21st. He was ordered to be bled yesterday, but an ounce only obtained, and the medicines with the exception of the cream of tartar were omitted; swellings much increased and the hands are now œdematous. Pulse 112. 22d. Feels very weak to day and swellings increased; pulse indistinct, urine rather more free, purged ten times by compound powder of jalap. Nitre in acetic acid. 23d. Swellings of hands and feet very much increased; pulse 116, slight heat of skin. " The swellings of the upper parts" of the body, however, have somewhat subsided. V. S. ad. ℥xxx. Cont. mist. potass. nitrat. Habt. haust. purg. 24th. The swellings are a good deal reduced, and he feels lighter; slight cough, pulse 120, small. 26th. Swellings gone, except a little in the feet and right hand : easier. Purgatives are frequently repeated, and he takes nitrous æther, &c. 29th. Is very weak : swellings have somewhat increased, with stiffness of the legs. Pulse very small. Purged by medicine. December 1st. The *face* and *hands* are very much swelled, but that of the feet has greatly subsided. Four thin green stools ; pulse scarcely perceptible ; does not complain of dyspnœa. Got rapidly worse and died at noon.

Liquor pericardii in excess, heart pale, flaccid, and very soft in its texture ; no effusion into the pleura. Lungs dark coloured at the posterior part, œdematous, and contain a great quantity of serum. Intestines very vascular, particularty the small ones. A little water effused into the abdominal cavity. The brain softened in texture ; vessels of the pia mater very turgid, and the lateral ventricles full of water. The blood quite fluid, except what was contained in the heart.

The increase of the swelling of the face and hands when that of the feet diminished, is an important fact; and the effusion on the brain may perhaps be ascribed to the same cause as the œdema of the face, obstruction to the circulation in the heart being a common cause of head affections. The curious circumstance of the blood being fluid as in cases of sudden death, is important in several respects, and should be carefully investigated.[79] In all those cases, where the blood was fluid from whatever cause, I have found the internal parts congested, often from the mere mechanical effect of pressure on the blood in the external parts, driving it into the larger trunks ;

[79] It is of frequent but not universal occurrence. Polypus concretions frequently exist in the heart, of which, I in one instance, found indications during the life of the patient. *Original note.*

and the neglect of this well known physical law, has led to serious errors in reports of dissections. Although in this case, the absence of the peculiar symptoms of œdema of the lung, shows that it had not proceeded to a sufficient extent to cause the swelling of the face, it will be satisfactory to put this out of question, by the following history.

Case 23d. D. Polygadoo, ætat. 40, 13th October. Admitted with sense of numbness and loss of motion of right lower extremity, which did not affect the left, in a perceptible degree, for some days; *dyspnœa on the slightest exertion.* Face full and bloated; stools dark and fetid. 15th. Has been well purged, and had calomel ℈j at bed time twice; swelling of face and body the same. Torpor has ascended above the thigh. Stools dark. Rept. calomel. Emplast. vesicator. pectori. 16th. Numbness and loss of motion somewhat relieved; breathing more free. From this period to the end of the month there was little change, except a very sore mouth, and total loss of power of the lower extremities. On the 1st November, diarrhœa supervened and continued till two days before his death; which took place suddenly and unexpectedly, on the 7th.

The pericardium was found completedly distended with water, and was firmly adherent to the pleura. The lungs were sound.[80] There were numerous

[80] The following case which occurred to Mr. Geddes is important, as illustrating the observations in the text, and the difficulty which occasionally exists, in this country, of distinguishing between hepatic disease and water in the pericardium. Dr. A. Nicoll of H. M. 80th regiment, in a valuable report on diseases of the liver, notices beriberi as an occasional complication of hepatitis, and two cases will be found in a subsequent note, in which the treatment was directed to remove disease of the liver, and on dissection, the pericardium was found to be distended with fluid.

" P. Farrell, Madras European regiment, ætat. 30; thirteen years in India. Was admitted into hospital at Masulipatam on the 19th November, " 1828, the case being named *liver*. Had on admission in the evening, a " pain in the right side and the part was swelled as far as the stomach; had

blackish spots, at intervals, throughout the whole course of the colon. The other viscera were healthy. The diseased colon does not appear to be an accidental circumstance, other examples having occurred. Another case with the same symptoms, will be found in a subsequent page.

The diminished and altered urinary secretion, although evidently an important agent in the production of the anasarca, is not so closely connected with it, as the diminished nervous power, for besides the instances which occasionally occur of its being healthy, the œdema is sometimes not removed by a copious flow of water of a natural quality; and in other instances, the œdema is entirely removed by the treatment which has restored the functions of the nerves, while the urine continues to be exceedingly scanty, and of morbid quality.

Case 24th. November 27th. Mrs. R. had some numbness of the lower limbs, and more slightly of the hands, for 3 months; face and legs became œdematous, action of heart strong and diffused over most of the left and part of the right side of the chest; uneasiness and weight at pit of stomach and under the sternum; lungs well traversed unless near the

" also cough. Sixty leeches were applied to the site of the liver, ten grains " of calomel given at night, and infus. sennæ next morning. On the 20th " his pulse being full and quick, his skin heated and dry, and the pain of the " side as before, he was bled to a pound and a half, the leeches repeated, " and he had in the course of the day two scruples of calomel with a warm " bath. 21st. In the morning 2 ounces of ol. ricini were administered, and " at this time his mouth was sore, but a dose of calomel and colocynth was " given in the evening and pulv. jalap. comp. next morning. 22d. P. M. His " face was much swelled, and from this date till the 1st December there is " little worthy of remark in the statement of the case, excepting that on the " 26th he was still salivated and had a great tendency to perspiration, and " vomited occasionally. On the 1st December, the last symptom is stated to " have been very violent, and in the evening his face was discoloured with " extreme difficulty of breathing; his urine was scanty, and he was very " restless. Died at ½ p. 10 P. M."

" On dissection, much water was found in the cavity of the chest, and more " than a pint in that of the pericardium. The liver was sound."

heart, where the sound on percussion is dull. Dyspnœa on any exertion; pulse very quick; walks rather unsteadily. Fell a month ago; had nursed a child and on its death menses returned. Ascribed the complaint to cold. She took ten grains of calomel, and next day a dose of jalap which she vomited, and not being purged she was violently salivated; but the action of the heart and pulse became natural, the œdema of face disappeared, as also the numbness and œdema of the extremities. The urine, which was previously scanty, was voided with more difficulty, and she passed in the night only two ounces of red urine, containing a little of the mucus of the bladder, which was increased by the irritation. It was not coagulable by heat,and the opalescence caused by muriate of mercury, readily disappeared on adding a little nitric acid. It was powerfully acid. She has taken the treeak farook with advantage for 3 days. December 4th. Urine is now exceedingly scanty,red,and made with pain,although all the symptoms of beriberi are gone. 12th. Cream of tartar was drank freely, and she recovered rapidly. Has now some bowel complaint. 14th. Well.

In another woman, the treeak removed the large œdematous swellings and the numbness together; the last more slowly, without increasing the urine, which was not at any time remarkably diminished.

In a few instances on the other hand, the œdema has appeared to precede the other symptoms, and it is not improbable that this may sometimes be the case; as spinal affection frequently exists sometime, before it is recognized by loss of power or numbness; but in the great majority of such apparent exceptions, careful enquiry will discover, either of these to have precedcd or come on at the same time with the swelling; and in others, pain of the description formerly described as often preceding the paralytic symptoms, or a slight tottering in the walk is observed, when the patient is not aware of any loss of sense, or of power of motion. Now and then, the œdema seems more connected with the nerves of sensation than with those of motion, and does not ascend above the knee to which the numbness extends, while the muscles of the thighs are rigid and painful; and in a few examples, where sense is little impaired and the palsy great, the subcutaneous cellular substance is nearly free of fluid, while that between the muscles is loaded with it.

The superior extremities are also occasionally more swollen than the inferior, but they are then also more or less paralytic, although I have not observed, that they were more so than the inferior; and interesting examples sometimes occur, in which the arms suffer in the manner the face has been seen to do, when there is severe thoracic affection. As the following case illustrates several other facts, it is here inserted.

Case 25th. Narroydoo, sepoy. Admitted 9th October, 1826. Face and feet much swollen and pit on pressure; complains of great difficulty in breathing and sense of suffocation on the least exertion; pulse very small and extremely quick; arms also slightly swollen, skin cool, tongue whitish, a slight cough. Complaint first perceived three days ago, and has increased remarkably since yesterday; sits up in bed; was discharged a month since, cured of chronic rheumatism. V. S.ad. ℥x, postea habt. pulv. jalap. comp. ʒj. ℞ Spt. æther. nitric. ʒj bis die. Vespere. Relieved by bleeding, lies down in bed; only one stool. Enema purgans stat. ℞ Calomel. gr. x, antimon. tartar. gr. ss. Fiat pilul. h.s. et primo mane sumend. 10th. Three stools, swelling the same, but breathing easy except when he is on his back. Pulse still very small, coughs a good deal and complains of pain about the stomach, where there is swelling; urine still high coloured but passed freely ℞ Calomel. gr. x, antimon. tartar. gr. ss. Fiat pilul. ter die sumend. 11th. Frequent stools; breathing easy when lying on the right side, but cough is very troublesome when lying on the left, or on the back; feet less swollen, arms more so. Cont. calomel. et antimon. tartar. ter die. Emplast. vesicator. sterno. Vespere. Hands feel hard, as if the swelling were not from water effused. Pulse less frequent and not so small, mouth not sore, no pain in chest. Habt. h.s. tinct. opii gtt. lxxx. 12th. Slept well and had little cough, swelling subsides, urine free, mouth sore. Cont. pilul. ut heri. Habt. spt. æther. nitric. ʒj ter die. 13th. Mouth sore, swellings subside, cough and breathing much less troublesome, tongue white, skin cool, pulse small and of natural frequency. 14th. Swellings almost gone, pulse weak. Cont. spt. æther. nitric. ʒj ter die et h.s. tinct. opii gtt. lxxx. Habt. mist. scillæ cum tinct. opii. 15th. No complaint but of gums being tender. Cont. mist. 19th. Convalescent. Decoct. cinchon. cum acid. nitric. 21st. Discharged to duty.

The hard swelling observed in the arms of this patient has been seen in a few other examples, and probably suggested the opinion, that the disease was allied to elephantiasis, which however is little known in the circars. It depends on effusion of lymph instead of fluid into the cells, but does not always indicate a severe disease, nor in every instance, much inflammatory action; although in one case, there was a blush on the skin when the swelling had become hard, and thoracic inflammation was present at the same time.

The subject might be illustrated by numerous additional facts, but as they all tend to the same inference I shall omit them, and briefly advert to the evidence of others, as to the relation of the œdema to the nervous affections. The accounts of most authors are indistinct from careless grouping of the symptoms, but the details of cases seem to support the view here taken; and the conflicting opinions advanced by most writers, when weighed in their connections, confirm it still further. Bontius, Tulpius and others have accordingly classed beriberi with palsies, and Good with an allied affection of the nerves; but more valuable testimony is found in Dr. Herklots' experience, and in the observations of Dr. Wight (which were particularly directed to this question), who observed the previous accession of palsy. Dr. Rogers, formerly superintending surgeon of the northern division, indeed, considered the complaint a dropsy, on the removal of which the cure depends, but the opinion does not appear, from the records, to have been adopted on any recent experience; and an instructive case by Mr. Bond, in the same sheet, demonstrated the error of the last part of the opinion; the patient being cured of the anasarca while the numbness and loss of power increased.[81]

[81] I am indebted to Mr. Adams, superintending surgeon of the northern division, for access to this report, and for the use of the returns of the division, and of the journals of several hospitals deposited in his office at Masulipatam. The statement regarding the prevalence of the disease in the circars, given by Mr. Hamilton, appears to have been furnished by Dr. Rogers.

A few examples however are met with, in which the paralytic symptoms are hardly to be detected, and in others, they appear to come on after the œdema, but the majority of these exhibited other marks of nervous disorder, or were otherwise satisfactorily accounted for.

It has been clearly ascertained, that dropsical effusion depends much more on the capillary arteries than on the absorbent system, and that the minute ramifications of these vessels, are influenced in all their actions by the nerves distributed to their coats; and the occasional profuse exhalation from the surface of the paralytic parts, also, demonstrates that this happens in beriberi. The same separation of fluid taking place into the cellular membrane, would cause the œdema which was generally present with it.[82] The capillary arteries being more under the influence of the nerves than the great trunks, which we shall afterwards find to be often remarkably affected in this disease, and the effusion being occasionally coagulable lymph, sometimes separated from beneath an erythematous surface, there can be no difficulty in admitting, that the altered action of the extreme vessels, in consequence of diminished or altered nervous influence, is the immediate cause of the œdema, as Home long ago remarked, in the chapter of his Principia on palsy, that "œdematosa devenit." The apparent exception, in the curious case mentioned by Dr. Herklots, of the insulated benumbed parts being dry, is a confirmation of the exhalation being under the influence of the nerves, and is analogous to the dry withered appearance of the paralytic limbs, both in this disease when great-

[82] When the face is œdematous from obstructed circulation, it is sometimes covered by a profuse moisture, while the rest of the body is dry. *Original note.*

ly protracted, and in inveterate palsies. But at the same time that I state, what has been suggested by the course of the symptoms in numerous cases, I would wish to be understood, as being anxious to avoid founding any positive practical conclusions, on what may appear to others to be a hasty generalization, when this is not supported by other circumstances; and to repeat the observation previously made, that the state of the urinary secretion, and other causes, (as visceral disease, and even the operation of a purgative which sometimes removes the œdema), are important elements in determining the degree to which it takes place.[83]

[83] That the capillary vessels take on the diseased actions ascribed to them, in consequence of disorder of the nerves distributed to the parts, on which they are ramified, is confirmed by several of the histories in the appendix to Bell's work on the nervous system. Thus, at page 113, there is a case in which the side of the face affected with numbness and pricking pains, from tumor at the root of the 5th nerve, became swollen, red, hot and livid; and in case 49th, morbid sensibility and puffiness was produced by affection of the same nerve. In case 37th, there were symptoms of disease of the 5th, and portia dura, of the left side; the muscles of that side of the face were paralysed, the skin insensible, and the cheek was *œdematous.* Professor Roux, who was subject to rheumatic pain of the back, was attacked in October 1821, with paralysis of the right side of the face, and when this was complete, he began to feel pain at the temple, *and there was œdematous swelling of the part.* The membrane of the tympanum was painfully sensible, and every thing tasted metallic on the right side of the tongue, and this was experienced even twenty four hours before the occurrence of the palsy: sensation was not diminished. That œdema accompanies palsy, or is easily induced in paralytic parts, will also appear by a reference to the histories at pages 373, 385, 393, and 417 of Abercrombie on diseases of the Brain and Spinal Cord. At page 377 a case is quoted from Portal, in which numbness of the inferior extremities was followed by *paralysis and extensive œdema. After some time the arms became affected, and the œdema extended over the whole body.* Serous effusion was found in the brain, spine, and centre of the cord.

In these examples, the origins of the nerves appear to have suffered more from *irritation*, than from pressure as in common paralytic strokes.

When the conclusions in the text were submitted to the Board, I was ignorant of the support these histories seem to afford. Neither of the authors make any observation on their occurrence, but if they had been met with, in writers less scrupulously accurate in their details of symptoms, the particular manner in which the œdema is noticed, would leave no doubt that they viewed it,as intimately connected with the affection of the nerves. The following case quoted by Abercrombie from Serres, is too important in its bearing on this subject, and on many of the phenomena of beriberi, to be abridged.

"A man, aged 20, in the beginning of 1815, had first impaired digestion, " then difficult breathing and palpitation; and, in the end of April, he had

I find no proof, that the anasarca is necessarily a result of inflammatory excitement, although often combined with local actions of that character; nor has the suspicion I once entertained, that high coloured urine would be found usually combined with such, been confirmed by enlarged enquiry, although the contrary state of the secretion has always been attended, even when local inflammation existed, with diminished vascular power. The division of beriberi, also, into two *stages*, according as there is an inflammatory or atonic state of the system is erroneous,[34] these being more advantageously considered, as va-

" anasarca of the legs, and such strong and extended pulsation of the heart, " as left no doubt of the existence of dilatation and hypertrophia of the left " cavities of the heart. He was relieved by diuretics, and continued better " till May, when he had pain, tenderness, and distension of the abdomen. " After free evacuation of the bowels, these symptoms subsided, and, about " the 18th May, it was first observed that he had weakness of the lower ex- " tremities, without diminution of sensibility. All the other symptoms now " disappeared. On the 20th of May, the paraplegia was complete, with re- " tention of urine; and he now, for the first time, complained of pain in the " loins. There was still no diminution of sensibility, but, on the contrary, " the limbs, when moved, were extremely painful. His digestion was now " good, his breathing easy, the action of the heart natural, and his mind en- " tire; and he continued in this state till the 22d of July, when the paraly- " tic limbs became insensible. Gangrene then took place on the sacrum, and " he died on the 10th of August."

" *Inspection.*—The bodies of the third, fourth, and fifth cervical vertebræ " were unequal and slightly softened, and the anterior ligament was destroy- " ed. The outer membrane of the cord at this place had degenerated into " a thick fungous tubercular mass, of the firmness of the pulmonary tuber- " cles not suppurated, and of a greenish yellow colour. This mass involved " in it the ganglions of the seventh cervical and three first dorsal nerves. " The portion of the cord covered by this mass was in a state of ramollisse " ment, which affected chiefly the anterior columns; but the posterior co- " lumns were also slightly softened, in a space corresponding to the three " upper dorsal vertebræ. The brain was sound, except a small tubercle in " the right hemisphere; the heart was quite sound, and the lungs, except " one small tubercle, not softened. In the abdomen there were adhesions " and some puriform fluid."

[34] It is not intended to deny, that in a great many cases of beriberi, vascular excitement and a tendency to inflammation exist at the commencement of the disease, and is followed by a state of debility, not admitting of active depletion; but to caution the practitioner against expecting to find these inflammatory actions, confined to the early period of the complaint, and, as is often done, from using bleeding, &c. as a general practice in the early stages, when they will often be injurious, and abstaining from them at other times, when they may have become necessary. The opinion alluded to seems to resolve itself into this, that beriberi is an inflammatory disease which produces debility. The peculiar atonic state of the system attending the phosphatic deposits, is not referred to, by those who adopt the above division.

riotioe in the form or complication than in the period; and our rules of practice can be guided only, by a careful reference to individual cases, and in these, only by the symptoms present at the time, when remedial measures are to be prescribed.

There is undoubted proof, of an opinion recently revived by Dr. Christison, after some years of neglect, that obstructed secretion of urine is a cause of dropsy; of which a striking instance was offered in an old havildar, subject to anasarcous swellings from beriberi, who was, when convalescent from slight fever, suddenly attacked with obstructed urine and swellings of the whole body, and died in a few hours.

There is another form of anasarca, which is not very uncommon in beriberi, and in every respect the same as that which follows exhausting diseases, and is truly a disease of debility: the legs are then much swollen, and the emaciation great. It often attacks those who have undergone severe mercurial treatment, especially, with the imperfect chemical compositions sold in the bazars. It presents no peculiar features.

Of the Cardiac Symptoms.

Of the morbid affections which occur in the course of this disease, the most important are those of the heart and pericardium, which give rise to much of the distress of the patient, are frequently the cause of sudden death, or more slowly, by inducing effusion either into the pleura or into the substance of the lungs, and lay the foundation, too often, for the most distressing class of chronic ails. Of the post mortem appearances, by far the most common, is a large quantity of straw coloured fluid in the pericardium, which was combined with adhesions of the heart to the pericardium, in the case of a sergeant in Good, vol. 4, page 498. A number of examples of water in the pericardium, will be found in different parts of this paper : in the following rapid and obscure case, no other viscus was diseased.

Case 26th. Chundoo, prisoner, ætat. 20, of unhealthy aspect, had fever intermitting at 3 A. M. with headach, dirty white tongue, and great debility. On the 4th day, he died in a sudden and unaccountable manner. The pericardium was completely filled with watery fluid, and no other morbid appearance could be detected.[85] The late Mr. Owen informed me, that he examined the bodies of several men in Ceylon, and found in the greater number, a good many ounces of fluid ; but his attention was not directed to the inflammatory symptoms. In case 10th, there were unequivocal signs of inflammation of the serous covering of the heart, without effusion into the cavity of the pericardium, and in Mr. Hamilton's case, the pericardium was inflamed both externally and internally, without effusion, but this is probably not a common occurrence. In one case the fluid

[85] The following case is extracted from the journal of practice, for June 1819, of Surgeon T. Forster of H. M. 46th regiment, then stationed at Madras.

" Richard Hill, ætat. 28, ordinary habit. Rheumatismus. Admitted 30th " November, 1818. It would be very uninteresting to detail this man's case " for so many months."

" At the period of admission into hospital, he laboured under a rheumatic " affection, and also had a gonorrhœa for which he bought medicine in the " bazar, and when I first saw him, he was in a state of salivation."

" He soon got well of the gonorrhœa, but the rheumatic affection never " quitted him, and for two months previous to his death, his limbs were quite " paralytic and much under the natural heat."

" 19th June. Died at 11 A. M."

DISSECTION.

" The pericardium was distended with water, and this was the only devia- " tion from health, in the thorax."

" The contents of the abdomen were in a natural state, except the gall- " bladder, which was wasted in size and did not contain a drop of bile, and " only as much colourless fluid as kept it in a state of moisture."

was of a bloody appearance. The diaphragm appears to be occasionally inflamed at the same time, but I am not aware of any observations, showing in what relation the diseased actions stand to each other. In other examples, of which case 19th is one, (andanother will be given), there is no affection of these parts, nor any morbid effusion; and in other cases, the fluid is rapidpidly absorbed, which should be considered, in the examination of bodies in which it was supposed to have existed, as in case 2nd, where there was no other mark of disease, than the doubtful one of a large white spot on the heart.

My attention was called to a subject, which I have little doubt, will hereafter occupy an important place in the history of beriberi, by discovering, in a respectable warrant officer, all the symptoms of hypertrophy of the heart, which had injured his general health and rendered him very subject to dyspnœa. The origin of the complaint was satisfactorily traced to an attack of beriberi, under which he laboured for a long time, and he had derived little benefit from the advice of several medical officers, but was afterwards cured in a few days, by native medicine, which I have reason to believe was the treeak farook. As this was not a solitary example of chronic disease of the heart, having followed apparent recovery from even slight attacks of beriberi, in which symptoms of affection of the organ had existed, there is reason to fear, that another formidable train of evils will be found to arise from it.[86] In no recent case

[86] The following case by Mr. Macdonell establishes the truth of the remarks in the text, and throws light on several other circumstances in the pathology of beriberi. This is one of those points, into which the vague method of grouping a variety of morbid appearances, without reference to the previous history of *individual* cases, has introduced confusion in the published accounts of the disease. It is evident that enlargement of the heart could not be the

have any signs been discovered of enlargement of the heart, but Mr. Ridley mentions it amongst the common morbid appearances, and in the case of Tallent, the pericardium was full of fluid and the heart enlarged. Tallent had been long ill, and had suffered from several relapses; and the same description applies to a case which was communicated to me, where the heart was enlarged and flabby, with four ounces of fluid in the pericardium; the stomach and intestines were inflamed. Both the officer and Tallent had enlargement with increase of substance, the other patient had enlarged heart, but its substance was not increased in thickness or firmness. In the following example, the same appears to have been the case, as the pulse was small and soft. Œdema of the lung was probably overlooked.

Case 27th. A sepoy, ætat. 18, had suffered from fever, with swelling of the legs and other symptoms of beriberi; urine is stated to have been natural, the

cause of a disease, which frequently terminates fatally in a few days or even hours, and fortunately, for the most part, ends in complete restoration to health. Another instance of enlargement of the heart in a protracted case of beriberi, in which its connection with the early cardiac symptoms can be traced, has been sent me by Mr. Davidson, and an abstract of the history will be introduced in a subsequent note.

"This man had been nearly two years in the Chicacole jail hospital, and died. "The symptoms were paralysis and numbness, these subsided but the irritability of the heart continued. Its sound was heard all over the chest, particularly in the right side, and the impulse of the left ventricle was distinctly seen through the chest. These symptoms were combated with digitalis and chalybeate tonics with milk diet, with partial success. Ten days previous to death his breathing became affected, there was a strong wheezing noise with copious frothy expectoration."

"Dissection. Body much emaciated. The left side of the thorax contained about a quart of straw coloured serum. The lung at the upper part, congested of a dark red colour. A few tubercles scattered through the general substance of the lung, slight frothy discharge from the lung when incised. The right lung attached to the pleura costalis by apparently old adhesions. The pleura dark and firm. The lung crepitated on pressure, and was loaded with a thick copious froth which unfitted it for inspiration; there was also effusion, but in less quantity than on the left side. The pericardium contained 9 oz. of fluid. The left ventricle thickened to the extent of an inch, the auricle very small; right ventricle flabby, and cavity enlarged, parietes attenuated. The auricle and pulmonary artery appeared enlarged. The liver much enlarged and of a yellow colour. The left kidney firm, enlarged, and very vascular; the right small, firm, and blanched. The other viscera appeared healthy."

stools green, and the pulse quick and small; he was treated with jalap, digitalis, and a scruple dose of calomel. The pulse got less frequent, and the swelling subsided slowly. In a month he was worse, and passed some firm white mucus by stool; the swelling had extended over the body, there was thirst and dyspnœa, which rapidly increased, with anxiety but without pain, and he died the day after. The heart was much enlarged; only an ounce of fluid in the pericardium. The lungs appeared sound; no water in the cavities of the pleura, and little in the abdomen. The abdominal viscera were healthy. In the distressing affections described by Mr. Ridley, as continuing for years after his recovery, there are indications of the heart being greatly weakened in its powers, and I have met with an example in some respects similar, following very slight disease. They are probably the consequence of that softening in the texture of the heart, noticed in several of the foregoing cases.

To discover symptoms which would clearly indicate, the morbid effusion of fluid into the pericardium, has occupied much of my attention; and I beg to propose the following observations, with the hope, that they will be confirmed by the experience of all my brother officers in the circars, as they have been by a few to whom I communicated some of them, a few years ago. It may appear presumptuous, to attempt to ascertain either general or stethoscopic signs of a disease, of which Laennec says he knows of no certain indications; but when it is considered, that hydropericardium is of very rare occurrence in Europe, and almost always complicated with hydrothorax and other disease, it will not be surprising, that the most extensive experience should be unable to separate the accidental from the essential symptoms, in individual cases, occurring at distant intervals and complicated in various ways ; while a little industry may unravel the slighter difficulties, occurring to one who investigates a disease of frequent occurrence, with few and simple complications. When I commenced the enquiry, I possessed no works in which the symptoms of dropsy of the pericardium were treated of, and the obscure and doubtful remarks of works formerly read had been forgotten. This disadvantage has been more than compensated by finding, after a number of years, on perusing the most recent papers on the subject, and still more, cases reported in various periodicals, in which water was found in the pericardium after death, although little suspected during life; that the greater part of those symptoms I had previously noted, were mentioned either singly or in combination; thus affording a confirmation more valuable than any other, and together with more systematic enquiry since instituted, with the aid of the stethoscope, leave little room to doubt of the correctness of the earlier conclusions. The first symptom which attracted my attention, and has never been found wanting, is at once correct and obvious, viz. a diffused pulsation felt by the hand, in every part of a wide space around the cardiac region, often extending over the left side, sometimes as high as the clavicle, and some way to the right of the sternum and into the epigastrium. In general, this alone will detect the existence of fluid in the pericardium, even when there is no uneasiness to lead the patient to complain ; and as a preliminary measure to more minute enquiry, should never be neglected. A remarkable and melancholy confirmation of this occurred to me, at an early period, in an hospital where the disease had recently commenced. The surgeon informed me, that the disease was easily removed by very slight remedies, and he showed me two patients who, he said, were cured, and the men professed themselves well, with the exception of slight weakness of the lower extremities; on examining them, I found pulsation over the whole left side of the chest, and a small quick pulse, and declared them still labouring under this alarming affection. They both seemed to improve, but on the 6th day one was found dead about noon, and the other, a lad of 15, having complained to his mother of faintness was taken to the verandah, and at one, on bringing him his rice she found him dead; the termination being the same, as frequently happens in ordinary hydropericardium. But although numerous instances occurred to me, where this alone has prevented my allowing patients apparently convalescent, to leave the hospital, whose future history has justified my conclusion; and that in beriberi, it hardly ever happens that any disease exists which could deceive us, it is necessary to notice other valuable diagnostics, which have been found practically useful.

The sound on percussion is dull, over a space somewhat less than that to which the action of the heart can be felt with the hand, and the respiratory murmur cannot be heard, in consequence of the lung being pressed aside by the increasing fluid; while it is often perfectly natural in other parts; and in a few cases, where the recovery was rapid, I have had much pleasure in observing the restoration of respiration, in the parts around the heart, to keep pace with apparent diminution of the quantity of fluid.

One case of complication with inflamed lung has only been observed, with reference to this enquiry, and the disease was of small extent, and in the middle lobe of the right lung, and was easily detected. But it may certainly happen, that hepatization of the lung around the heart may cause diffused pulsation, but the progress of the disease, its gradual extension into the healthier pulmonary structure and perhaps the violence of the heart's action, would lead to a correct diagnosis. If the disease is recent, it is not likely to be either hypertrophy or dilatation of the heart. The absence of increased force in the impulse with a sound as loud as in health, has enabled me to ascertain that it was not the former, and the sound being no louder than usual nor the pulsations much diminished in force, that it was not the latter. It is probable, that complications of a nature difficult to detect may occur, but I have not met with them. There are several symptoms which occur, rarely, in water in the pericardium, which have not been observed, as yet, in the same affection in beriberi. 1st. Fluctuation and tumefaction, which have been perceived very seldom, and, as far as appears, in cases of long standing only.[87] 2d. The stroke of the heart

[87] In Mr. Dick's admirable paper above quoted, this symptom of water in the pericardium, in this disease, is particularly described. "When the pericardium was the seat of the water, the patient felt generally stitches and "shooting pains, with frequent palpitations of the heart, for a considerable "time before any swelling of the legs, or any other complaint seized him. "The swelling of the legs was not often considerable, the urine was seldom "scanty, neither was the appetite impaired, nor the belly costive; and, till "the last stage of the disease, the difficulty of breathing was inconsiderable. "Upon a careful examination, the ribs on the left of the scrobiculus cordis "appear more prominent than usual; a great tenderness, and often an acute "pain, is felt in the left shoulder under the clavicle, and at the pit of the "stomach. By pressing on that spot, a crackling noise, resembling that in "emphysematous cases, is also felt. I know not the cause of this, but have "observed it only in the worst cases; and then also the heart beats so strong "and hard that the patient becomes very uneasy, and the least motion produces such palpitations, faintness, and irregularity of the pulse, that immediate death is threatened. He cannot lie on his back a moment, and not "with ease on his right side; but can lie tolerably well, even with his head "low, on the left side." A strong man of intemperate habits, complained in October, that upon walkiug much he had pain and strong palpitation at the chest, and a month afterwards of some swelling, tightness and weakness of his legs; pain at the pit of stomach and under the left clavicle; and frequent

being felt to pass from one part of the chest to another, of which two examples have been recorded by Corvisart, and have been erroneously introduced into some recent works, as a common symptom. Of this one example, but ill recorded, was communicated to me.[88] 3d.

shooting pains about the heart. His appetite, bowels and colour were natural, but his urine was scanty. Had a drachm of nitrous æther with forty drops of antimonial wine three times a day, a light nourishing diet, and flannel clothing, and in three weeks his complaints went off, the palpitation diminished, and the bark and sulphuric acid entirely removed it; but in five weeks he returned with the same complaint, dyspnœa increased, and he was bled, in Mr. Dick's absence, two days before his death, without relief, and next day took tartar emetic which vomited him and made him worse. That evening he was in the greatest agony; his breathing almost stopped, his pulse weak and intermitting; his heart beating most astonishingly strong and irregular, the epigastric region swelled, the thirst unquenchable; the vomiting incessant, and the pain at stomach excruciating and he expired before fomentations, &c. could be prepared. The liver and spleen were greatly enlarged and tender in their substance, and so distended with blood, that hardly any was to be found in any other part of the body excepting the heart. The stomach appeared a little inflamed; but there was no water or any other morbid appearance, in the abdomen. On raising the sternum a large portion of the pericardium was cut away with it, and about a quart of water gushed out, and nearly the same quantity still remained. The heart was double its natural size, distended with blood; and the pericardium adhered so firmly to the sternum and pleura before, and had squeesed the mediastinum and lungs so closely to the sides and back part of the thorax, that nothing but one large cavity containing the heart, floating as it were in water, could be seen. The lungs were formed into two thin cakes, adhering firmly to the pericardium before, and to the pleura behind, of a greyish colour, hardly containing any blood, air, or water. There was a quantity of coagulated blood in the heart; but it did not appear to have been formed into a polypus before death. In a number of natives a pint or more of water was found in the pericardium, and in some of them the lungs adhered firmly to the pleura. (*Medical Commentaries, vol.* x.)

The crepitus remarked in these cases is a singular symptom, and was observed in a patient labouring under a greatly enlarged liver, in which a large abscess had formed and appeared to point a little above and to the right of the umbilicus, but no adhesion existed between the peritoneum of the liver and of the parietes, nor could any cause for it be detected, on a very careful examination after death, either in the abscess or cellular membrane.

[88] In one of Mr. Davidson's cases (Syed Nubbi), the impulse of the heart was not felt by the hand constantly in the same spot, but the report notices that this did not seem to affect the sounds as heard by the stethoscope. The patient had suffered from rheumatism, to which pain, stiffness, and tenderness in the calves of the legs, and ultimately numbness of the feet and hands, succeeded. The auricular and ventricular contractions seemed equally strong. The impulse was difficult to count, appearing as if broken into two and not equidistant: the pulse strong, at first 80, sometimes irregular, and not always corresponding to that of the heart, which was more frequently irregular and usually 2 or 4 beats quicker, although once, the pulse was 58 at the wrist while the heart was 54. There were occasional throbbings of the carotids; and *after eating*, a sensation of a foreign body in the chest and stomach. A considerable time elapsed before the action of the heart became regular, and the numbness was for some time obstinate. Leeches to the region of the heart proved beneficial.

A sensation as if the heart were swimming in water, which is doubtful, and will be difficult to ascertain in India, except by one intimately acquainted with the native forms of expression.

Of the general symptoms, a sense of oppression and weight at the præcordia is almost always present, and is also often felt at the extremity of the sternum, and in the epigastrium which is now and then distended: this is also sometimes felt across the chest, and at others mostly to the right of the sternum. The respiration is always short on exertion, however slight, and it is remarkable that the patient, if the fluid is not in large quantity, may be little distressed with dyspnœa when at rest, and is frequently easiest in the recumbent posture, which is never the case when the lungs are œdematous, the bronchi inflamed, or when the effusion is into the pleura[89]; and as the dyspnœa from these affections is more urgent than from water in the pericardium, the patient is obliged to keep in the erect posture, whenever those complications exist. These observations explain the opposite statements of Mr. Geddes and of Dr. Wight, the first of whom states, that the patients are easiest in the recumbent posture, and often die suddenly; and the latter, in the few

[89] The observations of Mr. Dick show, that when the water, exists only in one cavity, as is most commonly the case, the patient can lie *on that side*, with the head very low. A strong muscular man had anasarcous swellings in November and was salivated, but the œdema extended over the body, his breathing was much affected, his rest disturbed with horrid dreams and startings. Thirst great, urine very scanty, belly costive, skin cold and clammy, a short dry cough distressed him and he could only sleep on the right side, which was more swelled than the other. He was easiest when his head was lower than any other part of his body. He took purgatives, cream of tartar in gin and chamomile tea, which brought on a free discharge of urine. The anasarca was so great as to induce the use of free scarifications, and in the hope that these would relieve the dyspnœa, paracentesis was put off till next day. A blister to the chest gave relief for a few hours, but in going to make water in the night, he stumbled on the threshold of the door, fell down and expired. Two quarts of water were instantly drawn from the right cavity of the thorax, and stimulants were applied, but in vain. There was no water in the left cavity, and Mr. D. was not permitted to open the body.

cases he had witnessed at the time of drawing up his report, had found them unable to lie down and had met with no instance of sudden death. In one example only, did the patient suffer more on lying on the left side, and in him this seemed to arise from affection of the lung.[90] The appearances on dissection clearly prove the frequent existence of inflammation, and careful enquiry will often detect the usual symptoms of pericarditis, obscure as they are, but considerably modified by the peculiar nature of the disease before us. Effusion of fluid is very often the direct result of inflammation, but when it is severe, there is usually flocculent deposit and a turbid appearance, but with the exception of three cases to be related hereafter, the fluid has always been clear and yellow into whatever cavity effused; this however is no proof, of there having been no inflammatory action. In a very remarkable case of pneumato-thorax uncomplicated with fistulous bronchial communication, which occurred to me lately, there were effusion into the right pleura, numerous adhesions, and a thick layer of lymph evidently just formed, and the result of inflammation; there was also a good deal of fluid in the pericardium, in which there was no vestige of previous excitement: both fluids had exactly the same appearance to the eye, but on examination, the former condensed into a solid mass on being heated, while the latter exhibited only the usual turbid appearance, caused by the coagulation of its natural proportion of albumen. I have reason to believe, that an examination of the quantity

[90] On this point, the observations I have had an opportunity of making are very imperfect. Mr. Dick states, that when the pericardium contains water, the patient lies easiest on the left side, and in one of Mr. Davidson's cases, an abstract of which will be found in a subsequent note, walking and attempting to lie on the left side brought on palpitation. There is reason to believe, that fluid is most frequently effused into the left cavity of the pleura, which will prevent the patient resting on the right side.

of albumen in the morbid fluid, compared with that in the natural secretion of the particular cavity, would lead to some important pathological results. The weight in the præcordia and epigastrium occasionally amounts to pain, where there are no indications of the stomach being the part which suffers.[91] I observ-

[91] The following cases illustrate this fact, and several other circumstances connected with the symptoms of water in the pericardium. The first is extracted from a report for 1825 of Mr. Macaulay, then staff surgeon at Quilon, who informs me that beriberi is little known in Travancore, notwithstanding that its climate is such as has been considered to give rise to that affection. "The first case was one of hydrothorax in a strong muscular gunner of "dissipated habits, 31 years of age, and 9 in India. He had been more than "once in hospital, complaining of dull pain and sense of weight at the "scrobiculus cordis, with an irregular state of bowels. It was then regard-"ed as chronic hepatitis, and he was each time discharged, relieved, after a "slight alterative course and purgatives; but on his last admission, which "was on the 4th of September, the case was more distinctly marked; he com-"plained of a "shocking weight" at the pit of the stomach, and an oppres-"sion at his chest, increased in the horizontal position, his countenance was "leucophlegmatic, and his ancles œdematous; he had thirst and scanty urine, "but his pulse and bowels were natural. He admitted that this attack was "preceded by more than usual dissipation. He was immediately blooded to "the extent of 25 ounces, and his bowels freely acted on by calomel and "jalap, and this was followed up by a course of pills containing calomel, "squills, and digitalis; he thought himself relieved after the bleeding, but "the following night was passed without sleep, being unable to lay down "above a few minutes at a time, and his breathing became more laborious, "consisting of a succession of slow deep inspirations. Fifteen ounces of more "blood were abstracted, and at his request a large blister was applied to the "epigastric region; but he derived no relief from this, and he continued in "the most deplorable state, unable to lay down and calling out for more air, "until the night of the 11th when he expired. On opening the body an ef-"fusion of a yellowish serum was found in both cavities of the chest, and the "pericardium was so distended by it, as to have the appearance of a full "blown bladder. A remarkable circumstance in this case, was the undisturb-"ed state of the pulse, notwithstanding the other symptoms were so urgent. Abstract of a case in the journal of surgeon Browne of H. M. 80th regiment for April, 1812. The regiment was then stationed at Seringapatam. Mr. Colhoun Stirling says, that beriberi prevailed there during both the last Mysore wars, (*Hunter on Diseases of Lascars*,) and Mr. Geddes met with the disease at the same place, *in natives of the circars*. H. Blandford, sergeant, ætat 32. of a full habit. Was admitted April 12th complaining of debility, pain at epigastrium, nausea, loss of appetite, foultongue, costive bowels and thirst; skin cool, pulse 100, headach. Bilious stools were procured by jalap and calomel. On the 14th his pulse was 110, tongue covered with a brown crust, and he had slight headach. Pain at epigastrium continued with some dyspnœa. A blister was applied to the epigastrium which gave no relief, and two grains of calomel twice a day and mercurial frictions were ordered, apparently under the impression that the disease was hepatitis. On the 17th he was emaciated, and very low and weak, he complained of restless nights and of uneasiness in epigastrium. Thirst was urgent, urine scanty, and pulse 120. His medicines were continued, with the addition of half a bottle of wine daily. The symptoms increased, and on the 22d his pulse was 125, small, and intermitting every third stroke; the pain at epigastrium had left him, but respiration was laborious. 23d. Mouth not affected, and his breathing continues laborious, he is not able to sit up, but feels no particular

ed in a very few instances only, tenderness between the ribs, which has of late been found to occur, when the pericardium was inflamed.

Case 28th. A man was admitted with pain at the sternal extremity of the left 6th rib, constant palpitation, dyspnœa and cough. Pain was increased on pressure. Pulse 120, strong and full; very restless. A purgative and sulphuric æther did no good. He was bled to 16 ounces with relief, and with the exception of slight œdema of the feet, was pretty well in five days. Digitalis was given and a blister applied; the latter quickened the pulse. He was discharged on the 12th day. A more important and peculiar symptom, the cause of which is yet obscure, is a burning heat in the chest, most commonly rather diffused, but most felt about the cardiac region. It has been observed along with other pericarditic symptoms: no opportunity of examination after death, of a patient who had recently suffered from it has occurred; but a sensation in the abdomen, in every respect similar, has been ascertained to have been caused by diffused inflammation in

pain and is perfectly collected, his countenance is sunk, his voice hollow, tongue and mouth parched, urine high coloured, pulse 130 and intermits, no stool. Rept. enema. Cont. vin. ad libit. Omitt. alia. 24th. Pulse scarcely to be felt at the wrist, breathing very laborious. Cont. vinum. 25th. Delirium in the night. 27th. Died at noon.

On opening the body the abdominal viscera were found of the natural appearance; as also those of the thorax, with the exception of the pericardium which contained a considerable quantity of water.

The distended pericardium appears in many cases to press down the diaphragm, and thus to embarrass respiration; hence the dyspnœa frequently induced by eating the bulky meals of rice used by the natives, and the feeling of a foreign body in the chest in Syed Nubbi (note 88). In one or two of Mr. Davidson's cases, this appeared to be the result rather of the excitement of digestion; at least, in one case, the slightest exertion had the same effect, and there was no diffused pulsation; the heart's action was slow, irregular, and communicated a grating feeling to the hand as if sand were interposed. One patient had no dyspnœa when lying down, or when *standing*, but it came on when he walked or attempted to *sit*; and another was free of it when standing, but lying down, eating, or walking brought it on. In Mr. Ridley's second case, also, respiration was, on the 2d day after admission, difficult only on stooping or suddenly changing position. In the case of Meer Kumroodeen alluded to in note 68, the heaviness in the chest and dyspnœa were induced by moving in bed, and by the exertion of sitting up or lying down.

beriberi, and in other diseases;[92] and it has been observed to come on with febrile heat, quickened pulse, and to necessitate the omission of stimulants. It is

[92] In one example it was only a modification of the neuralgic sensation formerly described, and on dissection no thoracic inflammation was found. *Original note.* This symptom was present during the fatal relapse which carried off the patient, an abstract of whose case is subjoined. The latter part of the history was recorded by Mr. Davidson, and it is much to be regretted, that the funeral being unexpectedly ordered the evening of the patient's death, prevented that minute examination of the body, which Mr. D. would otherwise have made.

F. Gouge, assistant apothecary, admitted 19th October 1832, from the outstation of Ragapoor. States that he has been labouring under swelling of the limbs for the last month, and has also had some pyrexia, but no distinct paroxysm of fever. The local affection was not preceded by pyrexia. His face is now somewhat bloated; lower extremities swollen, and tense except at the feet, upper extremities also swollen but rather puffy, especially at the hands; trunk is generally puffy, and, along the spine, œdematous. Pulsation of the heart is widely and strongly felt, but corresponds with the pulse which is, after rest, 116, rather firm and moderately full; difficulty of breathing on the least motion; is somewhat agitated. Slight dry cough. Urine scanty and high coloured, bowels costive except when moved by medicine, abdomen pretty natural. Tongue sodden, appetite impaired; not much thirst. Skin warm and dry; sleeps pretty well at night. Calves a little stiff but has no numbness. He was bled to 18 ounces which induced faintness. Five minutes afterwards the pulse fell to 100 and was fuller and soft. Blood drawn not buffy or cupped. 6 P. M. Skin warm and moist. Feels lighter about præcordia, and is able to sigh without inconvenience. Purged four times by a powder containing jalap, cream of tartar and nitre. Urine scanty, of a deep amber colour and clear. Gums and roof of mouth dark, but has taken about two scruples of calomel with aloes, before admission. Capt. h. s. aloës gr. xij. Rept. pulv. jalap. &c. cras mane. 20th 7 P. M. Five deep yellow stools from the jalap powder. Pulse easily accelerated, 108, soft; pulsation at heart 112, firmer and fuller than the pulse at wrist; feels no inconvenience except from throbbing at the heart. Urine deep brown, yellow, and a little turbid. Admoveant. hirudines xij regioni cordis. Capt. cras mane pulv. jalapæ gr. xxv, potass. subcarbon. gr. xx. 22d. Pulse at wrist and pulsation of heart both 102, soft and full. Skin warm and dry. No stool, having omitted to take the medicine. The powder was repeated, and small doses of digitalis, squills, and æther prescribed. 22d. Twelve stools, liquid and offensive. Pulse at wrist and pulsation of heart both 100, smaller and weaker; *the latter perceptible at epigastrium.* Œdema and tenseness of legs gone; arms still swollen and rather tense. 23d. Continues the purgatives and draughts. Forearms alone are tense, and he says that they also feel heavy; face is stiff and puffy. About 20 ounces of urine in twenty four hours. 25th. A drop of croton oil prescribed yesterday; severely purged in the night, stools liquid, bright yellow, with an admixture of mucus. Pulsation at wrist 98, smaller and weaker, of heart 104. Short cough. Skin of moderate heat and soft; tongue dry, furred, pale yellow and rough; thirst. The croton is omitted, and he takes treeak farook and digitalis. 26th. Slept comfortably. Pulse at wrist and pulsation of heart 100. *Upper part of body generally pits on pressure and the forearms are tense; lower limbs natural.* Urine 14 ounces in the night. 27th. Took an ounce of oil which purged him, and he felt much exhausted, mucus in the stools. Pulse 96, pulsation of heart 100. 28th. Pulse and heart beat 96 times in a minute but smaller and weaker. 28th Vespere. Pulse 104, firmer, pulsation of heart 106, irregularity approaching to intermission observed in both. 29th. Pulse at wrist 88, much smaller, softer and intermitting; pulsation of heart 92, stronger in proportion than the pulse at the wrist, but also intermitting; purged in the night before taking oil. 30th. Pulse and

therefore probable that it depends on the same cause, and it has in every instance been a symptom of a serious disease. Feverish heat over the body in the af-

stroke of heart regular and 96. Stools mucous, of different shades of orange with streaks of blood. Oppression at chest towards evening. Twelve leeches were repeated and the medicines continued. 31st. Pulse 94, soft and regular, pulsation of heart 90, firm, jerking and intermitting. Urine pale brown, yellow and turbid. The oil is repeated. Vespere. Seems faint. Pulse at wrist 96, firmer, fuller and distinctly intermitting. Pulsation of heart 108 with disjointed and redoubled stroke, skin rather hot and dry, frequent greenish stools with streaks of blood. Is subject to piles. 1st. November. A blister applied and has relieved the oppression of chest. 3rd. Nights restless, sighs frequently, respiration abdominal, audible and oppressed. Pulse 86, weaker and not very steady; heart corresponds but its stroke is still jerking and redoubled. 7th Bowels still loose, and takes purgatives which seem to exhaust him; pulse and heart correspond and are a little irregular, respiration is a little laboured and abdominal. Says he does not suffer from dyspnœa, and can lie in any posture. Takes a pretty full inspiration but hastily. 24th. Considerably improved. No dyspnœa, pulse and pulsation of heart 72 this morning, but the latter is impatient, jerking, and stronger than the pulse; both occasionally intermit and, sometimes, are irregular in strength. Palpitation on exertion; complexion darker; urine copious. Takes a grain and a half of digitalis four times a day, which make him giddy and he sometimes vomits them. Has half a drop of croton oil in the mornings. 17th December. Continued much as at last report till yesterday, when he was seized with purging, griping, and straining; stools composed of reddish fluid and mucous shreds, with some deep brown feces. No tenderness in any part of the abdomen. Pulse 84, moderately full; tongue moist and a little furred; little or no palpitation at present; urine more scanty: relieved by calomel and opium, and stools became natural in two days. 3rd February, 1833. Has improved greatly in appearance. Is free from œdema. Is still conscious of *palpitation on attempting to lie on the left side*, or on moving quickly; heart otherwise quiet. Pulse 84, rather weak; skin, tongue, and bowels pretty natural; urine by account only in moderate quantity. 1st March. Has had no occasion to take medicine since last report. Feels now merely irritable, his pulse becoming accelerated on locomotion. He wishes to return to his station, and is discharged with instructions to take medicine,should any symptoms of the disease recur, which he neglected to do, and on the 9th April he returned to Ellore,and was readmitted complaining much of oppression about his chest and pain of its lower part, and of the epigastrium which was very tender and in some degree distended. He complained much of *internal heat and that his inside appeared to be burning*. Pulse 120, irritable, and not full. In great distress. Has taken a dose of compound powder of jalap, and twelve leeches were ordered to be applied to the epigastrium, but he did not put them on till next morning. He passed a bad night,and at noon of the following day he was found in a dreadful state, labouring for breath, lips quite black, pointing to the cricoid cartilage and entreating to have his wind-pipe opened, or that if relief could not be afforded, that he might be shot. Mr. D. states that he could afford him no relief, and that he feared what had been done had been injurious. The pulse was felt to get weaker and intermitting till it ceased at the wrist, and he died at ½ p. 2 P. M.

An hour and a half after death the body was examined. It was not emaciated nor the face sunk. While dividing the ribs near the sternum, black blood poured out copiously which proceeded from a cut accidentally made in the liver, and was found in large quantity in the abdomen. The liver enlarged and very vascular in all parts. Gall bladder filled with very dark bile. Stomach vascular; the small intestines greatly contracted, feeling doughy, thickened, and firmer than usual; the mucous membrane was very red, much thickened and softened,and easily broken down and removed by the fingers:

ternoons, or constant low pyrexia, deserve attention, although I cannot state in how far they depend on the affection of the pericardium. They are sometimes absent, and more commonly assume the form of the prevailing intermittent. The action of the heart has frequently been violent, sometimes tumultuous and fluttering; and, as well as the pulse, has had in one or two instances the hardness of rheumatic inflammation of the heart, a little before the effusion could be detected; occasionally the pulse is full and the heart's action regular, but more frequently its stroke and that of the pulse has been small and very rapid, an effect of the fluid by which it is surrounded, and is most remarkable when that is in greatest quantity.[93] Irregu-

its folds were increased in size. Nothing unusual in the large intestines. Both kidneys and the bladder quite healthy. An inconsiderable quantity of serum in the abdomen, in which floated a handful of clear jelly. The lungs were collapsed, of healthy grey colour, without tubercles or adhesions, the crepitus, when squeezed, not quite so loud as usual, and when cut into no fluid oozed out. About a pint of water in the chest of a red colour, perhaps from the blood from the liver. Between 5 and 6 ounces of water in the pericardium. The heart seemed to be enlarged, but when cut into seemed healthy. A large quantity of blood in the right cavities of the heart. Large blood vessels healthy. Mr. D. regretted excedingly not being allowed time to examine the spine, as he did not see any thing to account satisfactorily for the fatal termination.

In Mr. Ridley's first case, the legs and hands were benumbed, heavy, and œdematous, the throat swollen and face bloated, respiration difficult with great oppression at the præcordia. The patient complained of a *sensation of great internal heat as if his breath burned his throat.* His head was slightly confused; his urine scanty, high coloured and hot. Under the use of purgatives, calomel, diuretics, &c. he was better on the 2d day, and his breath had lost the intense heat before complained of, but dyspnœa continued and he had a distressing sensation at epigastrium, which was relieved by laudanum. In 3 weeks he was discharged. The " pain and tightness at the lower edge of the sternum" was so distressing in several of Mr. R's patients, as to induce them to solicit that the *part might be cut open.* The extraordinary congestion of the liver in the assistant apothecary was similar to that in Mr. Dick's patient, J. Briggs, (note 77) and appears to have been caused by the blood being obstructed in its passage through the right side of the heart, which in this example was not the effect of the state of the lungs; and perhaps to those instances in which the " enlargement of the liver itself though accompanied with " some swelling, seemed to occasion death; at least, the quantities of water " in the thorax were not sufficient to produce such effects alone."

93 Many other causes of frequent and small pulse are in operation in different cases, as general nervous irritation, abdominal disease, prostration of the powers, &c. As is now and then the case in ordinary hydropericardium, the pulse may be slow; and oppressed brain and even dyspnœa in which the respirations are long and deep, have caused slow pulse. *Original note.* The

larity of the pulse is a frequent occurrence, and, according to my observations, most commonly takes place when the cardiac affection has existed for some time. When the pulse is hard, full and frequent, bleeding gives great relief, but the hardness may remain when the strength is gone; and bleeding is occasionally required, when the pulse is small and very frequent, with symptoms of copious effusion into the pericardium. The blood is seldom buffy, the serum is in large proportion, in some instances perhaps from the firm coagulation of the clot, and in others from the

two following cases *(first half yearly report of 1825, of asst. surgeon J. Thomson, of the 29th regiment N.I. stationed at Samulcottah)*, confirm the inference from the symptoms which accompanied slow pulse, in the cases alluded to in the first part of the last sentence.

"The fatal case placed rather improperly under the head, pneumonia, was "in a subject ætat. 18, of a robust habit. Admitted with difficult respiration "and oppression in the chest; severe cough, and copious expectoration of mu- "cus. Pulse very slow and soft, and at times irregular; appetite impaired; "bowels slow. He said the complaint attacked him 3 days ago, and that he "had been very much subject for some years, to a disease in the chest. A "dose of opening medicine and expectorants were administered, and a blister "applied to his chest, but these had no power over the disease; and on the "third day after his admission, the oppression and difficulty in breathing be- "coming very urgent, face flushed, and a strong palpitation of the heart, an "attempt was made to bleed him, but only four ounces could be obtained, "and he died on the 9th day after his admission. On examining the thorax "a few hours after death, the right portion of the lungs was found adhering "to the pleura costalis and in a collapsed state, but no tubercles or abscess, "and did not particularly indicate recent inflammation; the left portion ap- "peared quite sound, but *the blood vessels were very turgid*, and *the pericar- "dium was fully distended with serum.* No other morbid appearance was ob- "served, as it was rather a hurried dissection."

"The fatal case of anasarca was in a private, ætat. 26, of a full habit of "body. Admitted on the 20th April with an œdematous swelling of his feet "and weakness, pulse slow and soft, appetite a little impaired, urine rather "high coloured. The swelling had continued about 8 days, and he had been "previously taking bazar medicine on account of fever. He got a dose of "opening medicine, and his feet rubbed with a liniment; but on the even- "ing of the 23rd, the swelling began to appear general accompanied with great "debility; loss of appetite, and a slight difficulty in breathing. Pulse full "and soft; urine scanty and high coloured. He was bled to 16 ounces, and "calomel and squills prescribed, as the disease assumed such a marked ap- "pearance of beriberi. On the 26th he was reduced to a very debilitated "state, and had great difficulty in breathing accompanied with a strong pal- "pitation of the heart and an irregular pulse; and he died on the following "day. No dissection could be obtained."

From Mr. Davidson's cases it appears, that the pulse frequently becomes slower than natural, soon after the patient has been under treatment and removed from all causes of excitement, even when the heart continues to be irritable; and both when its actions are irregular in strength, and intermitting. In *one or two* of these cases, it may have been the effect of two beats run-

hydropic character of the blood.[94] As in common cases of pericarditis, hydropericardium and hypertrophy, the increased or disordered action of the heart, as well as the feeble powers of the softened texture, are apt to end in interrupted action, often suddenly fatal; sometimes however, I have seen the patient pass from one fainting fit to another, or he feels faint and his countenance is very anxious; the heart may flutter as if terribly oppressed, the carotids and jugulars pulsate, and the pulse almost ceases for two or three hours before death. I have not been able to determine except in a few cases, when this was to be ascribed to the water in the pericardium, to the state of the muscular substance of the heart itself, or the tendency of abnormal muscular action, whethter from functional or organic disease, to intermit or cease.[95]

ning into one, as in a sepoy whose pulse was 34 with a sort of double beat, and the sound and impulse of the heart not uniform in strength. On the 23rd the pulse was 39, and on the 28th 70, with a sudden stroke. The sleep was disturbed, the face puffy, and respiration accelerated. The following important observations are by Messrs. Geddes and Macdonell. "In a few, the pulse "has been observed to get more slow before death, but in general its getting "less frequent is to be considered the most favourable symptom which can "take place, and until it attains the natural standard both with respect to "number and softness, the patient can scarcely be considered free from the "disease, or secure from relapse at some early period. In slight cases where "the approach of the disease is gradual, and the symptoms have not become "urgent, the pulse is to be found little accelerated, and in these as well as in "others, on the œdema becoming removed, it falls occasionally below the na-"tural standard in frequency, descending to 46, or below it, in the minute."

[94] The clot is sometimes soft and the serum too plentiful. *Original note.*

[95] This subject is one of great interest and peculiar difficulty, requiring for its successful prosecution the minute detail of every symptom, both of thoracic and general disease. Even where the accumulation of water in the pericardium, appears to have been the principal cause of the anxiety and other symptoms, the functions of the heart have been disordered before the effusion could be detected, or have continued to be so, after it had disappeared, and exertion would continue to bring on the dyspnœa. In Mr. Turnbull's valuable observations (appendix) on a disease resembling beriberi, that proved very fatal to the prisoners at Bellary the end of 1832 and beginning of 1833, the orthopnœa and anguish preceding dissolution, was traced to obstructed action of the heart arising from violent inflammation of the pericardium, of the muscular substance of the heart, and of its external and internal surface on which adhesive lymph was deposited. The effusion into the pericardium and pleuræ was insufficient to account for the symptoms, and although the heart appeared enlarged, it was from the distension of its cavities with blood. The same inference is also suggested by a review of Mr. Davidson's

It is in cases of this kind that sudden death most frequently[96] occurs, and when the symptoms we have

cases, in many of which a grating feel, as if sand were interposed between the heart and parietes of the chest, was communicated to the hand ; in several the impulse was strong, jerking, irregular in the rhythm and strength, without diffused pulsation or other symptom of hydropericardium, and the least exertion brought on dyspnœa, attended with great irregularity of the action of the heart, and of the pulse. In a sepoy named Permalloo, the body and face were swollen, the abdomen tumid, and the upper and lower limbs tense ; he could lie down without difficulty, the heart's action was irregular, the auricular and venticular contractions of the same length, and occasionally intermitting ; the pulse was 90 and not felt irregular, but *on the least exertion became so weak as scarcely to be felt.* On the 31st, the pulse was 64 at the wrist and the pulsation of the heart 62, weak and irregular ; next day, the pulse was 66 and the heart 64, the dyspnœa was felt only on walking, and the swelling of the face had nearly left him, but it felt heavy. In some other cases, liability to disordered action of the heart remained long after apparent recovery, and appeared to depend on nervous debility or irritation. Some remarks on spasms affecting the chest will be found in a subsequent page, but it may be useful to mention, that lessening the quantity of blood will relieve the dyspnœa from affection of the heart, even when antispasmodics may be used with advantage.

It is of great importance to distinguish between dyspnœa arising from œdema of the lung, and from disorder of the centre of the circulation, which are both greatly aggravated by motion. The latter is frequently the cause of the former, but when this is not decidedly the case, the respiration being more *uniformly* embarrassed, the pulse though small and frequent being regular, and the patient unable to rest in the recumbent posture, will direct attention to the other symptoms which distinguish that formidable state of disease, from cardiac affection. These remarks will also assist, in distinguishing that state of congestion of the lungs consequent on disease of the heart, which Mr. Wright observed in case 11, and was also present in Mr. Hamilton's case and in others, (and which will often be relieved by lessening the quantity of blood in the vessels,) from effusion of water into the cells of the lungs.

[96] The important remarks in the following extract illustrate this and several other observations in the text.

" It is stated occasionally to have terminated in from six to thirty-six hours, " from its attack, but in the shorter of these cases, there is reason to believe, " that the date of the person's illness had either been placed at the period of " the commencement of the fatal dyspnœa, while some slight degree of ana- " sarca had previously been present, but not particularly taken notice of, or " that the patient had become relieved from conspicuous symptoms, leaving " however some internal disorder, as water in the pericardium or the like, and " that a sudden aggravating cause had brought on the rapid dissolution. In- " stances indeed could be brought forward, of the apparent disorder, being " even of shorter duration than that above mentioned, as in the case of a fe- " male employed as a nurse, who died in twenty-five minutes after she was " supposed to be taken ill, but water was found in her pericardium, and her " limbs were swelled, a circumstance which previous to death had been refer- " red to her becoming more corpulent." * * * " Of twenty-four deaths from " this disease, three occurred on the day of admission, five in two days, and " two more before the fourth day, but of these ten, seven were relapses and " the remainder had been ill from one to two weeks before being reported. " Of the other fourteen, six took place within less than fourteen days, seven " in from twenty-two to fifty-two, and one after being one hundred and forty- " nine days in the sick list. In sixty recoveries, again, ten were discharged " from the hospital in less than ten days, eight in less than fifteen, fourteen in " less than twenty, nine were either sent out on the convalescent list, or trans- " ferred to another part of the country, and the remaining twenty went to " their duty in from twenty to fifty-six days, after being admitted into hospi- " tal." (*Messrs Geddes and Macdonell's paper.*)

been considering are present, the patient is never for an instant safe, and I infer on a review of my cases, that not less than one half of the casualties occur in this way. I may be thought to reason in a circle, in considering this fact as confirmatory of the previous views ; but as the bearing of each class of symptoms was separately enquired into, by recording the inferences from separate examinations of numerous cases, and as they all tend to the same conclusion and are in every respect analogous to well known phenomena, the united evidence is as strong as we can expect to have in affections of this nature; and therefore the opinion of a writer of last year, which I have just met with, is no longer correct, viz. "that we know little or nothing of the immediate cause of death."* In no complicated affection, am I so confident in predicting the probable manner of the fatal termination as in beriberi, when the visceral affections have developed themselves.

The diagnosis is often obscured by the supervention of effusion into the pleura, but if the dyspnœa is moderate except on exertion, and the recumbent posture agreeable, the general symptoms present in the following case will be found, in general, to arise from hydropericardium.

Case 29th. Vanaloo, ætat. 60. Admitted 5th August, complaining of sense of numbness and loss of power of motion of the lower extremities, attended with extreme restlessness, oppression at præcordia, and difficulty of breathing ;[97] expression of counte-

* Article Beriberi, in the Cyclopædia of Practical Medicine.

[97] Oppression at præcordia, and feeling of distension and weight under the sternum were present in J. Briggs, in whom the lungs were distended with fluid (note 77), and in Mr. Hamilton's case, in which the pericardium was inflamed ; there was no effusion into the pericardium in either. The following account of these symptoms by Messrs Geddes and Macdonell is valuable.

nance peculiarly anxious; cold clammy feel of the body. Pulse small and rapid, tongue dirty white. Has been ill three days; at noon he got much worse, and died. There was considerable effusion, both into the pericardium and cavity of the pleura. (Compare this case with that of Kiser Naík.)

It appears to have been demonstrated by Dr. Elliotson and others, that inflammation of the pericardium is a common cause of enlargement of the heart with increase of substance, and of simple dilatation; and many facts render it probable, that the fibre of the heart loses its firmness and powers from the same cause; it will not then be surprising, that similar actions should lead to the same termination in beriberi, and we have seen that hypertrophy, passive dilatation, and degeneration of the muscular fibre are caused by the disease. But I have reason to believe that this happens, when there is no inflammation of the heart or its covering, but merely a certain degree of excitement of its vessels causing effusion.

Dr. Wight, the distinguished botanist, paid considerable attention to the singular irregularities in the action of the arteries, which sometimes occur: some of his observations I have been enabled to confirm. The pulsation in the carotids was strong in patients whose heart beat feebly, or in whom the pulse in the limbs was weak; and the impulse of the heart was sometimes strong, while that of the arteries was weak.

"The pulse has also been sometimes found irregular or intermittent, but "this is unusual. Connected with this state of the circulation, is to be refer- "red the sense of anxiety, which is often felt in a very urgent degree in the "varieties of this disease. This is described by the patient as a sense of ful- "ness in the chest, feeling of uneasiness, heaviness or oppression over the "belly, a sense of tightness, or of a collection of something at the scrobiculus "cordis; and in some instances, palpitation of the heart or sensations of alarm "appear particularly to attract attention. The veins of the surface are also "observed to be distended, and present a blacker hue than natural in the lat- "ter stages, and in the European, along with the severe dyspnœa, a lividity of "the countenance is observed."

This might be explained in some cases (as it was in a patient of mine), by the inflammation of the heart, of which strong pulsation in the carotids is a symptom,[98] and the pressure of the fluid on the organ obstructing and rendering its impulse indistinct. But for the phenomena in the following case,in which the strength and number of the pulse in different arteries varied, the only explanation that can be given, is, that the arteries are muscular, and influenced by the nerves distributed to their coats.

Case 30th. A man supposed to eat opium, was admitted 4th May with symptoms of beriberi, headach, wildness in his look, pulse 100, irregular, oppression at chest; bilious evacuations with febrile paroxysms in the night. 6th. Pulse in wrist and temples 100, strong and full, in lower extremities 120, feeble; heat

[98] Mr. Dundas found the carotids acting violently, when the heart was enlarged but not increased in power, and a fact in some respects similar occurred in case 10th. *Original note.* The pulse was weak when the heart gave a strong and grating impulse to the hand, in one of Mr. Davidson's cases, in which numbness and œdema of the upper and lower extremities, with afternoon fever, followed rheumatism. The periods of repose were too long, there were occasionally a number of rapid beats, and the pulsation was felt on the right side of the chest. In others, the action of the heart has been tremulous, unsteady, and broken into two, with a full and strong pulse ; in Syed Nubbi (note 88) this took place along with pulsation of the carotids, and symptoms of water in the pericardium. In Mahomed Khassim (note 68) the pulse and action of the heart were at first unusually full and frequent, in three days the pulse was 72 and rather strong and full, and the pulsation of the heart could not be felt by the hand, but its sound was regular and even strong. Laennec states, that pericarditis may be suspected, when, in a patient who had never had disease of the heart, the contraction of the ventricles yields a greater shock (and, sometimes, a more marked sound), than usual, and at intervals feeble and shorter pulsations are experienced, which correspond with intermissions of the pulse : the smallness of the pulse, also, contrasts remarkably with the strength of the heart's pulsation. The pulse in Mr. D's patients was often regular when the heart's actions were irregular, frequently from the contractions of the different cavities not corresponding with each other.

In one example (Syed Moortuzah), the impulse was felt on the right side of the chest, and as well as the pulse, was irregular and weak, and dyspnœa was excited by the least exertion. In a few days the stroke of the heart could not be detected by the hand and its sounds were irregular, that is, the rhythm was regular for a little, and then the venticular sound was alone heard. Three days afterwards, the impulse of the heart was stronger but did not then extend into the right side : after this the patient's recovery was rapid. In this patient, the face, belly,and legs were swollen, and the œdema of the latter diminished, with the improvement in the heart's action, disorder in the centre of the circulation being a usual cause of general anasarca.

heat natural. Takes calomel. gr. x morning and evening. 7th. Hiccups and bitter taste of mouth ; pulse 104 in the wrists, 96 in the ancles. Treatment continued with leeches to temples, and cold to the scalp; and anodyne draughts relieve the hiccup. 9th Pulse 120 in all the arteries. Dark stools removed by cathartics : and ptyalism does no good. 12th. When sitting up, pulse in radial artery 140, full, in the ancles very small ; on lying down for a short time, in wrist 120, in the ancles 130 and stronger. Took 30 drops of digitalis thrice a day, which Dr. Wight looks on as a stimulant. In the evening, pulse was 130 in all the arteries and full and strong, skin very hot, face tumid, dyspnœa, slight delirium. Ten ounces of blood were drawn, and removed the delirium and relieved the dyspnœa. 13th. A good night, pulse 120, soft and equal in all the limbs, very weak but easy. In consequence of Dr. W. being detached, there is no report till the 22d, when the patient was found labouring under dyspnœa, tumid face, swelled belly and legs, scanty red urine, and numbness of the surface, and he died in two days.

Abdominal pulsation[99] is in some instances violent; this occurred to Baillie in palsy, and I have seen it cause great alarm, in remittent fever in which effusion had taken place on the brain. To such examples Dr. Dwyer must allude, when he says that cases of beriberi have been mistaken for aneurism. There can be little doubt, that these examples are to be referred to injury of the nervous system, as in irregular pulse in cerebral palsy, or in that peculiar affection so well described by Dr. Bateman as occur-

[99] It should be stated, that this is generally in the epigastrium and sometimes arises from the distended pericardium pressing down the diaphragm. *Original note.*

ing to himself, and in which the irregular arterial action, was complicated with constriction across the chest.

In experiments on animals it has been found, that the effect on the circulation has been trivial, however severe the injury was, if it affected but a small part of the cerebro-spinal axis; but that if it were applied to an extensive surface, however slight the injury might be, the actions of the heart and capillaries were disordered and quickened, and if the surface was still greater, instant death from cessation of the heart's action was the consequence. The sympathetic which supplies the heart and capillaries, being intimately connected by means of numerous nervous fibrils sent to its plexuses and ganglia, with the whole extent of the spinal marrow, irritation of the spinal cord acts not only by exciting contractions, but also by exalting or depressing the vital power.[100] The ex-

[100] In some analogous examples, the circulation may be depressed while convulsions are induced in the voluntary muscles, the same cause being to one a stimulant and to the other a sedative: affording a probable explanation of the apparent transfer of the spasms from the external parts, mentioned as a cause of death, by a friend of great experience in the disease. *Original note.* The cases of Dauniah and of Mootoo-Roydoo, pages 82 and 115, illustrate this remark: the subject however requires to be again examined, and the different forms of dyspnœa above described, carefully distinguished from spasms of the muscles; which has not been done, sufficiently, in the following valuable observations by Mr. Christie. "One of the symptoms of beriberi, which "I lay considerable stress upon, as accounting for the rapid progress of the "disease, and sudden death, is spasms of the muscles of the chest, heart, or "large vessels; for although in none of my dissections have I observed a total absence of effusion in the pericardium, pleura, or cellular substance of "the lungs, yet the quantity found is, in general, inadequate to the extreme "violence of the dyspnœa; the spasms are, in many cases, evident externally, "and in other cases, the irregular action of the heart is plainly indicated, by "irregular and intermitting pulse." *Hunter on Diseases of Lascars, page* 80. Spasms of the gastrocnemii are common amongst the convalescents and are important "as if it is allowed, that these spasms may occasionally seize "the vital organs, they may serve to explain, why death happens, in many "cases, so suddenly, although there is but little effusion." *Ibid. page* 85. "I have "reason to be confirmed in my opinion, that a spasm of the vital organs is occasionally the cause of the sudden death; from a very particular case, where, "after the effusion was removed, the patient, for many weeks, was subject "to violent spasms of the external muscles of the chest, attended with "intermitting pulse, and excessive dyspnœa. These symptoms were repeatedly removed, by large doses of laudanum and æther, &c. but their frequent

planation thus afforded of these curious facts, (and probably of some examples of sudden death), is as satisfactory as of most others, in which the nervous power exerts an influence over the functions of other parts of the economy.[101] But besides this general effect, other more peculiar ones are observed to take place from affections of the spinal marrow; of which the inordinate action, inflammatory condition, and in-

" recurrence occasioned great exhaustion, and he was at length carried off by " one of those spasmodic attacks." *Pages* 87 *and* 88. To this cause he ascribed the death of two of Mr. Holloway's patients, who after the removal of the œdema died suddenly in their sleep. One of Mr. Colhoun's patients had beriberi attended with violent convulsive symptoms, and ultimately sunk dropsical, exhausted, and delirious, and in another, who died suddenly after taking a full meal, on landing from a small vessel in which he had suffered from exposure and starvation, there was little œdema or effusion into the chest, and Mr. C. therefore ascribed the fatal termination to the stimulus of the food, which would favour the opinion of its being connected with the state of the nervous system. Bontius found the disease tedious but not mortal, except when it seized on the muscles of the breast and thorax, and thereby stopped respiration. *Bontius on the diseases of the East Indies, page* 3.

The importance of the subject will easily be appreciated, by attending to the following remark by Mr. Christie. "That the dyspnœa is frequently occa- " sioned, or increased, by spasms I am convinced, from the external spasms " sometimes accompanying it, and from the immediate and almost instanta- " neous relief afforded by strong stimulants; but it must also be, in many " cases, dependent on effusion, as the quantity of serum found in the cellular " substance of the lungs, and cavities of the chest, is often considerable." *Hunter on Diseases of Lascars, pages* 100 *and* 101.

[101] Since the above was written, I have met with a longer review of Mr. Teale's work, than that given in the Lancet, afterwards alluded to, in which, angina pectoris and sudden death are ascribed to spinal irritation. I am happy to find, that similar views had been suggested in the analogous phenomena of this disease. *Original note.* Sir Charles Bell has expressed himself to the same effect. " The frequency of sudden death, where no corresponding ap- " pearances are exhibited in the brain or heart, leads us to consider more " attentively the only part of the system through which life can be directly " extinguished. In angina pectoris, we witness the agony of suffering in this " system when the patient survives; and when he dies suddenly we can ima- " gine it to proceed from an influence extending over the nerves, and in- " terrupting the vital operations." In Abercrombie's work instances of sudden death will be found, in which the only morbid changes detected on the most careful examination, were collections of pus, &c. in the spine. The muscles or nerves of the extremities did not always indicate disease of the cord; in one, the patient complained only of general weakness and depression, he was free from pain and fever, and his appetite was good. He grew fat in hospital, kept his bed constantly, and was suspected of feigning. On the approach of winter, he got thin and cachectic, and in February his legs became paralytic, and *he died suddenly* in March. The only morbid appearance was much bloody sanies in the spinal canal, and marks of inflammation and suppuration of the cord. In a case from Morgagni, acute pain and sense of weight in the vertebræ were followed by palsy of the lower limbs, dyspnœa, vomiting, convulsions of the upper and lower extremities, and *sudden death*. Much fluid was found in the spine. Pages 350, 372, 376, and 403.

creased and altered secretion of the kidneys and bladder, is the most striking example; and the inflammation and increased mucous secretion of the bronchi when the 8th pair is divided, affords an additional illustration. At page 126 I have referred to the important investigation lately entered into, regarding various visceral affections which arise from disease of the spine, all the important tendencies "of which de-" pend on the direct influence of the nervous on the " sanguiferous system, on the fact that continued " nervous irritation always tends to produce inflam-" matory action." That the pericardium suffers in this way in beriberi is exceedingly probable, the symptoms of cardiac affection seldom appearing, when there are not unequivocal symptoms of the part of the spinal cord, above the origin of the nerves which assist in forming the cardiac plexuses, being more or less diseased ; and in the same patient, it may frequently be observed, that the lower part of the body may suffer much, and recover from several relapses, but on a return of the disease, in which symptoms of the affection of the spine having extended upwards are apparent, effusion or irritation of the cardiac region, carries off the patient. In other instances, only the lower cardiac nerves are involved, those of the arms being but little or not at all impaired in their functions.[102] We shall also find, that treatment which cannot be supposed to have any very sudden effect, except through the nervous system, removes the car-

[102] This was the case in Mr. Hamilton's patient (note 49), but the thighs were paralytic, and the patient previous to death, had vomiting, *spasms of the abdominal muscles*, and increased dyspnœa. The engorgement of the cord was most remarkable in the dorsal region. See also case 10, page 111; and a history quoted by Abercrombie p. 419, from Olivier, in which there were frequent pulse and strong action of the heart, and the only morbid appearance was slight infiltration of blood in the cellular tissue on the *outside of the dura mater of the cord, especially about the lower part.*

diac affection in a very short period ; and that this happens, in that relation to the other symptoms, which we should expect to find, if the latter were an immediate consequence, of disorder extending up the spine to the roots of the cardiac nerves. Analogy of a very direct nature, also, supports this view. Olivier found the pericardium inflamed, in consequence of inflammation within the upper dorsal vertebræ, and Corvisart states, that water is only accumulated in large quantity in the pericardium, when the affection is local. But besides the effect of nervous irritation, and the tendency to inflammatory actions of the part, when urea is deficient in quantity, the nature of the tissue of which the pericardium is composed, probably exerts a certain influence, in producing the diseased actions in question. It is a compound fibro-serous membrane, and enters readily into the same train of morbid action, as other tissues of this class, or of either of those of which it is compounded. If, then, we were right in considering, that the fibro-serous envelopes of the spinal marrow are diseased, it will not appear improbable, that similar actions will be readily excited in the pericardium, *(See Bichat Traité des membranes, pages* 163,219*)*. We have seen that a curious affection of the joints, may, in some measure, be explained in the same way ; and the great tendency to inflammation of the pericardium in rheumatism, especially when the joints are affected, *(Dublin Hospital Reports, vol.* 4*th),* will leave little doubt, that in beriberi which has so many things in common, causes of the same kind are in operation. The nature of this metastasis in the better known disease, is still so little understood, that although it is legitimate reasoning to infer, in a general way, that analogous actions will have complications of the same kind which should be carefully observed, any minuteness of detail would be entirely useless. It however deserves enquiry, how far the union of the fibrous and serous portions of the compound membranes, being imperfect in early youth, and the sympathies between them probably less powerful, is the cause of pericarditis, and many of the complicated phenomena of rheumatism and beriberi, being nearly unknown in childhood. The pericardium is closely united to the diaphragm in adults, and inflammation of the former usually spreads to the latter, but how far this is commonly the case in beriberi, I have had no opportunity of observing, and from the little progress yet made in the investigation of the same subject in rheumatism,it is likely to elude our enquiry for a long time. There seems however to be little doubt, that the diaphragm in some instances takes on morbid actions from irritation of its nerves, as various facts show it to be much under their influence as irritants. I know no symptoms by which it may be detected during life. Inflammation has, in one instance, appeared to have extended from the diaphragm to the stomach, and in another to the pleura. Hiccup very seldom occurs, and when it does it is uncertain on what it depends.[103] We are nearly as

[103] Hiccup is an alarming symptom, and has, for the most part, been observed in connection with affection of the stomach and pericardium. The following is an abstract of the only case, in which Dr. Herklots met either with it or nausea. " In one case (Narraidoo), when all the symptoms were reliev-" ed and the patient complained of nothing but weakness, he had one day " much nausea; an emetic was ordered. Next day a slight hiccup superven-" ed. Took magnesia and chalk but they did not relieve that symptom. Pulse " 70 and weak. ℞ Tinct. opii et æther sulphur., āā, gtt. xl et repet. pro re " nata. Hiccup goes off after taking the draught, but returns every hour or " so. Shortly afterwards he continued growing worse, and expired."

Serjeant Brown of M. H. 35th regiment had symptoms of beriberi for some time, and on the 3rd April was admitted with oppression at chest and inability to stand. Was treated with calomel in 5 grain doses with squills, at short intervals, a bottle of wine a day, &c ; gets ague followed by sweating ; pain

much in the dark with respect to the state of the pleura in this disease, which has been found inflamed after death; a short dry cough but with hardly any pain, is the only symptom I have found in any number of cases. The hydrothorax is of very different characters; it is occasionally acute and the effect of inflammation of the latent kind, and is sometimes nearly confined to one side, indicating local excitement.

Case 31st. Purmeser Naik, admitted November 13th, with swelling of the feet, legs a little rigid, urine high coloured and scanty, pulse 126 hard, loss of appetite. Is treated with purges of croton; and with cream of tartar, nitrous æther, and calomel and squills. 17th. Swelling not much diminished, complains of vertigo, pulse very small, 108. Died that night.

The pericardium was much distended with water of a bloody colour. Heart pale and flaccid, and right ventricle contained a polypus. Several pints of fluid in the cavities of the thorax, the greater part being contained in the left side. Much adipose substance on the parietes of the abdomen; slight effusion into that cavity. Great vascularity of the mesentery, and vessels turgid. Intestines slightly inflamed, particularly the small ones, which exhibited a dirty discoloured hue.

In one example carefully watched, where the numbness had ascended slowly to the breast, with œdema of the cellular membrane, in which the lower lobes of the lungs afterwards participated, fluid was effused into the thorax in the same slow way, and ægophonism, and afterwards dull sound without respiratory

of left side; obstinate vomiting and severe hiccup. Was severely salivated and appeared better, but died in the night with violent oppression. ***Dr. Holloway, in Hunter on Diseases of Lascars, page*** **125.**

murmur, varying in its extent according as the patient was sitting or recumbent, was observed. In this example, the hydrothorax was, perhaps, like the œdema, the consequence of the imperfect nervous influence. In many instances it arises from the state of the heart and its coverings, and in others, the water is effused only a little before death, in the way well described by Corvisart in his treatise on diseases of the heart. Of this, case 5th seems to be an example, and along with the fluid, air was separated, which enabled the patient to distinguish the water moving in his chest; which I have found the patient sensible of in pneumato-thorax, when succussion of the living or dead body could not detect it. In one case which ended favourably, this symptom, which Laennec, Dr. Duncan and other eminent writers, consider to be a certain sign of water and air in the pleura, was several times observed.[104] In a few examples, mostly during the rainy weather, bronchial inflammation occurred, but in these also, there were indications of the extension of the nervous affection high in the spine. In one case the excitement ran high, requiring free bleeding, but in general, the symptoms are mild and offer no peculiarity.[105]

[104] Mr. Dick *heard* fluctuation, but he suspected that the fluid was in the stomach, it being a difficult matter for the most skilful to distinguish the difference. It was only by placing the patient on his back, in a palanquin, that he could plainly hear it. In the cases of beriberi above referred to, there was no pretence to the accuracy which this observation shows to be necessary.

[105] In a case quoted by Abercrombie from Olivier, uneasiness at the heart, difficulty of swallowing, and pain of the nape of the neck, were followed by fever, dyspnœa, and vomiting, to which palsy of the arms succeeded, and extreme difficulty of breathing and swallowing proved fatal. The upper part of the cord was inflamed and softened, water and some blood were effused in the spine; the lungs were *dense and loaded with blood* and the *bronchial membrane unusually vascular*. Dr. Alison ascribed the dyspnœa, choking sensation, accumulation of fluid in the bronchiæ, and the inflamed appearance of the bronchial lining, in the case of Peter Elder referred to at page 141, to irritation of the roots of the dorsal nerves, corresponding with, and below the carious vertebræ.

The spasmodic affection of the larynx formerly mentioned, appeared in a few cases to depend on irritation of the branches of the 8th pair, distributed to the heart and stomach, and to be excited by irritation of the extremities of that nerve, communicated along its trunk to the recurrents, ramified on the muscles which move the cartilages of the glottis; in conformity to that law, by which the different extremities of a continuous chain of nervous fibres partake most readily in diseased actions, as irritation of the phrenics is sometimes only known, by pain down the arm in the branches of the axillary plexus. It has also been found, that a less degree of the same cause has produced a change of voice, before the alarming symptoms of aphonia, or of constriction of the glottis threatening instant suffocation; these are always symptoms of great danger, and seldom occur except together with others of a very serious nature. These affections appear also to arise, from the cervical nerves being directly injured, and in such examples, great benefit has occasionally been derived, from blisters to the back of the neck.

The pharynx and œsophagus have only suffered in a few of the very worst cases, near their termination, where the upper part of the cord and the base of the brain had partaken of the morbid actions.[106]

[106] One of Mr. Colhoun Stirling's patients, who had been long ill, was admitted with loss of muscular power and œdema. He used calomel, squills and opium, camphor, arrack, small doses of tartar emetic, blisters, and frictions, with temporary diminution of the symptoms, but the swellings soon began to increase again and he became universally anasarcous, nothwithstanding the use of large doses of calomel and squills. Two days before his death he lost the power of articulation, but this symptom went off in a couple of hours; and he said that while it lasted, he had considerable pain about his throat; his pupils appeared somewhat dilated. For a day or two before death, he was subject to vomiting, and complained of an universal sensation of cold. Some dyspnœa supervened and he died during his sleep. The body was not examined, but Mr. S. suspected effusion on the brain. *Hunter op. cit. page* 92.

The loss of speech sometimes occurs without any difficulty of breathing, and in these cases the recurrents, which are distributed to the crico-arytenoideus

There are some affections of the abdominal viscera which still remain to be considered, and although less common and dangerous than those of the chest, are of great importance ; and for the most part, the symptoms can be more easily recognized, notwithstanding the statement of the author of the article on beriberi, in the Cyclopædia of Medicine, "that the account of the morbid appearances in the abdomen are stated in too vague a manner to be understood." Over no part of the system, do the nerves exert a more direct and powerful influence, than over the viscera of the abdomen, but this is almost entirely exerted through the 8th pair and the sympathetic ; ac-

and thyro-arytenoideus muscles which distend the opening of the glottis, are probably principally affected ; and when the glottis is spasmodically constricted, the superior laryngeal branches. In the case of Cumboo (note 30), the *voice* was entire, but the associations necessary for speech were deranged, by the state of the muscles of the jaws, &c. In the following case the symptoms were more complicated, and illustrate several circumstances mentioned in the preceding pages.

Charles Cooper, ætat. 45, October 19th ; complains of great numbness and pain of the lower extremities, which are œdematous ; some dyspnœa, great debility, pulse frequent and irregular, tongue white and dry, and face somewhat swelled ; urine very scanty and high coloured, thirst urgent, arms and head ache a good deal. Has been almost constantly drunk since he was discharged the hospital, sixteen days ago. He took purgatives, calomel, squills, tamarinds in punch, and on the 24th gums were sore, the urine increased and the œdema gone, but he was very weak. The same night he complained of great numbness and heaviness of the whole right side, together with a partial loss of motion in the right arm ; unable to articulate, deglutition seems difficult, and he makes a motion as if to intimate that his jaws were painful or fast, and exerts himself to open his mouth wider and cannot Pulse more full and regular than before ; he perspires profusely and has made a good quantity of water. Mercurial frictions are continued, blisters applied, and antispasmodics administered. On the 26th his eyes have a shining appearance, the pupil of the right is dilated, nostrils are drawn in, and some degree of strabismus is observable in the right eye. The jaw continued closed, the pulse became irregular, and he died on the 27th.

" On dissection, the heart was found larger than usual, some water in the " abdomen and a little more than usual in the pericardium. Nothing more " particular in chest or abdomen. The head was not opened." Mr. Christie had little doubt that effusion existed on the brain. *Hunter op. cit. page* 119.

In Abercrombie's 146th case, *difficult deglutition, dyspnœa, and hoarseness* with pain of the back of the neck, were followed by palsy of the tongue and upper eyelid, and subsequently of the upper and lower extremities, and he died after suffering greatly from difficult breathing. A fungoid tumour, attached to the dura mater, was found within the foramen magnum and upper cervical vertebræ. Portal also asserts that difficulty of speaking and swallowing, frequently depends on engorgement of the cervical portion of the spinal cord. *Abercrombie op. cit. p.* 408 *and* 414.

cordingly the stomach often suffers but little directly, from injury of the lumbar nerves, sufficient to paralyse the abdominal muscles. The intimate connection of the 8th pair, through its branches[107] joining the lower cardiac plexus, will lead us to expect that the parts directly supplied by this nerve, will correspond in its morbid actions with the pectoral affections; and similar actions will in many cases be extended, through the solar plexus and the direct inosculations of the sympathetic with the lumbar nerves, to other organs.

The stomach is the organ which suffers most severely and frequently, and there is no period of the disease, when it may not take on disordered actions. In many instances of the acute form of the complaint, the pericardium and diaphragm are inflamed, and it is occasionally difficult to discriminate, in what cases the affection of the stomach is a symptom of, or an extension of inflammation from these; or an original complaint arising from the same series of causes. The patient complains of a burning heat in the epigastrium, the part is tender to pressure, severe and frequently uncontrollable vomiting comes on, often lasting for days and only ceasing with the death of the patient. The tongue is usually clean and red, or it is

[107] In a case of palsy and spasmodic affection of the face from carious teeth, (*Medico-chirurgical Transactions*, vol. IV), there were uneasy sensations at præcordia and darting pain in the direction of the diaphragm, and spasms at pit of stomach; thus, showing the ease with which morbid actions are propagated from nerves of distant parts, to those allied in function or origin. An opposite series of actions occurred, in an officer (whose case at first simulated intermittent fever) who got severe pain low in the loins, coming on with violence in the night, and attended with darting pains of hips, thighs, &c. The vertebræ of the loins were tender. He was cured by leeches and blisters, after the failure of various remedies, but relapsed on returning to his duty; there was now tenderness of the dorsal vertebræ, and pain shooting along the intercostal nerves; then those of the shoulder blade suffered, and at length pain near the articulation of the lower jaw, shooting to the lips and in some degree obstructing mastication, came on. Issues to the loins were of great use. This case and several other anomalous affections, appears to me to have had some connection with beriberi. *Original note.*

furred with fiery edges. The state of the pulse has not been ascertained; so many grave symptoms of different kinds, having usually been present along with those of abdominal inflammation, as to throw difficulties in the way of ascribing its changes to any one in particular. It has often been quick and small, but has also been full and strong.

Dr. Bond had a patient who suffered from *acute pain*, *oppression*, and *numbness* at the epigastrium. Dr. Dwyer says that some cases are referred to gastritis; Mr. Ridley that the vomiting is often excessive, and such as not to admit of the exhibition of medicine, which Messrs. Rogers and Stevenson state, in one of their manuscript reports, to have been found by them, after death, to be connected with an inflamed or congested state of the stomach. In a case communicated to me, the patient felt acute pain as if a coal were in his stomach, he vomited incessantly, and was much purged. The stomach especially near the pylorus, and the transverse colon were inflamed, as was the peritoneal coat of the small intestines, which was of a fine pink colour. More accurate enquiries are still to be desired. In the following example, the vomiting appears not to have depended on inflammation.

Case 32d. A stout man complained of œdema of the middle of the legs, hot skin, pulse 124, small and hard. Was bled to twenty five ounces, and took purgatives, calomel and antimony, and the nitre and acetic acid mixture. In three days the urine was increased, and the swellings were nearly gone, but the pulse was 140 and small; no uneasiness or dyspnœa; cold skin and vomiting came on, the pulse was not perceptible, and he died. The only morbid appearances were much water in the pericardium and general cavity of the chest. But the frequent connection of the symptoms with inflammation is sufficiently proved,and suggest many important cautions, both in the diagnosis and treatment.[108] Inflammation of the stomach exists in a

[108] Several cases will be found in the preceding pages, in which the vomiting and pain in the epigastrium appeared to be caused,by the state of inflammation and distension of the pericardium. The following case by Messrs. Geddes and Macdonell is an additional example.

" Payadoo, prisoner, ætat. 24. Admitted 5th April, 1828. Prisoner under " trial. Was in hospital last January with symptoms of beriberi. Since two " days has again been affected with smarting in his feet, heaviness of the " lower extremities, slight swelling about his feet, vertigo on rising, bowels " costive and occasional pain in the belly, urine scanty and high coloured, " passed with scalding. Pulse 129, rather small and oppressed,tongue clean, " walks steadily. To have half a drachm of jalap,and the treeak farook with " its diet. 6th. Three stools yesterday, no urine in the night, and that to-day " is extremely scanty, scarcely an ounce and a half, and thick. Pulse 120, " very small. Complains of much giddiness on rising, otherwise much as " yesterday, appears languid, no dyspnœa. Had the treeak farook last night " and this morning, no stool. 5½ P. M. No stool to-day, complains of pain in " the belly like griping, appears altogether very low, no urine,and pulse as in " the morning,skin a little warm. Has had a little while ago, ol. ricini ℥iss, " and now, an injection. 7th. Enema and oil operated five times, pulse 112 " while lying down and very small, skin cool, complains of pain or an uneasi- " ness in the epigastric region, and there is pulsation felt in laying the hand " on the region of the heart or stomach; œdema of the feet much as yesterday, " giddiness as before, passed some urine along with his stool last night, but " what he has passed to-day scarcely exceeds half an ounce, not quite so high " coloured as yesterday. Continue, and apply a blister to the region of the " heart. 8th. Vomited once or twice yesterday, and having no stool and com- " plaining of pain in the belly, had a dose of oil at 5 P. M. which operated at " 8 P. M.; did not however take any food yesterday. Died at 2 A. M. to-day.

" On opening his body nothing unhealthy was discovered, excepting a collec- " tion of serum in the cavities of the abdomen, thorax, and pericardium, in " considerable quantity; the same, in a less degree in the cellular membrane " of the skin ; the various veins of the body and the right auricle of the heart " full of blood."

The case of John Halketh at page 117 of Hunter's work is very similar. He had œdema, pain, and numbness of the lower extremities, for a long time previous to his admission, the end of September. On the 1st October he was affected with dyspnœa, inclination to vomit, and great debility ; pulse irregular and frequent: on the 6th,the dyspnœa was at intervals very distressing,and the pains and numbness in the thighs aggravated, the urine only 3 oz. and very high coloured. He died on the night of the 8th, during which the dyspnœa was very distressing. As in some of Mr. Davidson's cases and in several of Dr. Herklots, the left limb principally suffered. The heart was large and soft, and there was effusion into the pericardium, pleura, and abdomen. It is in such examples that antispasmodics appear to relieve the vomiting, and if spasms of the stomach occur, the indication will be more decided. Dr. Herklots met with this symptom in one case, and Mr. Davidson has communicated the history of a patient, in whom the upper and lower extremities were benumbed, the heart somewhat irregular, and the muscles of the thighs were subject to painful contractions. The tongue was excited,the papillæ red, and there was a whitish fur on its substance ; there were also irregular febrile attacks, yet laudanum afforded relief. In a chronic case, regarding which I was lately consulted, burning sensations in the feet,pain in the lumbar region, and some degree of hemiplegia, was followed by severe spasms at the scrobiculus

chronic form in old cases, especially when the urine deposits the phosphates, and is marked by tenderness on pressure, loss of appetite, and a very red tongue. The pulse is not altered. If the patient is using stimulants they must be immediately omitted, as they easily excite the disease in a predisposed subject. This last affection is easily removed by a few leeches, but the original cause remaining, it is liable to recur from very slight irritation. In a case, already several times alluded to, in which the pain in the spinal canal was severe, there was, in addition to these symptoms, flatulency from secretion, and occasional pyrosis, symptoms stated by Mr. Teale of Birmingham, to be attendants on affection of the stomach from disease of the nerves. When the pain in the back and paralytic symptoms disappeared, the pyrosis and flatulency also ceased. The stomach is sometimes weak and easily excited to reject its contents, when no evident disease exists. The peritoneum of the intestines and general cavity of the abdomen are sometimes inflamed, and in Tallent's case in Ridley's paper, the violent pain in the bowels with irritable stomach, was fully explained by the inflamed state of the intestines, and the dissection noticed above (page 215), establishes the same fact in the disease of the peninsula. He states adhesions to be frequently found in their course, which we would ex-

cordis, great tenderness at epigastrium, and some irregularity of the heart's action. Leeches and blisters were the only means, from which any great benefit was derived.

The necessity of accurate discrimination in these cases is further illustrated, by the case of O'Callachan, (*Hunter, page* 123), in which after being relieved by calomel and squills, oppression at epigastrium came on, and the limbs continued paralytic, he was costive, weak, and the breathing was difficult. Nineteen days after his admission he was seized with irritability of stomach, his skin was hot, his pulse quick and hard, and "*his drams make him vomit.*" Vomiting was relieved; but he died with spasm six days after. This case was unknown to me, when the remarks in the text were written.

pect in serous membranes highly inflamed. I believe that the mucous membrane is more frequently affected, and that in general the abdominal affection is latent, and the symptoms obscure, their being no pain or only a little uneasiness, tenderness, tightness [109] or other slight sensation, difficult to distinguish from those caused by the paralytic state of the integuments. Occasional tension and pain induced by irritating secretion,(generally disordered bile),throw some light on the state of the parts, and although immediately removed by purging, are never to be neglected when there is any appearance of fluctuation. Of ten dissections,there were traces of inflammation with abdominal effusion in five, effusion without inflammation in one, inflammation unattended with effusion in another, and in three there was no abdominal affection. To these, the following account of a dissection communicated since this paper was finished, may be added, and is the most accurate account of

[109] Dr. Abercrombie insists, on the importance of a sensation as if a tight band were tied across the stomach, generally accompanied with a feeling of distension in the lower part of the abdomen, as if the bowels had, in part, lost the power of propelling their contents, as among the first indications of a dangerous affection of the spine. The following abstract of a case of beriberi by Dr. Herklots, illustrates the observation in the text.

Mahomed Moosa was admitted, 20th January, with pain and numbness of the upper and lower extremities, and of the body as high as the neck; œdema of the legs with sense of weight. Pulse natural, bowels costive, tongue clean, appetite good. Ill fifteen days; but much worse during the last three. Takes calomel and jalap, and next day the black oil. On the 27th the œdema was diminished,but the numbness and costiveness continued. 29th. Œdema gone. Numbness the same. *Has had a sense of tightness from umbilicus to stomach since admission.* February 1st. Numbness now from navel downwards only, and there is less tightness at the epigastrium. No pain except in the lower extremities, in which he has cramps at night. The black oil is omitted, and the wheat diet continued. 5th. Less numbness of abdomen and thighs; pain and cramps only in the calves. Tightness at epigastrium diminished. On 20th February, he had not recovered the free use of his limbs, but he was allowed to go to his duty.

In another case (Lutchanah), the numbness extended to the umbilicus,and the abdomen and lower extremities were swelled; there was no pain but the bowels were inflated after his evening meals, and he was not relieved by two doses of jalap. On the 3rd he took the black oil, and on the 5th the œdema and swelling of the abdomen were less. He now complained of pain in the joints. On the 21st he was discharged.

the abdominal appearances I have yet met with: the spontaneous separation of the jelly like albumen from the fluid, is such as I have observed in the product of inflamed membranes.[110]

Case 33d. A pauper, ætat. 18, was seen only in the last stage of the disease, and the previous history could not be accurately learned; examined two hours after death. Between four and five pounds of limpid serum in the abdominal cavity, from which on being put into a vessel, a pellucid jelly separated. Between three and four ounces of fluid, tinged with blood, were found in the pericardium, and four pounds of brownish serum in the chest, also spontaneously coagulating, but like that in the abdomen, the coagulum disappeared in twenty-four hours: no marks of disease of the lungs or heart, except an adhesion of the pleura pulmonalis to the pleura costalis of an inch square, near the heart. The kidneys although of their

[110] It will, I believe, be found that indications of abdominal inflammation occur more rarely, than they would appear to do from the above statement. The case here recorded was sent me by Mr Davidson, before the paper was copied for transmission to the Board; had he had an opportunity of enquiring minutely into the symptoms during life, it would have been of greater value. The case of F. Gouge (note 92) since communicated supplies this deficiency, and Mr. D. has also met with similar appearances in other patients, who died of protracted beriberi. The examination of his detailed cases, confirm the account of the symptoms, derived from the less accurate histories which I was in possession of, at the time of drawing up the paper. In old cases, the secretions seem almost always to become disordered, and the patient dyspeptic. A certain relation between the abdominal symptoms and those of the nervous system, could also generally be traced. In a patient in whom the numbness extended as high as the umbilicus and the arms were similarly affected, the thighs and the skin of the abdomen (chiefly the lower part) were œdematous, with feeling of fulness in the latter. There was some pain on striking the parietes with the tip of the fingers, and the muscles started into action in an unusual manner. It was remarkable, that œdematous tumours formed suddenly over the epigastrium and hypogastrium. In another, in whom the upper and lower extremities were palsied, the abdomen was tumid and felt heavy, and the colon was found contracted and tender in left iliac region. The skin was dry and unhealthy, and the tongue smooth, moist and blanched, an appearance Messrs. Geddes and Macdonell thus describe: "in some cases, especially where the disorder is more chronic, the gums as "well as the tongue present a pale bloodless apearance, as if they had been "soaked in water, and natives often point out this peculiar appearance in "describing their disorder."

natural colour both externally and internally, were diseased. They were less round and plump than usual, almost flat, and were remarkably softened and were torn with the slightest force, that is, an end being held in each hand, by slightly digging into it with the point of the finger, a portion was removed without almost any force. The mucous membrane of the stomach was pale, except a spot of the size of an inch, which appeared as if sprinkled *with red pepper*, each particle distinct and in the substance of the coat. This blush was found in a much higher degree half an inch below the pylorus, and occupied the whole circumference of the duodenum and some part of the jejunum. It then became very slight and occasionally disappeared entirely; towards the lower end of the ileum, the mucous membrane was of the same red granulated appearance as in the duodenum, but more deeply so, and was besmeared with a substance of the colour and consistence of treacle, of which a quantity lay in the intestine. This did not continue into the colon, which contained yellow feces. There was a slight blush of the head of the colon, but the rest of the large intestines was natural.[111]

The effused fluid is not often in great quantity, and frequently fluctuates in this respect without evident cause; it sometimes bears a certain proportion to the œdema of the abdominal parietes, and the fluid is usually clear and yellow. It is only found in the scrotum, in worn out patients in whom the common anasarca of exhaustion has supervened. From these

[111] These appearances correspond remarkably with the state of the mucous membrane in case 10; with the exception of the part of the small intestine affected. The nature of the action seems therefore to be the same, but the situation accidental. *Original note.*

facts it is probable, that the ascites is a result of increased action of the capillaries, although neither the pulse nor the appearance of the patient indicates the presence of inflammation, nor will active treatment adapted to this view, be often admissible to any extent, but the fact will afford many very important hints in the choice of remedies. The following abstract of a case, in which the fluid had all the characters of inflammatory exudation, is of considerable value, notwithstanding the want of explicitness in the details.

Case 34th. January 1st. Mahomed Nebbi, ætat. 30. Has had œdematous swelling of the lower extremities for several days, the legs pitting deeply; numbness and weakness of the limbs preceded the swelling; œdema of abdomen, no fluctuation; face puffy and sallow, eyes yellow, no dyspnœa in any posture, dry short cough, tongue clean and moist, pulse quick, small and irregular, skin cool. Has been ill two months and has used native medicine. Pulv. jalap. comp. ℥ss. 3rd. Four stools, urine now copious. Rept. pulv. jalap. comp. 4th. Worse, cannot breathe in a recumbent posture. Pulse indistinct. Temperature below the natural standard. Died at noon.

Sectio cadaveris. Two ounces of fluid in the pericardium, none in the cavity of chest. The lungs appeared healthy. (The gentleman to whom this case occurred, seems never to have suspected œdema of the lung.) Liver, spleen, and intestines said to be natural. Four pints of fluid in the abdomen, which seemed to have deposited a thick puriform fluid, which was found lying under the bladder; the state of which is unfortunately not observed.

The bowels are usually slow;[112] and the evacuations are frequently composed of disordered bile, sometimes greenish; at others black, like clay, white, or lumpy. Thick mucus of an altered quality is occasionally mixed with the feces; the mucous membrane being probably inflamed, either primarily or by extension from the peritoneal coat, and this has been sometimes attended with purging; which also happens from various other causes, in this as in most other diseases affecting the chylopoitic viscera. The colon has also in several examples been inflamed, and when no decided inflammation could be detected, distension of the veins and ecchymosed spots have been observed, on different parts of the intestine and stomach.[113] When the stools are natural, in bad chro-

[112] "The tendency to constipation of the bowels was coeval with the paralysis, and no doubt depended on it." Bell op.citat. appendix, page 61.

[113] The following quotation from Laennec cannot be too strongly impressed on the minds of those, who may have opportunities of examining the bodies of persons dead of beriberi. "On examining the bodies of persons who have "fallen victims to organic affections of the heart, besides the organic lesion "and the serous effusions which almost always accompany it, we find all the "marks of congestion of blood in the internal capillaries. The mucous membranes, especially those of the stomach and intestines, are of a red or violet tint; and the liver, lungs, and capillaries situated beneath the serous, "mucous and cutaneous tissues, are gorged with blood. The augumented "colour of the mucous membranes varies much in degree and extent. Sometimes it is observed only here and there, under the form of small points or "specks, disseminated over the surface of the membrane: at other times it "occupies the whole extent of the surface, and has the appearance of being "attended by some swelling of the part. These two latter appearances are "sometimes so considerable, that, if we looked to them merely, without examining the condition of the heart, and without reference to the history of "the patient, (who had been found capable of taking into his stomach wine "and other stimulant matters without experiencing any pain, even up to the "period of his death,) we might be tempted to believe that the fatal disease "had been a violent inflammation of the stomach and bowels."

It is not often, that the distinction between inflammation and congestion can be so clearly traced, as in the following case from the journal for April 1815, of surgeon R. Bellers of H. M. 86th regiment, stationed at Masulipatam.

"Sergeant Henderson, ætat. 35, admitted 11th April, with fever. 12th. "This patient came into hospital with erysipelatous inflammation in the legs "and shoulder, this gave way to antimonials, and keeping the inflamed parts "dusted with fine flour; complains at present of much weakness of body and "*inability to move*, and a sense of weight or oppression about his chest. Had "a dose of salts yesterday, which operated well. ℞ Liquor. antimon. tar-"tar., tinct. scillæ, āā, ʒss, spt. æther. nitric. ʒss, aquæ fontan. ℥j. M. Sum-

nic cases, the muscles of the abdomen have not power to expel them, and medicine is required to keep the stools soft. Hard lumps of feces have, in one or two instances, been found to lie in the upper part of the right lumbar region and to take the form of hard tumours, exciting apprehension of great organic disease.

Few organs suffer more frequently than the liver, although there are seldom any severe symptoms. The most usual are a yellow eye, sallow complexion, and feces of much disordered bile, usually in too great

"at ter quotidie. Habeat cinchon. officinal. ʒiij in sex dosibus et vini "Madeirensis ℥viij. 13th. Had a considerable eruption of prickly heat during yesterday on chest and other parts of the body, finds himself much better since; has less oppression at the chest, and feels stronger. Tongue "whitish. Pulse full and a little hard. Cont. medicament. Vespere. Continues better but bowels costive, tongue foul, and has some oppression at "chest. ℞ Calomel. gr. vj, pulv. antimonial. gr. iv. M. statim sumend. et "cras mane sulphat. sodæ ℥j. Applicet. emplast. lyttæ thoraci. 14th. Blister "rose well and relieved the oppression at chest, had also a considerable diaphoresis in consequence of the antimonial powder, during the night. Calomel "gently purged him but salts have not commenced operation. Contin. medicament. ut antea. 15th. Feels himself much relieved and much better since "the salts operated, feels scarcely any oppression about the chest, but is "weak and scarcely able to stand, though without much pain. Pulse full and "soft, tongue clean. Cont. medicament. ut heri. Vespere. Exceedingly ill "this evening with oppression about chest, profuse perspiration, and an immense quantity of vesicular eruptions chiefly the about chest and abdomen: "as he said that he had no stool since the evening before, directed an ounce of "acetas potassæ to be dissolved and given to him, this, however, he did not "swallow; had a purging glyster which procured a small stool. 16th. Saw "him during the night twice, his pulse had become so quick as scarcely to be "counted, was also bathed in sweat. Tongue white and thirst excessive, felt "a sense of suffocation on laying any other way than with his shoulders raised. Feels at present an inclination to vomit. Skin not very hot, and pulse "now low aud rather weak; passed no stool during the night. Tongue very "foul. Has pain across his brows. An injection and antimonial solution were "ordered, but he died at 8 o'clock A. M.

"On opening the abdomen the epiploon appeared void of fat, *the veins on "stomach and intestines filled with blood, but no appearance of any disease in "any one of the abdominal viscera.* The liver had several white patches on it, "which when cut into appeared firmer than the other parts, but exhibited in "nothing else the least appearance of disease, On opening the chest the "right lobe of the lungs adhered to the pleura costalis over its whole external surface, was dense, inflated and of a blueish black colour, when cut into "a quantity of frothy purulent matter issued from the bronchiæ; the heart "was immersed in a large quantity of fluid contained in the pericardium, and "externally had no appearance of disease, but when cut into, the right ventricle contained a thick coriaceous substance extending into the pulmonary "artery, weighing an ounce and a half; this appeared to have been formed "previous to death by a deposition of coagulable lymph."

abundance, but occcasionally the stools are nearly white. I have never detected symptoms of hepatitis, nor fulness below the ribs.[114] The liver has been found after death enlarged and soft, as in case 2d, perhaps from other disease, or congested and full of black blood. The hepatic symptoms are more remarked when the thoracic viscera also suffer, they seldom last long, and except by the irritation of disordered secretion, appear to have but little influence on the disease. Neither the symptoms nor the appearances on dissection are sufficient to prove, great internal congestion to be generally present. The spleen was greatly enlarged in one of Mr. Ridley's patients, but it is not often at all unnatural.

Diagnosis.

Were it my intention to write a systematic treatise, it would be proper to enter at some length on the diagnosis, a subject of considerable difficulty in practice, however simple it may appear to a writer of limited experience, more conversant with the history of the disease in books than with its appearance in nature, (*Cyclopædia of Medicine page* 270), but I have too little time at my own disposal, to do more than record such observations, as may have occurred on obscure or doubtful points.

To distinguish beriberi from rheumatism, the observations previously made will, in general, be sufficient if carefully attended to, but it must be borne in mind, that many rheumatic complaints are in ordinary practice extremely difficult to discriminate from

[114] See case of Payadoo, (note 108). In one of Mr. Davidson's cases, there was pain in the hepatic region on breathing, walking, or coughing. The bladder was tender, the stools disordered, pale, and brownish; the tongue red, tremulous, moist, and clean ; he felt confused at times, and a purgative never failed to relieve the numbness and affection of the spine and partial palsy of the hands, although it caused pain above the umbilicus.

affections of different nerves, and that when rheumatism prevails along with a mild form of beriberi, the cases will often be of an intermediate character, the symptoms of the one running into those of the other.

As in other endemics, various diseases have a tendency to take on the prevailing form of morbid action, and hence it frequently happens that men admitted with fever remain in hospital, and die of beriberi. In these instances the fever merely acts as a predisposing cause, as I have known various local diseases, as caries of the tibia, scrophulous sores, and rheumatism do, and in such examples, the beriberi is often severe and rapidly fatal. It is not uncommon, however, to see an intermittent or remittent fever attack a patient with beriberi, and go through their usual course as if no such disease existed. But I have often seen the irritable fever from internal disease in beriberi, so modified by the prevailing febrile influence, as to assume the appearance, and be mistaken for and treated as intermittent or remittent fever. The error is one of great danger, and too apt to arise when fever is prevailing, to which both patient and surgeon are, at such times, apt to refer many complaints. The following is an abstract of a case of beriberi mistaken for remittent.

Case 35th. Mahomed Gollib, ætat. 40 Admitted 9th August, with a continued fever, remitting slightly in the morning. Purges and calomel are prescribed. On the 11th, pain at stomach with tenderness to pressure, vomiting, and sense of internal heat are complained of. Pulse quick and full. On the 13th, these symptoms are rather better, but a sense of weight in the chest with quick pulse are observed; next day the attention was called to pains in the limbs, and on the 17th it is noted, for the first time, that the legs are paralytic. Œdema afterwards occured. His gums were sore at this time, but this did not check the progress of the complaint. He was transferred, "no better." It is probable, that the fever depended on inflammation about the heart and stomach, and would have been more benefited by bleeding, &c. than by mercury, which, if it exerted any power over the inflammation, was useless as far as the palsy was concerned, which was much aggravated when ptyalism was procured. The palsy often exists sometime before it is discovered, the circumstance of the patient's not moving off his cot, being ascribed to the languor of the fever, to weakness, indolence,[115] &c.

Slight evening exacerbations are ever an object of

[115] The importance of a careful diagnosis in these cases, is confirmed by the following valuable observations. "In other instances, again, and those are "the most severe cases of this variety of the disease, the patient states that "he has had one or two attacks of fever, before his admission into hospital. "These have usually been ushered in by a rigor, but the paroxysm seldom "terminates by perspiration. Sometimes the pyrexial type assumed is con-"tinued, while at others it is of a paroxysmal form, the time of exacerbati-"on being irregular, but generally the skin is observed to become hot and "dry in the evening, without any rigor preceding the later paroxysms. "With this state, there is pain felt in all the limbs, which the patient compares "to the feeling of being well beaten, and generally about the second or third "day the paralytic symptoms discover themselves, in the man not being able "to rise from his cot without assistance. At the same time or within a short "period, the skin is observed to be tense and shining, and the other symp-"toms soon develope themselves." *Messrs. Geddes and Macdonell.*

"The first, and by far the most frequent form of beriberi usually commences "in the following manner. A person having had a febrile attack of the de-"scription before mentioned, finds immediately afterwards that his legs have "suddenly become swollen and pit on pressure, he feels a degree of numb-"ness of the feet and legs, and of the hands and forearms, with a tightness "in the muscles of these parts; he experiences also a general feeling of lassi-"tude, and hebetude of body with an indisposition to use exertion, the parts "affected with numbness become shortly after more or less paralysed, and "the muscles are soft and flabby to the feel."

"These symptoms continuing a few days, he becomes unable to rise from "his cot without assistance, and if supported in the erect posture, and made "to walk a few steps, the disease is immediately recognized by the peculiar "method of moving the limbs, and from which circumstance it has received "its Indian name. This form of beriberi, as well as all others that I have "seen, is frequently attended with most distressing pains in the limbs, and "dragging of the muscles, particularly of the calves of the legs, the pain be-"ing generally most severe in the tendo achillis; the muscles of the extre-"mities may also be affected with spasms, but this is not so frequent, or so "troublesome a symptom in native as in European patients, in whom it is often

suspicion with me, when beriberi is prevailing. In a few instances, the patient has experienced painful sense of heat over the body, without fever. The nature of this feeling I do not know.[116] The skin is frequently dry and rough, without fever.

It is much to be regretted, that no account of the disease said to have been beriberi, which proved so fatal to the Madras troops at Rangoon, has been given to the public. Mr. Weddel did not see any thing of the kind amongst the men from Bengal, nor was it observed at Arrakan, by the writers who have described the diseases of the force, employed in that quarter. What little I saw of the affection amongst

" the most urgent, and distressing attendant on the complaint. The pulse " in this form of disease is strong, vibrating, of increased frequency, beating " from 100 to 120 in a minute, feels full, cord-like, and imparts a somewhat " fluttering sensation to the finger. The action of the heart is felt over a " larger surface than natural, and imparts a thrilling sensation to the hand, " when applied on the chest. The conjunctivæ and tongue are pale and ex- " sanguineous, the nails white or bluish, and the countenance assumes a leu- " cophlegmatic aspect. The urine is observed to be high coloured and scan- " ty, in some cases slightly coagulable by acids, but for the most part no tur- " bidity is produced."

" Anasarcous swellings extend to the upper parts of the body, and even to " the face and head, and often in a very extraordinary, and rapid manner, " but I have never been able to detect fluctuation in the abdomen, as occurs " in ascites; the action of the heart, and arteries, with thrilling and vibrating " increases, breathing becomes oppressed, the countenance assumes an anxi- " ous and distressed look, the pulse is reduced to a thread, and death " from apparent suffocation, and effusion into the thorax takes place, after " some slight exertion, as perhaps that of taking a little medicine, or food."

" The paralysis has never in any of the cases witnessed by me, extended " to the muscles of the trunk, nor have I seen any cases in which the patient " could not sit erect, even though the extremities, both upper and lower, " were so completely powerless, as to render a change of position an utter " impossibility, and the patient always retains the perfect use of his mental " faculties to the last." * * * 5th variety. The febrile paroxysms have been " found to recur, in some instances, after the setting in of the symptoms of be- " riberi, which are here of an insidious nature, and liable to be mistaken for " the debility caused by the previous fever."

" As it is a circumstance of the utmost importance to detect the early ap- " pearance of the disease, an examination of the state of the limbs should fre- " quently be made, where suspicion is excited either by the arterial excite- " ment, debility, or indisposition to use exertion, continuing after the subsi- " dence of febrile symptoms, in situations where beriberi is known to prevail." " * * * It is of the utmost importance to know, that beriberi coming on insidi- " ously may simulate the debility of fever. and run on to a fatal extent before " it is attended to." *Dr. Pearse.*

[116] It would appear from the dissection in the appendix to be neuralgic, and caused by disease in the spine. *Original note.* See case 10th.

the native troops in Ava, although considered at the time to be beriberi, I was convinced, after seeing the disease in the circars, to be a complaint of a different character, and apparently a complication of anasarca with a modification of scurvy, and perhaps, of the complaint known under the name of "burning in the feet." There was usually great distension of the abdomen, forcing the patient to lean back in a constrained position, a thing never seen in beriberi. An intelligent conductor who had suffered severely from what he called beriberi at Rangoon, and again in the circars, pointed out to me the great extent of the ascites, and the slight weakness of the limbs and want of numbness, as distinguishing his former sufferings from those of the other disease; and this is confirmed, by what I observed amongst the European and native troops on their return from Ava and Arrakan.

These imperfect hints are thrown out, from the hope that they may lead some of those who yet survive, and are well able from extensive experience and acquirements, to give an accurate description of the Rangoon disease.[117]

In deference to the opinion of a friend of high authority on all professional questions, and of great ex-

[117] Mr. Heward, superintending surgeon of the Madras army in Ava, and late 1st Member of the Medical Board, thus describes these affections. "Some cases of fever continued occasionally to appear among both the European and native troops, during the month of August, (1824), and some sporadic cases of the disease are still seen in the hospitals, but the cases are few in number and for the most part unimportant in themselves, and the disease would appear to have nearly run its course; but the disease which is now found so generally to afflict the European soldier, and with such fatal visitation is dysentery, combined with a scorbutic taint of constitution."
"The disease does not appear to possess any other striking peculiarity in its character, but the extreme fatality which attends it; and which may reasonably be accounted for, from the combination with scurvy, aggravated no doubt by the previously debilitated and exhausted constitutions of its victims. When the patient does not sink suddenly under the disease, he falls into a dropsical state, the swelling generally commencing in the feet, extends upwards, the belly becomes tumid, respiration laborious, deglutition painful, the countenance bloated, and his sufferiugs continue to increase, until death closes the scene." *Report dated 29th September*, 1824.

perience in beriberi, that the disease is scurvy, I shall make a few observations on the differences, which appear to me to exist between the two complaints; the general symptoms of which as found in books, have a considerable resemblance; but when studied, as I have had an opportunity of doing, with Europeans and natives labouring under both diseases before me, the distinction was sufficiently evident. I have already stated, that beriberi was unknown to the sepoys who returned from Rangoon to the northern division, after long exposure to hardship, a damp climate, and indifferent food, and a voyage in the most unfavourable circumstances of foul winds, heavy rain, crowded decks and numerous sick; but that after a residence of some months in the most plentiful districts, in the enjoyment of every thing desired by natives, it broke out with violence, when all the diseases connected with deficient nourishment had disappeared, and no class of persons suffered more, than stout young men in good circumstances. It must be observed, however, that worn out Europeans, natives, and Indo-Britons of both sexes (especially players on wind instruments), were the principal sufferers. In scurvy there is fatigue after slight exertion, and the palsy only appears in the latter stages, while in beriberi there is diminished power from the commencement, but the strength that remains is not worn out by exertions proportioned to it. There are no purple spots on the skin or spongy ulcerated gums in beriberi, as far as I have observed. In scurvy a hardness is usually observed in the upper part of the muscles of the back of the leg, over which the skin is livid, and as the extravasated blood is absorbed, yellow; and there are hard swellings of the tibia. In beriberi, I never saw any thing at all resembling this, except the general hardness of the cellular membrane described at page 177; or the contraction of the flexors, which is entirely unconnected with physical change in the muscles. The pulse is frequent, small, and feeble in scurvy, but I found no symptoms of hydropericardium, in the few cases I have had an opportunity of examining, but on the contrary, indications of the muscular power of the heart being simply enfeebled. The difficulty of breathing is also of a different character, although I am unable to point out distinctly the peculiarities of the latter. In one instance it arose, merely, from the great acceleration of the heart's action on slight exertion. In beriberi, ulcers, boils and wounds go through healthy series of actions; and when the contrary happens, as in a case of compound fracture of the leg to which beriberi supervened, the mortification was such as would be expected to occur in a limb, the vital powers of which have been diminished by palsy and constitutional disease. In one instance only, did a sloughing sore form, and that was in a blistered surface over the loins, where injuries of the spinal marrow commonly cause it. The mucous membranes are very liable to diseased actions in scurvy, and the constitution gives way under any accidental complication; in beriberi on the other hand, this tissue is in most instances but little affected, and the bowels instead of being loose as in scurvy, are almost always constipated. The constitution is also able to withstand the most dangerous diseases, without any very remarkable aggravation of their symptoms; patients recovering from cholera and remittent fever, with which they were attacked, while in hospital ill of beriberi. I had an opportunity of seeing some lascars suffering under scurvy, several of whom died suddenly; and the disease had much of the appearance of the disorder described by Hunter, (judging from notices of his work in different authors). The feet and legs were far more swollen than is usual in beriberi, there was no marked *local* debility of the lower extremities, the gums were spongy and bleeding, the pulse small and feeble, and hæmorrhage had taken place from the lungs and stomach, in several of the fatal cases. The appearance of the urine differed exceedingly from that of any stage of beriberi, being from the first fetid, turbid "pellicula oleosa superne tecta."* To these, other observations to the same purpose might be added, but they are either unnecessary or I have not had an opportunity of examining them personally, and ascertaining that they apply to the disease in India.

Since the greater part of this paper was written, I have met with the third number of the Cyclopædia of Medicine, containing an account of beriberi by Mr Scott. He states, that it is important to distinguish that disease from barbiers, which he calls a chronic palsy, while beriberi is an acute affection. The grounds of the distinction are stated in a very confused and imperfect manner, from slight notices in authors, few of whom seem to have seen either of the diseases, and none of them to have observed it with much accuracy. There is no account of the origin of two names so nearly allied, of the authors by whom the diseases were first distinguished, and the symptoms are so imperfectly described and mixed up with those of local palsy from exposure, that it is impossible to judge,

* Home, Principia Medicinæ.

on what to found an opinion at variance with those of Christie, Good, and most other writers who have paid any attention to the subject. No practitioner in the northern division has ever adopted the distinction; but as admitting its justice would take much from the value of their observations, I have carefully examined all the cases in my possession with a view to the remarks of Mr. Scott, and have endeavoured to reduce them to either of his divisions, but in vain. The cases commencing in the most chronic form, and such as would be referred to the chronic disease of barbiers, suddenly taking on the most fatal and rapid form, and those commencing with marked symptoms of beriberi, having in the course of the same attack or in a relapse connected with it, all those of beriberi: and the two classes of cases prevail at the same stations, at the same seasons, amongst men similarly circumstanced, and certain specific remedies are equally useful in both. I have therefore come to the conclusion, that the differences observed in the symptoms, so far from deserving a separate place in nosology, are not to be classed as varieties, but to be kept in view, only as far as the treatment is concerned.[118]

[118] Even Mr. Marshall who has treated of the two forms of the disease in different parts of his work, and is the principal authority on which the distinction has been made, allows, that it is " probable that a much greater de-" gree of connection exists between these two diseases than is at present sup-" posed." *Marshall on diseases of Ceylon, page* 210. A comparison of the cases and observations in Hunter's book, in Marshall, and Bontius fully confirm the remarks in the text, drawn from my own experience. The following extract illustrates the remark, that the most acute and characteristic symptoms of beriberi (as described by Christie), supervene on that form of the disease to which the name of barbiers would be given. Dyspnœa " is present with little " exception in all the varieties before death, often occurring in a very sud-" den manner, and when presenting itself without evident anasarcous effusion " or any paralytic affection, it is generally found to be the relapse of an at-" tack of beriberi, the more conspicuous symptoms of which had at some for-" mer period been removed. In this case, as well as when occurring in the " progress of the other varieties of beriberi, its first approach is observed in " the sensation of a weight on the breast, which in the course of a day or

Prognosis.

The prognosis in beriberi is always exceedingly doubtful, and rather to be learned by careful study of the details, and prevailing form of the endemic, than from any general statement. A patient can never be considered safe till he is free from every paralytic symptom, nor even then, if the heart's action is at all disordered, or even if there is cracking in the joints on moving. If there is any effusion into the pericardium after apparent recovery, we cannot assure the patient an hour against sudden death. When the numbness extends to the hands, the case is always of a serious nature. Swelling of the face and hands are ever alarming symptoms, however slight the complaint may otherwise be, and however easily all signs of disease may appear to be removed by appropriate remedies; relapse, sudden death, dyspnœa from affection of the heart, œdema of the lungs, or hydrothorax coming on rapidly and carrying off the patient. This is so much the case, that many intelligent non-pro-

"two, changes into an unsupportable state of anxiety and sense of suffocation, "occasionally however the attack is much more sudden, and before the patient being brought into hospital, the dyspnœa has become fully established, "and is well marked by the great increase of the individual's distress, on being raised from the horizontal position. It is also much increased by conversation or any thing tending to accelerate the circulation, or impede the "action of the heart, and a fit of this nature excited by any exertion, or by "distension of the stomach by a meal, is often found to prove suddenly fatal. "The beriberi has been named by Dr. C. Rogers, formerly of the Madras "Establishment, in his inaugural thesis printed in Edinburgh in 1808 "Dropsical asthma," from the severity of this symptom, combined with dropsical "effusions, but the dyspnœa in this disease is very different from the spasmodic affection in asthma. The patient seems to feel the unpleasant sensation only when he distends the lungs. He occasionally takes a long inspiration, and then remains quiet until he is obliged to inspire again. As this "disease proceeds, the anxiety increases and the patient appears as if he could "not fill his lungs with a sufficient quantity of air; he generally lies upon one "side, most frequently the left; his restlessness does not allow him to lie long "in one position, and he keeps turning from one side to the other, his head "bent down to his breast, his nostrils distended, and his mouth wide open "and his tongue often out, by this time his voice only amounts to a whisper, "his limbs have become cold and death soon terminates the struggle." *Messrs. Geddes and Macdonell's paper.*

fessional men who have lived much in the circars, consider it a fatal symptom, and a native practitioner of experience informed me, that when it was observed, nothing but an early and diligent use of remedies could save the patient.[119]

When the disease has commenced gradually and no remedies have been used, the cure is often easily effected, but if it continues long without amendment, or if chronic disease succeeds immediately, or by relapse, on acute attacks ; or if considerable palsy remains long in any circumstances, the probability is, that the patient will die either from the supervention of the peculiar visceral affections of beriberi, or by the slow process of decay common to other forms of palsy; or he may drag out a long series of years a burden to himself and others. Much depends on the early use of remedies. When the phosphatic deposits have commenced, there is very little chance of ultimate recovery.[120]

[119] " Besides what has been already stated with respect to the native prac-
" tice in beriberi, it may be added, that the severe forms of the disease, par-
" ticularly of a relapse attended with fever and much paralysis, is generally
" considered fatal." *Messrs. Geddes and Macdonell.*

[120] To avoid repetition, I have condensed this part of the subject more, perhaps, than its importance admits of; but the following observations will more than compensate for the deficiency of detail in the text. " The prognosis of
" beriberi is chiefly determined by the state of the respiration, circulation,
" degree of anxiety, extent of numbness, secretion of urine, and in some
" cases by the tendency to stupor. The freedom with which respiration is
" performed affords the most certain prognostic, for few cases end fatally
" without this function being very much impeded. The least approach there-
" fore to dyspnœa, especially if the patient shows that he has more relief in
" the horizontal than the erect posture, is to be dreaded, for rarely is it pos-
" sible to cause any check to the disease after this symptom has shown itself
" in any great degree, that is, after the patient cannot without the greatest
" increase of anxiety raise himself to the erect posture. Frequency of the
" pulse, whether this is large and tumultuous, or small, contracted and irregu-
" lar, and feelings of anxiety or oppression about the præcordia, are also to
" be considered as unfavourable symptoms, but the prognosis from the former
" is more to be drawn from the degree of obstinacy with which the pulse
" keeps up at a rapid rate, or its increasing in frequency under the treatment
" employed, along with the severity of other symptoms, than from its frequen-
" cy alone." * * * " It may be necessary to repeat here, that nothing shows
" the progress to recovery so much, as the gradual diminution of frequency in

Treatment.

The opinions regarding the nature of the disease and its leading symptoms, in the early part of my own practice, and, as far as can be judged from the re-

"the pulse, and the patient can scarcely be considered as convalescent or "free from the chance of relapse, until this come down to the natural stand- "ard. The extent of numbness taken in conjunction with the other symp- "toms is an important feature of the prognosis, and when great, not only re- "duces the chance of recovery, but renders the convalescnce much more te- "dious, and during this period the patient continues very subject to a relapse. "With respect to the urine, it may be generally stated, that the danger is in "proportion to its scanty and high coloured state, and its becoming copious "under the treatment, is one of the most favourable changes which can oc- "cur. Any tendency to stupor is, of course, to be considered as of the same "nature as the fatal dyspnœa, giving evidence as it does, of the commence- "ment of serous effusion in an important organ like the brain."

"In ascertaining the value of different modes of treatment, however, it is "always to be recollected, that the disease is in some seasons, or in some "cases, much less violent, more slow in its progress,and more easily checked "than at other periods, or in other individuals, and that in like manner, pe- "culiar remedies in one season, from the prominence of certain symptoms, "may either not appear to do harm, or may even seem beneficial, while in "others, hurtful effects may be experienced from them." *Messrs. Geddes and Macdonell.*

Of the truth of the remarks contained in the last sentence, I have been fully convinced by the enquiries I have had an opportunity of making, since the paper was written; in so much, that I am satisfied that, in the present state of our knowledge of the disease, any inferences as to the benefit resulting from various modes of practice, derived from the comparative number of deaths to recoveries, would be erroneous. Mr. Christie referring to the very different success which attended similar modes of treatment pursued by himself and Mr. Colhoun, remarks, that "in general amongst Europeans the at- "tack of beriberi is more sudden, and the symptoms more severe, and dis- "tinctly marked, but that the proportion of cures is, with them, much great- "er than with natives." *Hunter op. citat. page* 100. The observation also applies to the disease as it attacks natives of robust constitution, as contrasted with its obstinacy and fatality in men of an opposite description. The rule is however far from being one of universal application. Dr. Pearse furnishes the following remarks relative to the prognosis. "When attended "with, or preceded by much fever, with strong, full, vibrating pulse, and a "disposition to œdematous swelling, extending to the upper parts of the body "or face, with a hurried manner and anxious countenance, even though no "paralysis of the limbs has yet commenced, the utmost danger is to be ap- "prehended, as such cases frequently terminate fatally in a few hours, if not "relieved by art; cases also in which patients had suffered from tedious at- "tacks of fever or rheumatism, and by which they were much debilitated, "are also of an unfavourable description, and if they do not end fatally, are "usually protracted, and recovery becomes tedious. Dropsical swelling ap- "pearing after the disease has continued for some time, is also unfavourable, "and dyspnœa coming on, may be invariably looked upon as the precursor "of death, no instance of recovery where a tendency to dyspnœa once ap- "peared, having been met with in my practice." He also observes that in certain cases of the chronic form of the disease, several months may elapse "before the muscles of the limbs are capable of much exertion,and are often "years before they gain their wonted powers." The following is his description of these cases. "The chief symptoms which mark the third form of "beriberi as a distinct variety from all others, are the following. Paralysis

cords of the hospitals, in that of others, have been uncertain and fluctuating, and the employment of remedies has in general been directed, by little more than some general principles, which, when applied to unknown complaints, are more destructive than other kinds of empiricism. As in the following observations, I have not been guided by the preceding remarks, but have cautiously examined every case, and noted down separately the apparent effects of each remedy used, with all those circumstances which could at all bear on the result; and then enquired into the connections of these with each other, and with the indications which were deduced from the symptoms viewed separately; I trust I may be justified, in admitting into the practical part of this essay, inferences derived from the phenomena of the disease: and that any incidental proofs of these views thus obtained, may be looked on as legitimate, having been arrived at, by a different and independent method. The access to the records of the practice of others has been of great use in this enquiry, by showing the effects of remedies used in various forms, and with

" of the extremities, excessive debility, wasting of the body, and flabbiness " of the muscles, coming on after a slight febrile attack more or less marked, " but unaccompanied by any tendency to dropsical effusion in the early stages, " as is met with in the two former varieties, nor does a tendency to effusion " show itself until a short time before death, should it end fatally, when there " is swelling of the legs succeeded by dyspnœa: partial œdema of the feet " may sometimes be observable during convalescence. The difference of " symptoms in this variety of the complaint from either of the two former, is " to be attributed to its being of a more chronic form, and there being less " vascular excitment present, the pulse all through the disease is weak and " soft, though sometimes quicker than natural, and after the disease has con- " tinued for some time, the artery at the wrist becomes so much reduced in " size, as not to feel larger than in a child of six or eight years of age, absorp- " tion of the solids continues to go on, wasting the muscles till they no longer " give form to the limbs, which are rendered perfectly useless, and unable to " sustain the weight of the body. There is always some pain complained of, " generally in the calves of the legs and tendons of the muscles of the lower " limbs, but it is never very urgent."

A remarkable case will be found in a subsequent note, in which the numbness had existed for six years, and had extended over the head; yet a cure was speedily effected by the use of the black oil.

different views from my own; but, while I believe, that I may have thus been enabled to add something to our knowledge of the treatment, I am sensible, that some most important agents can yet be used only with much uncertainty, as to the symptoms which indicate them, and to the extent to which they should be carried.

Bleeding. The very various forms in which the disease appears, will prepare us to expect, that any general plan of treatment will not be found to answer, and that the profuse evacuations recommended by Mr. Hamilton, on the unsupported principle of great congestion, and on very limited experience; or the more moderate though still free use of the lancet recommended by Mr. Scott, and grounded on a theory equally defective and on no experience, will be both dangerous and insufficient. Mr. Marshall justly observes, that more extended "clinical experience is "still necessary, before a due estimate can be made "of the true efficacy of the depletory means of cure;" and as, in recording a fact little understood, until it is ascertained what circumstances have nothing to do with it, we ought to omit nothing capable of being noted, I shall state at length the observations I have made on this important subject. Mr. Marshall found bleeding useful in a case where the chest was severely affected; and when it is so, and the pulse is strong and full, no doubt can exist as to the advantage of a free use of it. The following example illustrates the fact, in a stout European soldier.

Case 36th. James Wain, ætat. 30, in India 10 years. 14th December, 1831, admitted last night complaining of pain under the ensiform cartilage, increased on pressure and preventing full inspiration, the attempt causing much pain. Complains also of weakness of the knees, and of slight numbness of the lower limbs as high as the middle of the thigh ; says that he feels as if he tottered in walking, but appears to walk straight, numbness over the back of the hands (not in the fingers) and up to the elbows ; face is fuller than natural and feels slightly numb. Slight œdema over the tibia. The affection of the legs and arms came on ten days ago, the pain in the chest only two. The action of the heart is unusally strong and bounding ; skin moist, tongue clean, rather too red. Bowels costive, urine said to be natural in colour and quantity ; slept ill from starting in his sleep, and since he was taken ill is easiest on the left side. Was sent sick from Rangoon in 1825, for a bad ulcer and scurvy, but has otherwise had excellent health. V.S. Habeat pulv. jalap. comp. ℥j. Vesp. Pulse got small when 20 oz. of blood were taken away, pain at stomach relieved, dyspnœa and numbness continue, pulse 88 full and sharp, but not strong. ℞ Calomel. gr. vj, antimon. tartar. gr. ss, extract. colocynth. comp. gr. x. Fiat pil. h. s. s. 15th. No pain in chest but a slight oppression continues; slept ill and at intervals only, from shooting pain in knees ; walks worse and there is a cracking sound from his knee joints; numbness diminished, some anxiety of countenance, pulse 72, less strong; is easiest in the recumbent posture, and now lies turned a little to the left side; stethoscope detects slight inflammation in the middle lobe of right lung. Habeat tinct. digital. gtt. xxx quater die. ℞ Pil. hydrarg. gr. iv, pulv. scillæ gr. j. Fiat pilula ter die sumend. Emplast. vesicator. magnum pectori. 16th. Blister did not rise till 10 P. M., no pain in breast and there is less difficulty in drawing his breath, less numbness but pains and weakness rather increased. Pulse 70 and a little sharp, urine said to be of a dark colour but made freely, slight cough, three stools, tongue clean, slept from 8 to 10 but hardly any rest since, limbs feel "tired". Cont. medicament. 17th. Three draughts yesterday, hardly any oppression of breathing and no pain of chest, slept well, less numbness of hands and face; feels comfortable, very weak on the knees, and joints of hands and toes feeble. 18th. Same; slept well, pulse 76, was 86 at evening visit, no stool. ℞ Pulv. jalap. comp. ʒj. Cont. alia. 19th. Physic operated well, slept well, walks more steadily, the left leg is the worst, relieved by frictions; no complaint of breast, pulse 76 strong, action of heart more natural. Cont. medicament. 20th. Vespere. Feels better; very little pain in knees, weakness continues, no thirst, bowels open, no pain or uneasiness in chest except on pressure, and a tightness across the breast on making a deep inspiration, urine of a deep red colour. Cont medicament. Applicet. emplast. vesicator. parti dolenti pector. 21st. Free from pain, weakness in the knees much the same, blister rose well, bowels open, pulse 86, soft and full; no tightness across the chest, urine passed easily but in very small quantities. Cont. medicament. Vesp. Some difficulty in making water. Two pints of extra tea. 22d. Better, and walks much stronger, urine free and scalds him a little. Cont. medicament. 23d. No complaint but of weakness in his knees. Pulse 98, full and soft, urine free and light coloured. The improvement was progressive, and he was discharged on the 5th January, permanently cured.

The following case is selected, to show its beneficial effects, in similar circumstances, in removing the pectoral symptoms in natives, and also the great tendency to relapse, a fact which forced itself very unwillingly on my attention when less familiar with the disease, the successful termination of a few cases, having led me to be very sanguine in the success of the remedies here employed.

Case 37th. Budday Khan, a stout sepoy. 15th January. Complains of swelling of the feet, and of his limbs having almost entirely lost their sensibility, and of stiffness and want of power in them, they pit on pressure, face is also swollen. Breathing oppressed, slept well. Insensibility extends to the abdomen but there is no swelling; urine scanty, high coloured and scalds in passing. Bowels natural. Pulse full, frequent, and hard. Tongue clean, no appetite, thirst; took calomel. gr. x last night, from which four stools. V. S. ℥x. Vespere. Breathing much relieved by bleeding. Pulse as before. ℞ Calomel., pulv. scillæ, āā, gr. ij. Fiat pilula, omni nocte sumend. Tinct. digital. gtt. xx ter die. Habt. pulv. jalap. comp. ʒj. cras mane. 16th. Breathing perfectly free, swellings of limbs rather less, urine a little more copious, insensibility the same. Pulse of natural frequency but full, has had two stools from physic. Rept. pulv. jalap. comp. ʒj. Cont. liniment. et alia. 20th. Mouth sore, and makes more urine which is now light coloured, insensibility and weight of limbs continue. Pulse full. Cont. liniment. Omitt. alia. 26th. Pains of limbs rather better; on pressing the parts about the tibia there is slight pitting, complains of the hands being also affected with partial insensibility. Habt. mistur. camphor. ℥viij, guaiac. gum. ʒss, tinct. opii gtt. xl in die. 28th. Limbs rather better from rubbing them with hot sand, otherwise free from complaint. 31st. Complains of his limbs feeling more heavy and senseless, they are slightly swollen, face is also swollen again, urine free, pulsation of the heart can be felt over a considerable part of the left side of the chest. Habt. statim pulv. jalap. gr. xxx, calomel. gr. v. Vespere. Only three stools, says that since morning the urine has been high coloured and scanty. Pulse very full, hard, and frequent. V. S. ad ℥x. Habt. stat. tinct. opii, tinct. digital., āā, ʒss, mist. camphor.℥j. 1st February. Much serum in blood drawn, the coagulum pretty firm, no buff; feels better. ℞ Calomel., pulv. scillæ, āā, gr. ij, antimon. tartar. gr. $\frac{1}{4}$. Fiat pilula ter die sumend. et h.s. rept. haust. 2d. Says he is better, skin warm, pulse full and hard, 80, does not sleep well. Cont. 3rd. Urine sometimes scanty and red, sometimes pale. Bowels regular He suffered from repeated relapses after this; had severe pains in his limbs, and was sent to another station for change of air but without much benefit. He sank under a relapse many months after.

In these cases the pericardium was the part principally affected, the pulse was full, strong, and frequent, the action of the heart violent, and the disease recent; but when the symptoms return, the same treatment may be repeated with equal advantage while the strength is yet little reduced. The effect of the bleeding was assisted and the urine increased by digitalis, squills, and touching the mouth with calomel, but the constitution being under the influence of mercury did not prevent a return of the symptoms.

When there is no dyspnœa, if there is evidence of much excitement about the heart, a free bleeding will be very beneficial, as in a patient (Guntaloo) under treatment at the same time as the last, who complained of numbness and heaviness of the lower limbs from the middle of the thighs, with œdema, and followed by evening fever and some rigors. No dyspnœa, but the heart was felt to beat strongly over the lower part of the left side of the chest and in the epigastrium, and the pulse was quick, full, and hard. He was bled to 20 ounces which were nearly natural, but had rather too much serum. The pulse fell to 70, was easily compressed but still hard, he had no return of fever, and the urine was in 3 days of the natural quantity. The affection of the limbs remained unaltered under the use of frictions, salivation, mezereon and diuretics. On the 16th, the pulsation of the heart was "felt over the whole left side "of the chest, and there seemed to be water interposed "between the heart and ribs:" he could not sleep from feeling of deadness over the body. Pulse small, two stools daily. Œdema could barely be detected. He did not improve for two weeks, and was sent to Vizagapatam for the benefit of change of air, but died during the first march. Nor is it in recent cases only, that venesection may advantageously be employed; in case second, palsy had lasted for many months and anasarca and affection of the chest had several times occurred previously, yet a moderate bleeding was necessary to relieve dyspnœa, oppression, and violent action of the heart with a quick, full, and strong pulse. A more remarkable case occurred in a sepoy, aged 53 but robust, who had numbness and pains of the lower extremities for three months. He got fever, mostly in the night, violent action of the heart; pulse was 130, strong. He was bled to 10 oz. and fainted, it was repeated to 6 oz. next day, and with a purgative reduced the action of the heart and arteries to a natural state, the œdema of the face left him, and he was allowed to leave the hospital. The power of the legs was not restored and he was readmitted with anasarca of the abdomen and legs, increased action of the heart, breathing more oppressed, although not complained of by the patient. Pulse quick and weak, tongue dry and white, urine high coloured and stools green. The hands and feet soon got cold, he was restless, and died, apparently from thoracic effusion and œdema of the lung consequent on the diseased pericardium. In one severe case of beriberi of some continuance, in a musician, remittent fever with high action came on, and notwithstanding the debility of the patient, the thoracic inflammation was acute, the dyspnœa considerable, and dry hard cough and strong pulse indicated bleeding, which I performed with anxiety, but as it gave relief both to the head and chest, freely, and with the best effects. The beriberi continued however, and was slowly cured by other means. In such examples it is certain, and in all it is probable, that bleeding is to be employed no further than is required for the relief of the local affection; and there is no ground to hope, that the nervous torpor and disorder will often be much benefited by antiphlogistic measures, and even over the disorder of the heart the benefit is far from certain or permanent, as may be seen in several of the fatal cases of which dissections are recorded. The following is a good example of the result which may too often be expected, even when the immediate good effects are well marked.

Case 38th. Shaik Modinah, ætat. 24, admitted on the 22d August, into the hospital at Vizianagram, complaining of stiffness and partial loss of feeling in the legs which are slightly œdematous, face and hands are also slightly swollen. Pulse quick and hard, action of heart felt over almost the whole chest, and its stroke is hard, tongue white. Has been ill six days. V. S. ad ℥xxiv.

Habt. h. s. calomel. ℈j, cras mane pulv. jalap. comp. ℈j. 23d. Frequent stools, swellings have lessened. 25th. Swellings gone, a little stiffness and insensibility of the left foot, complains of weakness of his limbs. Rept. calomel. ℈j h. s., et cras mane pulv. jalap. comp. ℨj. 27th. Cannot now walk without assistance, which he ascribes to the bleeding, although it did not become very remarkable till yesterday. Insensibility and swelling gone. Perspired from Dover's powder. Pulse still quick, not so full but rather hard, skin dry and a little warm, gums white. ℞ Carbon. ammon., pulv. Doveri, āā, gr. x. Fiat pulvis, ter die sumend. October 12th. Sent to the coast. 26th. Has returned improved, can walk and has appetite, but pulse and action of the heart still indicate the existence of disease. Ordered to return to the coast.

Keeping in view the important remarks of Dr. Bright, that in the disease described by him, in which the urine is scanty and the urea deficient, and the inflammation often latent; and the affections of the membranes in beriberi being in some degree analogous in their cause and progress, and that, although the urine is often scanty without inflammation, it is generally accompanied with a scanty secretion of high coloured urine; we shall be led to employ depletion where the pain is slight or absent, and there is no certain indication of the particular organ affected. In Beemanah (case 19th), the firm pulse as high as 96, slight pyrexia, and puffy face called for bleeding, the necessity of which was fully confirmed by the marks of inflammation found after death. Of a similar nature was the important case, noticed (page 128) when examining the nature of the urine in the early stages, in which the blood was strongly buffed.

In the case of Purmeser Naik (page 210), a quick hard pulse and high coloured urine, were the only symptoms of the internal inflammations found after death, indicated by the bloody fluid in the pericardium, and the redness of the intestines. Bleeding was not employed. A man named C. Nagalingum had dyspnœa on exertion, œdema of the *face and feet only*, high coloured urine, and the pulse was 120, hard and small; could walk between two men, but dyspnœa comes on and prevents him. He was not bled, and although the urine was increased by calomel and squills, cream of tartar, &c. he was not relieved, and died. This kind of evidence is, however, very uncertain in this disease. A man was admitted at the same time as the last patient, with dyspnœa increased on exertion, anasarca, dry cough, pains in limbs, scanty urine, pulse quick and strong, stools at first dark, then whitish; he recovered under the use of purgatives, digitalis, and cream of tartar, and a blister to the sternum.

It is much more difficult to determine, what circumstances demand general bleeding when the pulse is weak or small, as the other symptoms are not very obvious, imperfectly understood, or liable to be confounded with others, to which the words of Dr. Rogers are applicable, " quin et ad phlebotomiam tandem cursum ejus funestum celerius absolvit."

Mr. Abernethy has remarked, that water in the pericardium, being confined by a strong membrane not easily dilated, presses on the heart, and thus causes a small quick pulse; and therefore we may expect, that when there is little excitement of the muscular substance of the heart, the pulse will be but an uncertain guide. In a few, the pulse has been found hard or sharp, although weak and small, and when with this sign of inflammation of the heart there were indications of effusion into the pericardium, bleeding was borne well, and proved useful, for the time. As it seemed desirable to overcome the inflammation without permanent diminution of strength, the tartrate of antimony was given in large doses and with some apparent benefit, but notwithstanding the use of digitalis, squills, calomel, and purges, the effusion into the chest increased and the pulse for a short time, perhaps, indicated the propriety of repeating the bleeding; but the period when this was admissible was exceedingly brief, as in Purmeser Naik and others; the pulse getting rapidly feeble and small, and the debility extreme.

Case 39th. Shaik Emaum, ætat. 22, admitted 17th March, 1827. Face and lower extremities swollen and œdematous; has no oppression of breathing, action of heart can be perceived over the greater part of the left side of the chest, pains in calves of legs and all over the limbs, slight numbness in the feet and legs, pulse hard and sharp but easily compressed, tongue white, skin dry, two stools from a dose of jalap taken yesterday. Was discharged from hospital, cured of fever, on the 9th. ℞ Tinct. digital. min. lx, antimon. tartarisat. gr. iss, tinct. opii min. xl, aquæ ℥ij. Fiat mist. Half to be taken in the course of the day in divided doses. Habt. stat. infus. sennæ ℥vj. Vespere. V. S. ad ℥x. Habt. cras mane pulv. jalap. comp. ʒj. Cont. mist. 18th. Bore the bleeding well, much serum in the blood; no better; has a little cough which, he says, he has had for eight days, voice hoarse. Face and arms rather more swollen. ℞ Antimon. tartar. gr. xxiv, confect. aromat. gr. xij. Fiat mass. et divide in pilul. xij quarum capiat unam quarta quaque hora. Applicet, h.s. emplast.vesicator. magn. pectori. 19th. Blister rose well, took four of the pills, the first at 11 A. M. the last at 10 P. M., vomited once after each of the first three pills, and had several stools; no vomiting after the fourth pill, but had 5 stools, swelling rather less. Pulse hard, tongue nearly natural, urine not high coloured or scanty. Rept. pilul. antimon. tartar. 3tia quaque hora. Cont. mist. 20th. Took eight pills, was vomited yesterday morning, to-day no vomiting. Two stools after the second pill, one stool this morning. Feels better, pains in limbs easier, pulse nearly natural, still a little hard. Vespere. Habeat cras mane pulv. jalap. comp. ʒj. Cont. pil. antimon. tartar. gr. iij secunda quaque hora. Cont. mist. 21st. Took twelve pills, vomited at 12 after the third pill, having drank a quantity of fluid, swellings have lessened, urine as before. Vespere. Has taken 6 pills, vomited once after the third pill and was purged once; stool dark green inclining to red. Rept. pil. statim et habeat h. s. calomel. gr. v. Cras mane pulv. jalap. comp. ʒj. 22d. Physic has not yet operated, is better, skin still dry, and urine is not increased. Omitt. pilul. Cont. mist. 23rd. Three stools from medicine, yellow and as if mixed with curdled milk, breathing easy, swelling subsides, no pain in the legs, but complains of slight spasms, skin cool, pulse still rather sharp. Ol. ricini ℥j cras mane. ℞ Tinct. digital. min. lx, antimon. tartarisat. gr. iss, tinct. opii ʒss, aquæ ℥ij. Fiat mist. ℥j bis die. 25th. Improves, but cannot stand up without support from debility of limbs, tongue yellow. Cont. mist. digitalis. Habeat stat. pulv. jalap. comp. ʒj. 27th. Complains only of want of power in his limbs. Pulse full, tongue yellow and coated. Rept. pulv. jalap.

comp. Cont. mist. To bathe his legs three times a day in the nitro-muriatic acid bath. 28th. Frequent stools, some swelling of face has returned, pulse frequent and full. Cont. tinct. digitalis. ℞ Calomel. gr. iij, pulv. scillæ gr. ij. Fiat pilul. ter die sumend. 29th. Swelling of face increased, action of heart can be felt over the whole of the left side of the chest and to the clavicle; pulse very frequent but oppressed, tongue coated yellow in centre, skin dry. Applicet. emplast. vesicator. magnum thoraci. Cont. Vespere. Breathing laborious, face very much swollen. Pulse very frequent and small; appearance of great oppression. Omitt. scillæ. Cont. alia. Habeat h. s. calomel. ℈j. 30th. Breathing continued to become more laborious in the night, and was not relieved by sulphuric æther. Died at 5 A. M.

If the case is more chronic, the relief from bleeding is little marked, notwithstanding the hardness of the pulse; and the spasmodic symptoms whether of the legs, larynx, or other parts are not in the least alleviated. In cases where there is short cough with some sharpness of the pulse, and other symptoms of inflammatory affection, the relief from bleeding has been much less marked, than when the pericardium has been principally diseased, a fact probably depending on the direct benefit derived in the latter, from the diminished quantity of circulating fluid passing through the heart. My experience does not enable me to state any thing with precision, as to the circumstances accompanying the sensation of diffused internal heat which require evacuations, the symptom being often obscurely described by the patient, not of very frequent occurrence, and attended with such various combinations as render much careful observation requisite, to ascertain the effect of treatment on this peculiar symptom. But as it has been found to have been the result of inflammation, and as I have found it aggravated by stimulants of all kinds, the probability is, that evacuations will be required in many examples: but the rapid recoveries of patients in whom this symptom is present, which take place without the use of the lancet, will deter us from using it for this alone, or at least to any great extent. There are other cases in which evacuations may be cautiously employed, although the pulse is small, weak, and irritable. The case of Narroydoo (page 176) may be taken as a fair example of a certain class of cases, and of the extent of benefit to be expected. In that patient, the dyspnœa was distressing, principally after exertion, it had made rapid progress without much previous disease, the urine was scanty and high coloured, and the arms were œdematous. A small bleeding relieved the breathing, but the pulse and other symptoms remained unaltered. There being cough, and pain with swelling at the pit of the stomach, probably from distension of the pericardium (as noticed by Mr. Abernethy), and extension of inflammation, the bleeding was repeated and relieved the pain, and the pulse got slower and fuller. [121] It is remarkable that the dyspnœa, œdema, and quick pulse left together, and that the urine was increased at the same time; a circumstance which has frequently been observed. Ten grains of calomel and

[121] The following cases by Mr. Wright are very valuable. "J. Taylor, "quarter master serjeant, ætat. 56, of a strong habit. 22d October, 1831, "admitted. Has been unable to walk beyond the limits of his compound "during the last week, from a partial loss of the use of the lower extremities, and states that within the last six hours he has been affected with difficulty of breathing, fulness in the chest, loss of power in the lower and upper extremities, with general œdema, pulse at present weak and frequent "at the wrist, with full and hard pulsations at the carotids and large arteries, "bowels constipated, skin hot and dry, urine scanty, tongue furred. Mittat. "sanguis ad ℥xxx. ℞ Calomel gr. x., pulv. antimon. gr. iij statim. 23rd. Af-

half a grain of tartrate of antimony were taken thrice daily, for four days, and affected the mouth with marked benefit to all the symptoms, apparently from its power of subduing inflammation. In an interesting

" ter the abstraction of the blood the dyspnœa was considerably relieved, and " the pulse became quick and full at the wrist; at present states that he feels " much easier, there is a feeling of slight oppression at the chest, but the dys- " pnœa is relieved, skin moist, pulse 86 rather full, œdema and paralysis " much as before, bowels have been freely opened. ℞ Calomel. gr. x, pulv. " scillæ gr. iij mane et vespere, et infric. liniment. ammon. part. dolent. 25th. " The œdema has become less general, the lower extremities only being swol- " len, can walk a short distance with ease, pulse regular, free perspiration, " urine copious, bowels open, tongue furred. Cont. 27th. Continues to improve. " Cont. medicament. 28th. Convalescent. 2d November. Discharged.

" Humeron Sing, sepoy, B company, ætat. 25. 14th July, 1832. Complains of " having had a sensation of numbness in the lower extremities during the last " ten days, there was slight œdema at first which has been increasing gradu- " ally with pitting on pressure, pulse 84, skin hot and dry, urine scanty, bowels " constipated. ℞ Calomel. grs. vij, pulv. scillæ gr. ij ter in die. 15th. Passed " a restless night, œdema increasing, lower extremities becoming paralysed, " skin and pulse as before, bowels have been freely opened, urine dark co- " loured and more copious. Cont. calomel. et scillæ. Infric. liniment. ammon. " part. dolent. 16th. The œdema has become general, complains of a sensa- " tion of straightness across the chest, with dyspnœa, pulse 86 and wiry, skin " hot and dry, bowels open; paralysis of the lower extremities. Mittat. " sanguis ad ℥xx. Cont. calomel. et scillæ et liniment. Low diet. 17th. Com- " plained much of weakness after the abstraction of the blood, the dyspnœa " however was relieved and there is less œdema, paralysis as before, pulse at " present 78, of good strength, skin moist, bowels open. Cont. calomel. et scil- " læ et liniment. 18th. Slept well, œdema disappearing, less paralysis, pulse " of about the natural standard, urine copious, skin moist, mouth slightly " affected. Omitt. calomel. et scillæ. To have a grain of nux vomica morning " and evening. 19th. Less œdema and can walk with more ease, otherwise the " same. Two grains of nux vomica to be taken twice a day. Cont. liniment. " 20th. Much improved. Cont. medicament. 25th. Convalescent. 4th Au- " gust. Discharged.

" Remarks. The two abovementioned cases are instances of the occasional " acuteness and violence of this disease; the suddenness with which the drop- " sy became general, the arterial action, and relief occasioned by blood-let- " ting indicates an inflammatory tendency, which could, from the rapidity of " the progress of the disease, hardly have been removed by medicines alone."

" Ramoodoo, sepoy, 8th regiment N. I. A company, No. 28. 11th. August, " 1833, of rather a stout habit. Admitted with loss of the powers of progres- " sive movement, the eyes are suffused with red, bowels constipated, tongue " white, urine scanty, œdema of the legs and anxiety of the præcordia, pulse " 90, rather hard. Complaint of three days standing. Habt. calomel. gr. v, " pulv. scillæ gr. ij statim. 12th. During the night there was jactitation, rest- " lessness, and anxiety with general functional disturbance, and at present " there are symptoms of disease in the brain, occasional delirium, (not mutter- " ing), contracted pupil, slow pulse, laboured breathing, and heat of skin. " Mittat. sanguis ad ℥xx. Habeat calomel. gr. x, pulv. scillæ gr. ij statim. " Vespere. Much the same, restlessness, dyspnœa, slow weak pulse; bowels " freely open. Cont. calomel. et scillæ. Lotio frigid. capiti. 13th. Passed a " better night, at present no dyspnœa, anxiety, pain of head or restlessness, " skin moist, bowels open. Cont. calomel. et scillæ mane et vespere. 14th, " Gums affected, bowels open, pulse regular, skin moist, urine copious, no " œdema, and only slight weakness of the lower extremities. Habt. mistur. " camphoræ ℥ss, spt. æther. nitric. ʒj mane et vespere. Omitt. calomel. In-

case of an European, ætat. 31, who had œdema of the body and lower extremities, great oppression, pain in chest and tenderness to pressure, with a hard, strong and rapid pulse, and feeling of weakness from previous attacks, bleeding was unfortunately neglected at first, and diuretics, purgatives, and sulphuric æther prescribed. These in some degree reduced the swellings, increased the urine, and relieved the dyspnœa and increased cardiac action, but violent oppression at chest from disordered action of the heart came on at intervals, the stomach gradually became irritable, and the pulse small. On the 11th day, he had severe oppression at chest, dyspnœa, violent throbbing of the heart, quick and full pulse, and inability to retain any thing on the stomach. His eyes were blood-shot as if inflamed. He was bled to 48 oz. which relieved the dyspnœa and throbbing, but the oppression continued much the same till next day, when the swelling of the arms also decreased, the ascites and irritability of stomach being unaltered. Sulphuric and nitrous æther, tincture of opium, and spirits, with purgatives were used on the 14th and 15th days; oppression at chest kept him restless, but both this, the irritability at stomach and ascites diminished. During the 18th day, he observed the swellings about the chest, increase rapidly, bringing on oppression at his chest and dyspnœa. The pulse was rapid and small, he was greatly exhausted, and the above symptoms were aggravated. Sulphuric æther and ammonia gave no relief, and the œdema increased and

" fric. liniment. ammon. cruribus. 15th. Convalescent; regular exercise and " nourishing diet. Cont. liniment. 29th. Discharged.

" This is one of the few cases in which I have observed beriberi to be at- " tended with local determination to the brain, and is also an instance of the " occasional good effect of blood-letting, the habit of the patient and the ur- " gent symptoms being attended to."

extended up to his neck. Pulse was hardly perceptible, the heart throbbed greatly, and dyspnœa gradually increased to suffocation, and he died at 9 A. M.

It is much to be regretted that this case was not recorded with more care, and a dissection made by the gentleman to whom it occurred; it is however, still very instructive. A moderate bleeding at first would have enabled other remedies to have acted more effectually, and the termination would probably have been different.

When bleeding is required for the relief of irregular and violent action of the heart, it should be limited to such a quantity as may be sufficient to relieve the oppressed organ, without debilitating the patient and thus rendering him more liable to irregular actions, and putting it out of our power to repeat the evacuations when the symptoms return. The operation should probably be performed in the erect posture and in a full stream, but we must not produce fainting, which is always dangerous in diseases of the heart. I have been able to derive very little information as to the circumstances requiring the use of the lancet, from the information or cases of others, to which I have had access, a very general prejudice having existed in the northern division against its use; and when it has been employed, it has very frequently been in that form or stage in which it is injurious. I am informed that both Mr. Stevenson and Mr. Paterson employed it, in the early stages, when the pulse was full; but I have not learnt whether they pointed out any other guide.[122]

[122] I have since had an opportunity of examining some of the cases of the former, but they do not suggest any additional remark on this subject. *Original note.* (See note 76.)

The following extract from Mr. Paterson' 1st half yearly report for 1822, contains the most important observation on this subject, which I have met with. " The treatment I have found most beneficial in this disease, is at its com-

Dr. Wight speaks unfavourably of v. s. but without stating any specific reason; many others have also objected to it, as the disease appeared to them to be attended with debility; and to the *general* employment of bleeding, the objection is well founded, but we have had good reason to conclude, that it is also, like drop-

" mencement, one large bleeding, not less than sixteen ounces of blood; an al-
" most immediate subsidence of the swelling of the surface is the consequence,
" and the pulse is generally reduced with respect to the number of pulsations
" to its natural standard. Purgatives and blisters appear to me to be of con-
" siderable utility. I have administered calomel combined with squills in
" pretty large doses, but have never found them act as a diuretic, and ptya-
" lism does not ensure the patient's safety. To restore tone to the system,
" acids and tonics, particularly the Peruvian bark, have I think, been most
" beneficial."

" I may here observe, that I do not consider the disease as at all inflamma-
" tory, and that *the bleeding resorted to at the commencement of the disease, is to*
" *afford relief to the circulating system, merely by diminishing the quantity of*
" *fluid in the blood-vessels.*"

The same views appear to have guided Mr. Alexander Campbell in the treatment of the disease, in 1822. " If from the state of the pulse and strength
" of the patient, I thought bleeding admissible, I had recourse to the lancet;
" in some however, the powers of life were so far exhausted that I considered
" it a hazardous experiment. Calomel and squills united, were what I chiefly
" relied on, exhibited in such doses as merely to act on the mouth and kid-
" neys, stimulating frictions also, with a purgative now and then, and a blister
" applied to the chest, where the breathing appeared to be any way affected,
" (a common symptom), were found useful."

In the more acute forms of the disease, the experience of Dr. Pearse appears to authorize a freer employment of the lancet. " From the description
" given of the varieties of beriberi, it will be sufficiently obvious, that the
" symptoms in the two first forms are those of an acute, whilst in the other
" three varieties they are those of a chronic disease, differing both in the mode
" of attack, and in the early symptoms, though gradually assuming the same
" characters in the subsequent stages." * * * " When called on to see a pa-
" tient who has been suddenly attacked with swelling of his legs, gradually
" extending upwards, whose countenance is anxious and pale, his manner
" hurried, but who perhaps walks stoutly, and says there is little the matter
" with him, but a fluttering sensation about the heart, but whose pulse on ex-
" amination is found to be full, bounding, and imparts a vibrating action to
" the finger, experience points out, that if this state of excitement is not
" speedily removed, and the violent action of the circulating system relieved
" by depletion, a fatal termination from effusion of fluid into the pleuræ, or
" pericardium must probably soon be the consequence." * * * "Abstraction
" of blood being requisite in most cases of the second form, on account of the
" greater severity of symptoms, except when accidental circumstances, or
" previous debility, contraindicate its use, should seldom be delayed beyond
" the first twenty-four hours, it being constantly borne in mind, that whilst
" acute symptoms continue, hydrothorax or hydrops pericardii, are to be fear-
" ed, and that when symptoms of those affections once set in, recovery is, if
" not hopeless, a circumstance of the most doubtful nature; and as before
" remarked, no recovery from such symptoms has ever been seen by me,
" though others, perhaps, may have been more fortunate." (See note 3rd
" page 9.)

Dr. Herklots objects strongly to blood-letting, and the perusal of the three cases in which he employed it, certainly show, that it may be used without affording any relief, even when the pulse is strong and frequent.

sy, often attended with increased action requiring appropriate treatment. It is not however required in all examples of excitement in the cardiac region, as we fortunately possess remedies which exert a direct influence over the disease; but although we have other means, so well understood and efficacious a remedy is not to be neglected. Local bleeding from the chest has been used in a few instances with benefit, and might be more freely employed with safety and a prospect of advantage. The tenderness of the chest, (although not observed with sufficient accuracy), is analogous to that lately pointed out by Dr. Elliotson as a symptom of pericarditis, in which cupping over the cardiac region is found to be beneficial; and since this was written, a friend on whose judgment I have great reliance, has communicated two cases now under treatment, in which twelve leeches applied every second day, reduced the frequency of the pulse and the irritable, irregular, and increased action of the heart, which had been little benefited by a variety of other treatment.[123]

On the employment of general bleeding, when there are symptoms of abdominal affection, I am not able to communicate more than one or two observations. The stomach suffers less in the circars, than in Ceylon, and seldom until the disease has made great progress, and other dangerous complications have supervened. As it has been found to be inflamed, in some cases in which it had been irritable before death, it is probable that bleeding will be useful; and I have found it so in a few cases, although the benefit has not been so decided as in the cardiac affection. The pulse is

[123] Mr. Davidson, the gentleman referred to, has continued to employ local bleeding from the cardiac region with marked advantage. (See note 88, and Mr. Turnbull's report in the appendix.)

usually small, and the powers feeble, but this is not universal, and I have not had sufficient experience to justify my coming to a conclusion, whether the difference depends on the seat or nature of the affection of the stomach, or on those of the chest or other parts. In two examples, however, the fuller pulse depended on pectoral affection, and in one, where the inflammation seemed to extend from the pericardium and diaphragm to the stomach, the benefit was more remarkable to the former parts, than to the secondary affection. When the inflammatory state of the stomach is chronic and attended with only slight pain, tenderness, and fiery tongue, local bleeding and avoiding stimulating food and medicine, effect a certain and speedy cure, although relapse may occur in any period of the disease. Ten or fifteen leeches are usually sufficient, and may require to be repeated. I cannot state from experience, any thing regarding bleeding in the general affection of the peritoneum, but from the facts noticed in a former page, of the effusion being often attended with inflammation, and that the fluid in some instances partakes of the character of the product of inflammation, it is probable, that attention may discover symptoms which will lead to its detection during life. In the mean time, should pain and tenderness be absent, when the fluid is secreted in the abdomen in moderate quantity, the probability is that depletion may be cautiously employed. It has never been required for hepatic symptoms. When the bladder is very tender to pressure, or there is more than the usual degree of pain in hypogastrium; and when the irritation of the urine causes either some degree of strangury or retention, in the sequela I have fully described, bleeding by leeches is generally followed by relief, although it cannot be expected to be permanent. Some benefit has also been derived from cupping and leeches over the kidney, when there was much pain or tenderness in the lumbar regions.

The rheumatic pains in the limbs are often attended with pyrexia, and when the pulse was firm, a small bleeding seemed useful.

Having communicated what my observations have enabled me to add to the published information on this subject, which yet stands in need of accurate and more extensive investigation, I shall state some of the cases in which bleeding is injurious. The frequent employment of bleeding for the relief of the violent dyspnœa, especially by medical men little accustomed to treat beriberi, in cases which I have either seen or had the details communicated to me, has afforded undeniable evidence of its injurious effects, and justifies to a certain extent, the prejudice before noticed, against its use, and enforces the utmost caution in recommending or practising it. This was strongly impressed on my mind at an early period, by the unfortunate result of the measure, in a sepoy who had been long under my care and was convalescent. He was seen by another person during a paroxysm of dyspnœa which came on in the night, and as that was violent, a copious bleeding was ordered, and the death of the patient was the almost immediate result. He appeared to have œdema of the lung. Numerous examples of the same kind might be adduced, but as few who have had much experience in the disease, have given way to the temptation " to do something" for the relief of the urgent dyspnœa, the cases are not sufficiently accurate in the details. The following is a specimen.

Case 40th. A subadar, ætat. 56. Admitted 6th October having been a month ill with anasarca of the body and face, and swelling of the throat; dyspnœa, upper and lower extremities palsied; is nearly speechless. Pulse quick and small, tongue white. Had a purgative and ol. nigri gtt. xx bis die. On the 8th, œdema of the face and neck were nearly gone, but in the evening breathing became laborious and the pulse was hardly perceptible. He was bled and immediately after got rattling in the throat, vomited, and died.

There are three classes of cases in which bleeding has been uniformly fatal, but some further experience will be necessary to define them with accuracy. The first is that in which œdema of the lung, (and probably also where effusion into the chest) has taken place suddenly, characterized by symptoms previously described. These cases are most commonly fatal under any mode of treatment, but by the use of powerful stimulants assisted, if required, by antispasmodics, recoveries sometimes take place, and the immediate danger is more frequently got over, although the symptoms are apt to return in an aggravated form.

2d. In that form of spasmodic dyspnœa shooting from the limbs, or otherwise connected with the muscular affections, and attended with lowness of pulse, cold extremities and prostration of strength, the peculiar nature of which is likely to be but imperfectly understood, until that of long known analogous affections are better explained, bleeding has been a fatal measure; while recoveries have been brought about by stimulants; and warm frictions to the limbs, by restoring their temperature and natural actions, have appeared to be very beneficial. Of these cases, I do not possess details which would justify me in forming an opinion, as to the nature of the paroxysm. It has appeared to be, to some extent, connected with the peculiar affections of the heart to which many of the sudden deaths are to be ascribed.

3rd. These are of different kinds, but at present we can only class them as being a spasmodic, enfeebled, or obstructed action of the centre of the circulation arising from various causes, and indicated by tendency to syncope, sense of faintness, dyspnœa coming on in paroxysms, coldness of the extremities, cold sweats, anxiety and restlessness, a pulse hardly to be felt, a throbbing of the heart,[124] not always feeble, irregular

[124] Much accurate observation and nice discrimination is required, to distinguish these symptoms from those referred to at page 249, and of which Mr. Wright's cases (note 121) afford interesting examples. It is evident from his observations, that bleeding is sometimes required when with these symptoms, there is throbbing and increased action of the heart and great vessels, and that the pulse which may have been small and even weak, occasionally becomes stronger and fuller; but I am satisfied, that if the pulse is feeble, the utmost caution is requisite in practising it, and this opinion is confirmed by the following case recorded by Mr. Wright.

"Goorapah, sepoy, A company, ætat. 25. 1832, August 1st, vespere. Admitted with paralysis of the upper and lower extremities, dyspnœa, weak "and intermittent pulse at the wrist, full pulsations at the large arteries, general œdema, hot and dry skin, scanty urine and constipated bowels. States "that during the last week, he has had numbness of the extremities, and "was attacked last night suddenly with the above symptoms. Mittat. sanguis "℥xv. ℞ Calomel. gr. x, pulv. antimon. gr. iij statim et repet. post horas tres. "Habeat mist. camphor. ℥j, spt. æther. nitric. ʒj, tinct. opii gtt. x. 2d. After the abstraction of the blood the patient expressed himself much relieved, there being less dyspnœa, moist skin, and pulse more regular, he felt "inclined to sleep, and I imagined that he would probably continue free from "any urgent symptoms; they however returned suddenly with increased "violence at 2 A.M., and although I arrived at the hospital shortly afterwards, "he was in a dying state: could I have anticipated this and been in time to "repeat the venesection, I think that from the relief afforded by the first, "this might also have been attended with benefit, and perhaps been the "means of restoring the patient."

"Morbid appearances. On examination the lungs were found much collapsed, of a dark colour, being tinged with venous blood, and appeared to "float in water of which there was a considerable quantity. The venous "system of the brain and medulla were engorged, and there was about half "an ounce of water in the ventricles; no traces of inflammation were observable in the stomach and intestines; the heart appeared flaccid and enlarged."

Temporary relief may sometimes be obtained from the abstraction of a small quantity of blood even when effusion has taken place into the chest, but in such circumstances it must always be a doubtful remedy, and its repetition perhaps inadmissible.

The following case treated by Mr. Macdonell shows that the remedy is of uncertain efficacy, even when indicated by the symptoms.

"Goorapah, sepoy, 22d regiment N. I. Admitted into the Rajahmundry "hospital, 8th January, 1828; quite a young man. He says that ten days "ago he was quite well, he then first observed some swelling of his feet which "gradually increased, four days ago first felt some numbness of his feet, there

pulsations,&c. These have been traced to water in the pericardium and to softening of the heart, but many are related to the peculiar symptoms which succeeded beriberi in Mr. Ridley, and to that singular disorder of

" is now considerable œdema of his feet and hands, and his face is puffed. " Had fever for the last three days. The numbness is not much complained " of, and is felt from the middle of the thigh downwards, he has the power " of his toes and no pain in his limbs. His gait is staggering. Pulse 110, and " skin a little above natural. Urine high coloured and he says it is of the na- " tural quantity, tongue clean. His bowels confined for the last three days ; " took a purgative yesterday which gave him four large stools. The chest " sounds clear on percussion, but the action of the heart is full. Breathing " more hurried than natural. Had fever yesterday evening. Was on foreign " service and had dysentery from which he recovered. Extrahat.sanguis bra- " chio ℥xx. Frictions with unguent. hydrarg. camphor. to the spine. ℞ Scillæ " pulv. gr. vj, pil. hydrarg. gr. xx. M. Divid. in pilul. æqual. vj. One morn- " ing and evening. At 2 o'clock his breathing became distressed and at 5 " P. M. he died."

The opinion of so experienced an observer who had used it freely in the earlier part of his practice, that bleeding is likely to do more harm than good if not used with the most accurate discrimination,deserves to be carefully attended to. The following observations are valuable. " The first indication " is fulfilled by reducing the pyrexial excitment and venous congestion, and " restoring the energy and general tone of the system. Where the disease " has come on suddenly, where the patient is of a strong constitution, there " has been no general bad health preceding, or where it is accompanied with " considerable pyrexia, or along with the external dropsy there is much dys- " pnœa in the horizontal posture, one or more very cautious blood-lettings " may be performed, the effect of the operation on the patient being at the " same time watched, and care being taken that it is not prosecuted, so as to " debilitate, or after any appearance of aggravation of the disease such as " increase of frequency in the pulse or of œdema from its use, has shown " itself." * * *

" Thus the compound powder of ipecacuan has with advantage been given " in the paroxysm of febrile excitement, producing a remission of the pyrexi- " al symptoms, attended with profuse perspiration. A similar effect appears " to have been produced by the use of fumigation, and most likely the pedi- " luvium and fomentations may have acted in some measure in this manner."

" The digitalis however has been that medicine, which has been chiefly " used to restrain that strong action of the heart which has been mentioned, " and thus to control in some degree the irregularities of the circulation in " beriberi." * * * " Mr. Macdonell, surgeon of the 41st regiment, again, re- " ferring to the use of mercury, remarks with respect to digitalis as follows : " during the progress of the fever it will be found that the patient is gene- " rally unable to get off his cot, in fact is in a state of paralysis, he has some " little power in moving his limbs, but they are quite unable to support the " weight of his body. Sometimes he is not able to turn himself in bed, and " at the same time the heart is found beating strongly in the chest. To com- " bat this state of irritability, I have recourse to such doses of digitalis as may " be necessary to control the heart's action. The exact quantity of course " varies, but I have given as far as forty five minims every fourth hour con- " secutively, before a decided effect was produced upon the pulse."

" When symptoms have taken place which show, that the irregularities of " the circulation have gone on to decided congestion in particular organs, and " that serous effusion is either impending or has already, in a greater or less " degree occurred, experience appears to confirm what the opinions advanc- " ed in these pages would suggest, that a stimulant plan to restore as quickly

the nervous system under which Dr. Bateman laboured, the only relief for which was afforded by powerful stimulants, (*Medico-chirurgical Transactions, vol.* IX). These are to be used with great freedom, combined with large doses of laudanum, sulphuric æther, and warm frictions, in the circumstances here stated; and I can confidently affirm in the words of Mr. Ridley, "that in many desperate cases these medicines have "suspended those alarming symptoms, and thus time "has been obtained for the employment of other me-"dicines." Purgatives have been frequently prescribed in these forms of dyspnœa, but with invariable ill effects. An instructive but ill recorded case, is quoted by Good from Dr. Dwyer's report to the London Medical Board, in which bleeding was employed to relieve extreme dyspnœa, great anxiety, and loud fluttering pulsations not to be felt by the hand applied to the side, occurring in a relapse case, never perfectly cured. The patient seemed to be relieved by the first bleeding, but its repetition caused exhaustion, and he died in half an hour. There were adhesions of the heart to the pericardium, and seven ounces of fluid in that cavity, slight effusion on the brain and

"as possible the energy of the system, and the application of means for ex-"citing the action of the extreme vessels of the surface, are more likely to "afford relief and to impede the progress of the symptoms, than a different "mode of treatment. Where the violent dyspnœa of the more advanced stage "has taken place therefore, or a patient is brought into hospital gasping for "breath, with but slight external anasarcous effusion, little time is left for "the gradual restoration of the balance of circulation, and the immediate ob-"ject is to remove the extreme pressure on the organs of respiration and "circulation. The use of the warm bath, fomentations and fumigations, as-"sisted by stimulants of a quickly diffusible nature, antispasmodics and blis-"ters, should be had recourse to, such as are recommended by Mr. Christie; "and when the urgency of the affection is somewhat relieved, these should be "gradually diminished, while the more permanent and less vigorous means, "are in like manner substituted, in order to keep up an equally diffused "state of the circulation, by restoring the energy of the whole system. In "those cases where the congestive state is more evident in the brain and spi-"nal marrow, the same principles ought to guide the treatment, but here it "is probable that narcotic remedies should be entirely avoided." *Messrs. Geddes and Macdonell.*

into the abdomen, and great intumescence of the legs. The blood was buffy, yet I am convinced that the evacuation was a most injurious measure, and that the same symptoms occurring from the same cause (water in the pericardium), have frequently been recovered from, under a different plan of treatment. Should I ever have another opportunity of seeing the disease, it would be to this part of its history that I would pay most attention; but without very extensive experience nothing of importance could be added, on a subject so very difficult and in which little assistance can be drawn from the study of allied affections, which are themselves as yet very ill understood.

Both general and local bleeding have been employed where there was much pain in the spine, and in a case in which this and swelling of the abdomen were, at first, the most prominent symptoms, v. s. was used with advantage, although cupping over the pain ful part was more efficacious. The patient, an Indo-Briton, complained February 3rd, of partial palsy and numbness of the lower extremities, tottering in his walk, œdema of legs, abdomen swollen, with obscure fluctuation, pain in the course of the spine especially of lumbar vertebræ. Pulse 92, small but sharp, skin warm, urine passed frequently in small quantity, tongue white. To be bled to ℥xvj, and to have calomel and colocynth. 4th. Great relief to all the symptoms. Blood buffy and cupped. Pulse 88 full, skin cool, feet numb and cold. To be cupped over the spine and to take jalap. 5th. Much relieved by cupping. Pain in back slight, but extends down the legs, which still pit on pressure along the tibia; stools green. 6th. No pain, numbness extends no higher than the knee, but complains of great debility and cannot walk without assistance, the right leg being most paralysed. 15th. Has improved under the use of purgatives, calomel, squills and digitalis, but there is still some œdema of the legs; the abdomen is tense with flatus, and feels hard at the lower part. March 4th. Much benefit derived from blisters to the loins and sinapisms to the feet, and from walking on the heated sand, and he now considers himself nearly free from complaint. After this he was allowed to go out convalescent, relapsed, and became the subject of closer observation through an illness of many months, during which every symptom of beriberi were in their turn exhibited. In case 10th page 114, general bleeding removed the thoracic symptoms without having any effect on the chronic disease of the spine, which was immediately relieved by leeches. *(Report, December 2d and note 46).*

Mercury. From the very great number of cases in which I have had opportunities of observing the effect of this agent, as used by Europeans and natives, I am enabled to state more confidently its effects, and consider it unnecessary to enter into lengthened details, in support of inferences derived from multiplied and uniform experience. It has already been pointed out, that mercury in large doses to the extent of affecting the mouth, has in a few cases appeared to aid bleeding or other antiphlogistic measures, in subduing inflammation of the membranes, and that in some rare cases, the effect has been a rapid and perfect cure. But such a result is not to be looked for once in fifty cases, and it may be stated as a general fact, that mercury exerts no directly salutary influence over the nervous symptoms, nor prevents the accession or return of the visceral affections. Beriberi has made its first attack on men under the influence of mercury, administered for the cure of other complaints, and the paralytic affections have been remarkably aggravated by the medicine, when it seemed to assist in the cure of other symptoms. All debilitating causes render men more liable to the disease, especially to relapses, but from none has this been so frequently and clearly traced, as to the constitutional effects of mer cury. In my early practice I used it freely, though cautiously, but after some time the dangers to which it led attracted my attention, and every additional case the records of which I have had an opportunity of consulting, has more and more forcibly impressed the conclusion on my mind. I admitted it with reluctance, being at variance with my previous notions, and I therefore hope that my opinion may in some degree counteract the unsupported advice of Mr. Hamilton and others, to saturate the system with calomel in scrúple doses. I have seen the practice frequently adopted, and Dr. Wight has mentioned six cases in which it was employed, but although he speaks favourably of it, they, as well as others, lead to an opposite conclusion. Mr. Stevenson has seen gangrene of the mouth destroy the patient, without the least effect on the original disease; and on examining the case, I find it was one of no severity, and that the calomel was administered in ten grain doses every night till the mouth was affected. I have also seen several patients destroyed by violent ptyalism, produced by mercury prescribed by the lower class of native doctors. It is a common practice of the sepoys, especially when the disease is tedious, to take mercury, which I have never known to do them good, and I have received patients, who had been rapidly improving a little before, with greatly swelled mouths, profuse salivation, complete paraplegia, general anasarca and ascites, rapid feeble pulse,and debility under which they sank in a few days. The ill effects in one instance might be partly accounted for, by the imperfect composition of the preparation employed, but in none of the others. The superior class of native practitioners do not appear to use it, in beriberi: a respectable man of great experience to whom I owe some information, assured me that he never did; and several men (Europeans and natives) treated successfully by a celebrated Hukeemin the Masulipatam zillah, were convinced that no mercurial preparation was used in their cure. As in the form of dropsy described by Dr. Bright, the mouth is also for the most part easily and violently affected by mercurials, except inflammatory excitement is present. This view probably suggested itself to the reader of the preceding cases, but the two following, having other points of interest, may be inserted here.

Case 41st. 28th October, Omegadoo, ætat. 45, of sickly appearance. Face and body full and bloated, feet œdematous,numbness and loss of power of motion of the legs ; has exacerbations of fever in the evenings, urine scanty, bowels slow, tongue foul. Habeat calomel.gr.x ter die. Emplast.vesicator.sterno. 29th. Stools scanty, dark and fetid. Habeat calomel. gr. x, pulv. jalap. comp. ʒss. M. statim sumend. Calomel. gr. x h. s. 30th. Dejections still morbid,gums sore, œdema abates, loss of power of motion worse. Ol. croton. gtt. ij. 31st. All the symptoms worse, stools black, watery, and fetid,mouth sore. ℞ Calomel. gr. ij, pulv. scillæ gr. iij. Fiat pilula bis die sumend. November 2d. Mouth very sore since yesterday, is evidently sinking, pulse very irregular, dyspnœa, voice scarcely perceptible. Expired at midnight.

The viscera of the abdomen were found healthy; the pericardium completely distended with fluid, and a good deal of effusion into the cavities of the pleura.

Case 42nd. Pędma Naick, admitted September 2d. Sense of heaviness and oppression all over the body, especially of the chest: urine at first scanty and red, now light coloured. Pulse 130, full. Has been ill twenty days and used purges, calomel, digitalis, &c. Cont. tinct. digital. et potass. supertart. V. S. ad ℥xvj. 3d. Blood not buffy, some relief, pulse 120, full. 5th. Better, less heaviness, pulse 120, rather hard, would not allow himself to be bled, skin rather hot. 10th. Limbs scarcely support him, pulse 120, hard, tried to bleed him but got only 4 oz., totters in his walk and there is some rigidity of the limbs, gums sore. 14th. Mouth very sore, rigidity increased, takes jalap, æther, nitre, &c. 26th. Very weak, face and body much swelled, great dyspnœa which got more urgent and pulse very feeble, till the 28th when he died.

It has already been noticed, that the neuralgic pains resembling rheumatism affecting the muscles in beriberi, were not in the least relieved by the mercurial treatment, which is generally rapidly successful in the common rheumatism prevailing at the time, and even in rheumatic pains in the joints with which those of beriberi were combined; which is a strong proof that the nervous disorder is not under the influence of mercurial action. The spasmodic dyspnœa has in several instances come on the day after salivation and has proved fatal, which may in a few instances be ascribed to the known effects of mercury, on some constitutions, in causing irregular actions of the heart and blood vessels: an opinion rendered more probable by the fact, that in the best marked of these cases, the system was difficult to affect with mercury, which was taken in considerable quantity, the gums suffering much, but ptyalism could not be produced. Emaciation has been increased by the internal use of mercury; and fumigations of the lower extremities which I employed in a few instances, were suspected of having the same effect. Frictions with camphorated mercurial ointment have been a good deal employed, but I have seen no reason to believe, that they were equally effectual as other liniments of greater stimulating powers, and from the risk of constitutional affection, and the paralytic symptoms which have been induced by mercurial fumes, there is reason to believe that the free use of them may have done harm. As a purgative combined with jalap, calomel has been very useful in a great many cases, and as might have been expected, this is best marked when the biliary secretions are disordered, the eyes tinged yellow, and the abdomen tumid; but it has been remarkable, that the secretion of disordered bile and the yellow eye, have frequently continued after salivation until the death of the patient, and in some instances in which this was observed, ptyalism and diuretics had failed to restore the urinary secretion to a natural standard.[125]

[125] On a question of so great practical importance, I have much satisfaction in finding that observations similar to those in the text, have been made by other practitioners in the circars. So much attention is paid to the observation and record of hospital practice, that it can seldom happen, that the real effects of powerful medicines can continue to be mistaken, by those who have had sufficient experience to enable them to judge for themselves. The gentlemen whose opinions are given in the following extract, used mercury freely in their early practice.

" The experience of others does not confirm that of Dr. Wight or Mr. Ha-
" milton, respecting the value of mercury in this disease. The report quoted
" in a subsequent note shows, that it was tried at Ellore in 1822, (and many
" other cases of the same kind could be quoted), but profuse salivation took
" place without having any effect either on the paralysis or frequency of the
" pulse, and the patient died. Mr. Macdonell practising at Rajahmundry made
" use of mercury to affect the system, purgatives, diuretics, bleeding, blisters
" to the spine, and mercurial frictions, as in the subjoined case, but his pati-

Purgatives are often of essential service in beriberi, and the compound powder of jalap has been, almost universally, acknowledged to be the best. One or two doses frequently remove the œdema of the

" ents died, and he observed that the cases at Samulcottah were not more " fortunate. Mr. Price again, of the zillah of Chicacole, not only considered " mercury useless, but even prejudicial. He states in a report to the Medical " Board, alluding to beriberi, that ' as for a course of squills and calomel it " ' was not of the least benefit, even in mild cases, and the slightest approxi- " ' mation to ptyalism extremely aggravated the disease.' In short the failure " of the mercurial plan,led the medical officers in their helplessness, to enquire " into the native practice. * * * If to these observations we add,that although " mercury may occasionally check the progress of the symptoms, it can have " no effect in strengthening the constitution, or in preventing relapses, but on " the contrary that the tedious convalescence of the patient will, in many " cases, lapse again into a dropsical condition, enough will have been said, it " is hoped, to show that the use of mercury, generally, in beriberi is at least " of very doubtful propriety, and the greatest caution must be observed in " its exhibition."

" Shaik Chand, sepoy, 22d regiment N. I., ætat. 26. Admitted 22d De- " cember, 1827, into the Rajahmundry hospital. Says that last night he was " well, and that he attended drill. At 8 P. M. was attacked with fever which " subsided in the course of the night, this was followed by general pains par- " ticularly in the legs and arms, from his knees downwards there is consider- " able numbness but it diminishes towards the body, he is unable to move his " toes or to support his weight on his knees; is unable to grasp and the mo- " tions of his fingers are impaired. Pulse 120, soft; urine high coloured, " chest free. ℞ Pulv. jalap. gr. xv; calomel. gr. iv. M. statim sumend. Vesp. " Well purged during the day, no return of heat of skin, otherwise the " same. ℞ Calomel. ℈j, opii gr. ij. M. Fiat bolus statim. Apply thirty-six " leeches to his spine, half to his loins and half to the back of his neck. 23rd. " No fever, bowels moved three times, leeches bled freely, limbs much the " same, desponds much. ℞ Tinct. digitalis gtt. x, vin. antimon. ʒj, ex aqua. " To be taken every second hour. A blister to the loins. On the 24th the numb- " ness is a little better, and he can grasp more firmly than he did yesterday. " Pulse 120, soft, and easily compressed, urine of the natural colour, 17 " ounces in the night. One large stool, gums touched, blister rose well, de- " sponds. Cont. 25th. The numbness and pain less felt to-day and the power " of motion increased, mouth affected. Pulse 120 small and soft, skin soft " but above the natural temperature, one large stool in the night. Omit " the calomel. Cont. haust. On the 26th his mouth was more affected, had " some sleep, otherwise the same. ℞ Haust. salin. ℥iij, tinct. digital. gtt. xv, " vin. antimon. ʒj, to be taken every third hour. Frictions to his limbs with " camphor oil. 27th. The numbness and pain in his limbs is much relieved; he " says that he has no strength to assist himself. Pulse 120, mouth so affected " as to be kept from sleeping by it. Cont. medicament. The blister to be kept " open. 28th. Considerable ptyalism, pulse more full, otherwise the same. " Cont. medicament. A gargle for his mouth. On the 29th complained much " of the pain of the blistered surface. Pulse soft, as above, no stool, has " the power of moving his limbs freely, but the pain and numbness still re- " main although much diminished. Cont. medicament. Blistered surface to " be dressed simply. 30th. Yesterday evening he vomited twice some mucus, " and this morning he also vomited his food, had bilious scanty stools to-day, " his breathing slightly affected, and his pulse 100 at the wrist and weak " while his heart is beating strongly in the chest, a total failure of appetite, " took a gentle purgative this morning. Omitt. digitalis. Cont. haust. 3 P. M. " Breathing more affected, pulse at the wrist gone, extremities cold. 5 P. M. " died." *Messrs. Geddes and Macdonell.*

lower extremities, sometimes increasing the urine at the same time, but without benefit to the other symptoms; thus affording a clear proof, that the dropsical effusion is not the primary disease, nor even in all instances, a symptom of great importance.

The œdema thus removed, is very apt to return in the palsied parts, and if the urine is nearly suppressed or if the nervous symptoms are increasing, will be little affected by purgatives or mercurials, until the palsy is removed. The œdema of the face, shoulders, and arms are not much influenced except in a few cases, in which the pectoral symptoms on which they depend, are relieved by the purging. There are a few examples in which the rigidity of the limbs and other affections of the nerves, have been relieved by purgatives alone, or combined with a full dose of calomel, and in slight cases, perfect recoveries have been thus effected.[126] Four patients were cured by elate-

Mr. Colhoun Stirling in a letter to Mr. Christie (*Hunter op. cit. p.* 104), has the following important observation, which, it is much to be regretted, has been overlooked by the systematic writers, who have without exception recommended the practice pursued by the latter. "It is very unfortunate, "that the sepoys have invincible prejudices against the remedies generally "used in this disease by Europeans, and in consequence seldom report them- "selves sick while at all able to perform their duty; trusting to the promises "of cure which are always confidently made by their native doctors, who "certainly succeed in reducing the œdematous swellings very quickly, by "means of drastic purgatives. Perhaps it is in some measure owing to the "great debility thus induced, that I have not found the use of calomel so "effectual a remedy as it appears to have proved at Trincomalie. *Almost all* "*who have died*, at least the greater part, *had their mouths affected by it*, "and an idea prevails amongst them, that a sore mouth is frequently the "immediate forerunner of death."

The examination of the detailed cases in that work, will lead to the same conclusion regarding the effect of salivation on European soldiers ill of beriberi, however usefully mercurials may be employed in combination with diuretics. Mr. Hamilton salivates by scruple doses of calomel with laudanum every hour and a half or every two or three hours, and uses at the same time mercurial fumigations and frictions; and because mercury takes off determination from particular parts and is a diuretic and diaphoretic, has very little doubt of saving his patient. (*Edinburgh Medico-chirurgical Transactions, vol.* 2, *p.* 23 *and* 24.) Had he had an opportunity of treating a few more cases (he refers to three only), he would most probably have acted and expressed himself with more caution.

[126] Though the kindness of medical friends, I have lately had an opportunity of perusing the journals of practice of the hospitals of several corps, in

rium, in a station where beriberi seldom occurs; and examples are now and then met with, (most frequently when the paralytic symptoms are very slight), in which free purging by croton and other medicines, enable the constitution to throw off the disease.[127] It is necessary to repeat the important observation, that purgatives are injurious, in the species of dyspnœa described as requiring stimulants, and that the irritation and exhaustion they occasion, have appeared to bring on the symptoms described at page 257. As a general rule, I would only use mild and warm laxatives in advanced cases; rhubarb answers very well, and is also an important adjunct to a remedy hereafter to be described. Gamboge so much used by Mr. Ridley, does not appear to possess any advantage over more certain and less drastic purges, and has

which beriberi had prevailed, which afford abundant evidence of the efficacy of purgatives in removing the milder forms of the disease.

The following extract gives the result of Messrs. Geddes and Macdonell's experience. "Some of the remarks made with respect to blood-letting and "the exhibition of mercury, appear applicable to the subject of purgatives. "Some mild cases may be cured by them in conjunction with rest and other "circumstances, attendant upon removal to hospital. But where immediate "benefit does not follow their exhibition, their frequent use, (and the same "may be said of emetics), will tend to debilitate the patient, while the re-"moval of the disease is as distant as ever."

To the same effect Dr. Herklots remarks, that "in very slight cases I "have found the use of calomel and colocynth together with external stimu-"lating frictions to answer every purpose." He however is averse to much purgation, and states, that being ignorant of the prevalence of beriberi at Chicacole he considered the first cases he met with to be anasarca, and treated them accordingly, by cooling remedies such as saline purgatives, cooling diuretics, cream of tartar, lemonade for ordinary drink, &c. but he soon found that he was doing mischief; and adds that if a dose of salts is prescribed to a patient complaining of anasarcous swellings of his limbs, costive bowels, and somewhat scanty urine, he would expect to find his patient next day "to "have had stools copious and watery enough, but unfortunately the poor fel-"low will be found to have totally lost the use of his limbs, which are per-"fectly benumbed, and he will complain of not having had a wink of sleep "all night, in consequence of the severity of the pain and spasmodic contrac-"tions of muscles of his limbs, which will have come on since he took the "salts." I do not concur in this opinion, as here stated; Mr. Dick, however, is also averse to the use of saline purges.

[127] Croton has been much employed by some gentlemen. The tincture in whatever form administered, often excites distressing vomiting, and the oil given in pill is not altogether safe, if there is any intestinal inflammation. It has caused severe pain while operating, and left increased tenderness to pressure. *Original note.*

appeared to excite inflammatory action in the stomach and intestines. Oil of turpentine may probably be used with advantage, as it exerts antispasmodic powers, but the cases in which it has been used as a purgative, do not warrant any opinion. As an internal stimulant it has perhaps done some good, in small doses combined with æther; but it has appeared to have done harm in some other cases, and notwithstanding the recent opinion of Dr. Elliotson, I would dread its irritating effects on the urinary organs.[128] When the stomach is irritable, purgative injections are useful, to which æther, &c. may be added as recommended by Ridley, should the symptoms indicate them. When the disease is confirmed and the phosphatic diathesis formed, the disordered secretions of the bowels are best removed by mild medicine. When the costiveness arises from want of muscular power, laxatives are constantly required to keep the stools soft and prevent the accumulation of hard lumps in the large intestine, which injections cannot do, the collection taking place in the right colon.

Diuretics. From the intimate connection that appears to exist, between the deficient and altered urinary secretion and some of the most formidable symptoms, the indication of restoring it to its natural state is evident. The remark of Dr. Christison, that the urine when increased in quantity by diuretics, contains the same *proportion* of urea as before, and that the separation of that excretion is therefore increased in proportion to the additional quantity of urine

[128] Dr. Elliotson does not believe that turpentine irritates the urinary passages, because he has seen large doses retained, without this effect following. During a scarcity of copaiba, I treated many gonorrhœa cases with twenty drops of ol. terebinth. twice a day, and was in most cases obliged to intermit it, from the irritation (frequently amounting to bloody urine) caused by it. *Original note.*

passed, will probably be found to be true, in general, in beriberi; but I have had no opportunity of examining the subject with care, and the healthy state of the fluid has been frequently brought about by the same means which increased its quantity. Be this as it may, the use of diuretics is of essential importance to the removal of the œdema, and especially to prevent the extension of the anasarca upwards, and the effusion of fluid into the internal parts, particularly the cells of the lungs. To this their usefulness is limited, and we shall find that their effect is greatest when the spinal symptoms are slight, that these are not benefited by the removal of the effused fluids, and that the effect of diuretics is diminished or altogether prevented, by the dependance of the anasarca on the state of the nerves. It has already been observed, that bleeding and mercurial action have increased the flow of urine and changed its sensible qualities, and the same observation applies to purgatives, more particularly the compound powder of jalap; and that these were the means by which the change was brought about, was evident, from the return of the morbid state notwithstanding various diuretics were prescribed or continued. But this effect is not very common, except when there is inflammation of the internal parts, and is of too little permanency and importance, to justify their employment with a view to it alone. Mercury has been very much employed in combination with squills, and its diuretic virtues in this combination are very decided, without its being used so as to affect the mouth; which should not be done, unless with the greatest caution and in a few severe and obstinate cases: the small quantity of calomel which will affect the gums in this disease, therefore, renders it of importance to give it in small quantity, that it may be continued as long as the squills, &c. may be required. I was in the habit of prescribing about two grains three times a day, until I had the advantage of the advice of the late Mr. T. Owen,* who remarked in looking over some of my cases, when inspecting my hospital at Chicacole, that this was too large a quantity. His extensive experience in beri-beri, both in Ceylon and the circars, entitled his opinion to respect, and in my future practice I found it of great advantage. The blue pill, well rubbed up, or calomel to the extent of half a grain or one grain, may be prescribed along with squills with safety, and perhaps as much certainty of increasing the urine, as in most other hydropic affections. The employment of large doses of mercury as the primary means of cure, is inconsistent with this line of practice; and the repetition of two grains every fourth hour, as recommended by Mr. Ridley, can only be useful, in as far as general mercurial action may be considered as a cure for the disease, independent of its diuretic effects, or as salivation may be believed to increase the flow of urine. Three grains of blue pill three times a day, is the smallest quantity which has been found of use. If the powder of squills has lost its virtue, the tincture is to be preferred, but I have not found it more effectual, and have not often used it except for the convenience of combination with tincture of digitalis. Digitalis has been much used in the form of tincture, the only one in which its virtues are well preserved in India; and has been very useful as a diuretic, given pretty freely and with the usual res-

* First member of the Medical Board, and at the time referred to, superintending surgeon in the northern division.

trictions, at the same time that calomel and squills are taken. It may be advantageously combined with nitrous æther, and if there is much spasmodic action and dyspnœa, with large doses of laudanum, sulphuric æther, ammonia, &c. It has appeared to be more effectual in removing the œdema of the face than other means, which is probably to be referred to the moderation of the heart's action and lowering of the pulse, which frequently follows its exhibition. It has been of benefit when there was burning sensation in the chest, and of little use when the pulse was regular. I must not, however, fail to state, that this connection of lowered action of the heart and the removal of œdema of the face, has not been proved by a sufficient number of cases; and the same remark applies to another opinion, also probable enough, both from the general history of the drug and the experience I have had of it in this disease, viz. that its powers are greatest when some excitement exists, and as an auxiliary to, or substitute for more direct antiphlogistic treatment. Its power over the arterial system has been evident, but it is very difficult to find positive proof of the other connections, when the symptoms are complicated and several other medicines are used at the same time. Nitrous æther from its stimulating powers, and the advantage of variety in so uncertain a class of remedies, has often been used with some, though uncertain, advantage, and when there was heat in the chest and other symptoms of excitement, it has increased the urine without other benefit. Nitre has been employed in various combinations, but although not without efficacy, it did not appear to be possessed of any peculiar virtues.

But of all diuretics, none is so generally successful and universally useful, as cream of tartar, which has been very generally adopted by experienced practitioners (from evidence of its powers) in beriberi, and in ignorance of the remarks of others.[129] Thus, Mr. Ridley in Ceylon and myself and others in the circars, can bear testimony to the virtues ascribed to it. Its laxative effect, grateful taste, and consequent soothing qualities are powerful recommendations, in addition to the direct benefit from its diuretic powers. The thirst is often urgent, especially when the œdema is increasing, and the medicine can be given with much fluid, by which its effect is increased. I have not used it with punch as recommended by Mr. Ridley, and prefer prescribing gin by itself, in punch or otherwise diluted, as it is necessary to give a large quantity of the supertartrate; while gin or other stimulants are often inadmissible, and always to be used with cautious reference to existing symptoms. It appeared to me remarkable, that in some cases which lately occurred, in which the urine was examined and found to be highly acid, that this acid salt was particularly beneficial. The practical fact was certain, and a theoretical difficulty on a subject so little understood, did not deter me from continuing its use. An analogous observation was found in Scudamore's work on gout, in which he states that he found the acid qualities of the urine in that disease, counteracted by effervescing draughts of carbonate of soda and lime juice; which confirmed the propriety of the practice, although affording no explanation. In the Medico-chirurgical Review No. 14, 1827, which I met with a

[129] It deserves to be mentioned, that in that disease of the urinary organs noticed as in many circumstances analogous to this, Drs. Gregory and Bright have found cream of tartar the most effectual diuretic. I have, however, found the stomach unable to retain it, when not otherwise irritable. *Original note.*

few weeks ago, there is an account of a series of experiments on the urine, by Whoeler, one of which explains the fact, as far as chemistry can account for any phenomenon in the living body. He found that both the supertartrate of potass and the acetate, passed off by the urine in the state of carbonate, the vegetable acid being decomposed.[130]

The acetate of potassa has been used in a few cases, and was probably useful. In this place, two plants employed by the poorer classes for the cure of beriberi, may be noticed. I observed several persons pulling the leaves of two trees near my house, and found they were affected with beriberi, for which they used them. The one most usually employed is the " dursan-chettoo" or " dursunah" of the Telingees, in Duccanee called " soorinj", the " Mimosa sirisha." Two table spoonfuls of the juice of the leaves made into a paste with flour, are taken morning and evening, the patient abstaining from fish and acid food. It generally purges twice. The two cases I had an opportunity of observing treated with it, did not derive much benefit, although they were not severe, and were afterwards cured by the treeak farook. I am informed that it is also used in dropsy, and the celebrated Decandolle states, that the allied plants contain an extractive matter united with acetate of potassa, and possess a bitter, and often a laxative quality. The sirisha has the latter qualities, and I hope to detect the acetate, which would account for its virtues. The second was also a mimosa, called in Teloogoo, " sikeserum-chettoo," and in Tamul " wynarum chēēru," and was used in the same way.[131] The man I saw, used it

[130] I should have been aware, that Sir Gilbert Blane first pointed out, that salts containing a vegetable acid render the urine alkaline.

[131] Dr. Wight informs me, that the sirisha is more properly an acacia, and that the sikeserum-chettoo is the Acacia frondosa.

without benefit, and I had no opportunity of trying the effect of other remedies.[132] One gentleman used decoction of spogel seeds, but, as might be expected, without benefit.

By means of these remedies, the dropsical effusions are very often rapidly removed, and even that into the pericardium appears to be quickly absorbed, affording an example of a nearly general fact, that dropsies in India, as they are usually the result of less chronic and permanent disease, are much more easily cured than hydropic diseases in Europe.[133] But although an important indication is thus fulfilled, and the system freed from an oppressive and dangerous load, and is frequently enabled to throw off the disease altogether, it is unfortunately very common, for the nervous disorder to continue unalleviated, and too often ultimately destroys the patient, by inducing relapses of the previous symptoms, œdematous or spasmodic dyspnœa, or death by syncope; or he is gradually crippled and dies exhausted. The œdema of the extremities is sometimes removed, while the dropsy of the cavities remains or supervenes, of which instructive examples have been mentioned above; and the reverse of this also frequently happens. It is also true, that dropsy and every symptom of beriberi may be removed without the urine being increased, and in a few instances, it has even been diminished after the apparent cure of the disease. If the paralytic symptoms are slight in comparison to the anasarca, the benefit from diuretics is often permanent, and in other

[132] A case in which it was used without benefit, is recorded in a subsequent page.

[133] See Heberden's chapter on dropsies, where they are stated to be almost always fatal. In one author, dropsy of the pericardium is said to be "of course fatal." *Original note.*

cases the tendency to renewal of serous effusion is lost; although there is no period, even when the phosphatic diathesis is confirmed, in which the urine may not become scanty, the dropsy return, and diuretics be indicated. A most important connection has been occasionally observed, between a diminished and morbid secretion of urine and the inflammatory and dropsical affections of the chest, and when the kidneys can be got to act, the life of the patient will be often saved; although too many instances occur in which they run on to a fatal termination, notwithstanding a copious diuresis; or return, or attack for the first time, while the use and effect of digitalis, cream of tartar, calomel and squills, which have removed the anasarca, are still continued. The dropsy of the cellular substance will also rapidly increase, and ascend from the extremities to the chest, notwithstanding that the flow of urine is abundant, as in the case of the sergeant noticed at page 251; and in the following case, in which the nerves became more severely affected, as the kidneys were excited to increased secretion, the anasarca augmented at the same time.

Case 43rd. September 6th. Nursiah, a fat sepoy, ætat. 49. Admitted with intumescence of the feet and legs. Took a brisk purgative yesterday, which operated well. To take cream of tartar and tincture of squills,and blue pill at bed time. 7th. The œdema has increased in the feet and extended higher up the legs, and has attacked the hands. 8th. No better, had two or three stools, secretion of urine is increased. Cont. potass. supertartrat. et pilul. Omitt. tinct. scillæ, et capt. ter die tinct. digital. ℥ss. 9th. The œdema has much increased, and locomotion is impeded in consequence of numbness and rigidity in his lower limbs;

has had two or three stools, pulse nearly natural, his respiration seems slightly affected. Omitt. potass. supertart. et cont. tinct. digital. cum tinct. scillæ ℨss. Cont. pilul. 10th. Is much worse; locomotion is entirely impeded and the œdema is increased. Habt. stat. ol. terebinth. ℥j. Cont. haust. et pilul. 11th. Is worse; had several stools and made a considerable quantity of urine, the œdema is nearly the same as yesterday. Rept. ol. terebinth. ℥j. Omitt. pilul. h. s. 12th. Is worse; complains of a spasmodic rigidity shooting up to the chest and impeding his respiration. Complains also of an increased internal heat in the chest; the œdema of the feet and legs is increased, and the skin is very tense. Three stools. Rept. ol. terebinth. ℥j. Cont. haust. h. s. 13th. Is worse; œdema increased, took last night pulv. ipecac. comp. gr. x. Habeat ter die ol. terebinth. ℨss. Cont. pulv. h. s. 16th. Is much worse; the œdematous intumescence is become general all over the body, and the spasmodic rigidity is so much increased as to obstruct entirely the voice, and nearly the respiration. Pulse 70 and very feeble. Cont. haust. 17th. He continued in an insensible state until 12 o'clock last night, when he died.

The following case is analogous, in the death being independent of the dropsy which was almost removed, and could not endanger the life of the patient. It was mistaken for intermittent fever and anasarca, and was consequently ill treated.

Case 44th. Shaik Budday, ætat. 42. Admitted 4th January, 1826, complaining of quotidian fever and ague, coming on at night. General œdema of body and face, foul tongue, urine high coloured, pulse nearly natural. Has purgatives, and is salivated by pills of calomel and squills. On the 7th, numbness of the feet is noticed; œdema is rather diminished. 14th. Œdema gone, numbness no better. Pills omitted. 28th. Œdema returned to the face and feet; mouth still sore. February 8th. Less numbness, and swelling has nearly disappeared. 9th. Was seized last night with spasms of all the body, dyspnœa, cold sweats, tongue dry, thirst, articulation difficult, eyes sunk, pulse very feeble, loose yellow stools, and he died at 4 A. M.

But not only are diuretics often unsuccessful when they do act on the kidneys, but it is unfortunately true, that in bad cases most requiring them and to which they are best adapted, they often fail; an observation made by Mr. Ridley, and fully confirmed by my experience: and this appears to be dependent, rather on something peculiar to the disease, than on the usual uncertain effects of this class of remedies. The painful conclusion from all these observations is, that there are no remedies of a general nature, on which we can place more than a very limited or uncertain confidence, in the treatment of beriberi. To this result all practitioners of experience have at length been reduced, when like myself they have found their early success reduced by relapses, and their utmost efforts end in the death or bed-ridden state of a very large proportion of their patients. So deeply was this impressed on some of my acquaintances, that they viewed the disease with greater dread than cholera itself.[134]

There are however many other remedies, of use in

[134] The end of 1819 and beginning of 1820, a number of cases of beriberi, (most of them in a state of ptyalism) were sent into the garrison hospital of Berhampore, from a field detachment at Itchapoor. On being received there, they were treated with tincture of cantharides and squills, which acted powerfully as a diuretic. The doses used were from 20 to 40 drops of the tincture and from 2 to 5 grains of squills, as often, in severe cases, as once in two hours. Frictions with turpentine were useful. A dose of laudanum was occasionally allowed. Much of the success was ascribed, to the change of

various circumstances of beriberi, which must not be neglected. Some need not be specified, as their application is influenced by nothing peculiar, and others will only be alluded to, to mention their want of efficacy.

Stimulants, &c. In all paroxysms of dyspnœa coming on suddenly, especially when they are of a spasmodic character, and attended with feeble pulse and cold extremities, large doses of laudanum as recommended by Mr. Ridley, in combination with æther, spirits, aromatic spirits of ammonia, &c. as circumstances may indicate, are to be diligently employed. The extremities and body are to be rubbed with stimulating liniments, which of themselves have been found sufficient to restore the heat; and of these, turpentine, ammonia, and especially cajuput oil, have been the most effectual. In two examples they were continued for a whole night, and with unhoped for success. Gin, from its diuretic effects, is certaintly the best spirit, and should be given largely diluted. As far

weather from cold and damp to dry and temperate. Mr. Towell was of opinion that the mercury previously taken assisted in the cure, but from two of the detailed cases it appeared to have been injurious.

Bavah Sahib, 1st battn. of the 9th regt. N. I. received December 21st, emaciated, weak, and limbs powerless. Face bloated and watery, abdomen swelled and hard, feet œdematous. Bowels costive. There was some affection of his chest. The urine was increased by tincture of cantharides and squills, but the ptyalism continued, with frequent sudden aggravations of the disease, and he sunk exhausted by dysenteric purging, notwithstanding the removal of the dropsy.

Nursoo, admitted 8th January with swellings of the limbs, face, chest, arms, and of the scrotum. His limbs benumbed. Severe ptyalism and great debility. No uneasiness in chest. The diuretics acted well. (The skin over the sternum pitted half an inch.) He was relieved of the dropsy by the diuretics and gradually recovered. The convalescence was very tedious in all these cases, apparently from the obstinacy of the paralytic symptoms. It is in examples of extreme distension of the cellular substance of the trunk with fluid, that Mr. Dick found scarifications of the integuments of the chest useful. He says that scarifications of the legs are unsafe. Messrs. Geddes and Macdonell state, that "the removal of the dropsical symptoms has in a few "instances been tried by scarification; but the result has not been such as to "recommend a repetition of the practice." They are of opinion, that the operation of tapping the pericardium should not be attempted, except the patient is already in articulo mortis.

as my experience goes, the vomiting has not been relieved by tincture of opium, and the frequent dependence of this symptom on inflammation of the stomach, suggests the propriety of caution in its use; although I have had too little experience in the treatment of this symptom, to be entitled to object to the practice of Mr. Ridley, who states that it will often moderate the vomiting. In combination with sulphuric æther, it has removed distressing attacks of hiccup. After bleeding or other evacuations, when there is cough, or general symptoms of irritation, and mobility of habit, a large dose of laudanum will be safe and useful. When the œdema has spread upwards and involved the lung, and the patient cannot remain for any time in the horizontal posture, this treatment has been of little use; nor are we, in these circumstances, entitled to expect more than occasional success, and we must even then, for the most part, expect the patient to relapse and probably die. Many other observations might be made, but they are either not of a sufficiently general character, or too obvious to require to be mentioned here.

Many cases of beriberi from the commencement, and all chronic ones in their progress, are attended with low action and debility, and it has therefore been very useful to prescribe stimulants; nor is there any reason to doubt of their being frequently of use, although it is generally difficult to say to what extent, or in what manner they act. As they are necessarily continued for a long time, and a tendency to general or local excitement is always present, their effects are to be cautiously watched, and they should be omitted, whenever symptoms requiring antiphlogistic treatment present themselves; and as these are often obscure, stimulants should not be ordered on vague views of the nature of the complaint, or merely from anxiety to do something. This caution is to be more particularly attended to, when the chest is in any way affected, the heart's action excited, irregular, or frequent, when there is a sense of internal heat, tenderness at epigastrium, or vomiting, *or when any of these have been recently removed.* The most effectual is a moderate allowance of spirits at dinner time, which is very generally required by old European soldiers, who cannot be altogether deprived of their usual stimulus without injury, except when labouring under acute disease. The aromatic spirit of ammonia, and ginger in doses of one or two scruples answer well in natives, and have frequently been of great use; sometimes appearing to have tended materially to a favourable termination.[135] A friend who kindly communicated a number of his cases to me, was partial to the use of mustard seeds, which he gave to the extent of one or two drachms several times a day, but I did not perceive that they were of much advantage. The horse radish is stated by writers on materia medica, to be one of the most valuable of medical stimulants, of which the list is indeed somewhat poor. The root of the Moringa tree (Hyperanthera moringa) has been used as a substitute, possessing all its qualities, and has diffused a warmth over the abdomen, appear-

[135] The following preparations used by the Mussulmaun Hukeems, were found useful by Dr. Herklots.

1. " Urg filfiline" or Tinctur. Piper.long.comp.

℞ Piper. long. ℥iv, piper. nigr., rad.amom. zingiber., āā, ℥ss, arracci ℥xx. Digest for 7 days and strain. Dose ʒj two or three times a day. It occasionally produces excitement, heat of skin, and restlessness.

2. The second called the " Sont ka mooruba" is a " composition of dried ginger, black pepper, lesser cardamom seeds, cubebs, cinnamon, saffron and honey."

Dr. H. states, that guaiacum and the compound tincture of pepper together with stimulating frictions, have removed the symptoms in some rare instances; but that the disease, in general, requires far more active means.

ed to encourage a warm perspiration, and in the flatulent distension of the abdomen in confirmed cases, was a grateful tonic. I did not observe any laxative effect, and there was but little increase of the urine during its use, although it is not unlikely that it may possess both, as stated by Decandolle. Very offensive eructations, the smell of which was compared by the patient to that of the evacuations of a man dying of bowel complaint, were caused by it, probably from the extrication of some compound of sulphur, which has lately been detected in several plants of allied sensible qualities.

Cajaput oil is stated by several writers to be useful in dropsy and palsy, by its stimulating and diaphoretic powers. It was used internally a good deal by one gentleman, but its effects were not very evident. As an external application it is very useful, and from the singular effect on the nerves of the eye when rubbed on the temple, by which its qualities are tested in the countries where it is procured, it would appear to have peculiar powers of stimulating the nerves of distant parts.

Camphor, assafœtida, Dover's powder, mezereon and gum guaiac have been occasionally employed, but, as far as I know, without benefit, although probably adapted to some cases.[136] The aromatic tincture of guaiac was used in some cases of severe pains, but without advantage; and the China root (Smilax china) a popular remedy for chronic rheumatism and secondary venereal complaints, has not been of more

[136] Mr. Davidson has found the aromatic tincture of guaiac a useful stimulant and diaphoretic, when administered with mucilage. When given in draughts it was decomposed, and proved comparatively inert. The result of my experience with Dover's powder is given in the text, but I have since perused cases, in which its sedative and sudorific effects were beneficial. Mr. D. also employed the vapour bath with advantage.

advantage, in the hands of two of my acquaintances. Iron has been used in a good many cases, and is, as far as I have been able to judge, beneficial, principally as a general tonic. I fear the opinion of Mr. Ridley, that the tincture of muriate of iron is a powerful antispasmodic in the *acute* form of the malady, will be found to be incorrect, as indeed his own cases nearly prove; but its powerful tonic qualities have been beneficial in general debility, and in various abdominal affections arising in the course of chronic cases. There is no reason to doubt, that iron will act in some degree as an antispasmodic and assist the cure of the dropsical symptoms, but we are not to content ourselves, even in the early stages of the mildest case of beriberi, by prescribing carbonate of iron, &c. as I have known the urine become nearly suppressed in a few hours, the œdema extend upward, and the patient die from effusion into the lungs, while using it. The tincture of the muriate is useful in the irritable state of the bladder, when it has become diseased in the latter stages, and is alternately unable to expel the urine or to retain it for any time. That iron is beneficial in beriberi, is confirmed by its being one of the approved remedies of the Teloogoo practitioners, although not believed to possess virtues equal to the treeak farook and oleum nigrum. The preparation is formed in the following manner: a seer and a quarter of steel, or, if these cannot be got, iron filings are mixed with oil, and after two days are rubbed between two stones; the mass is then placed in a new earthen pot to the mouth of which another is luted, and is burned for a day, in a shallow pit filled with ignited cow-dung. When one hundred cakes of the fuel are consumed, this part of the process is completed.

The powder is then rubbed with the astringent juice of the bark of the jamun tree, of the mango and numerous others, and is then a black powder fit for use.[137] I have not ascertained the composition of the preparation thus formed, but it is probably an oxide united with gallic acid, and will possess those powers in disease depending "on leucophlegmatic habits of body as palsy," ascribed by Dr. A. T. Thomson to iron.

Bark has no power over the proper symptoms of beriberi, but is sometimes useful in those cases in which intermittent fever is combined with them, and also when the irritative evening paroxysm is modified by a prevailing febrile cause; but as this is fre-

[137] In a form, of which the other is probably only a less expensive modification, it is directed to calcine the powder *sixty* times before using it, which could only leave oxides and metallic iron, the latter of which is probably advantageous, as it is said that the preparation should have a blueish colour. This powder was examined for me by Mr. Smith, and appeared to consist of peroxide, mixed with particles of protoxide and metallic iron. No part of it is soluble. It is given with spices. The remedy is used when "the disease is rising" (beginning?), and differs from the treeak farook in curing more slowly, but requiring no regulation of diet. Colcothar of vitriol (peroxide of iron) was shown to the native doctor, who, after careful examination, said he thought it would answer as well, and he is to make experiments with it, but he says he must use it cautiously at first. *Original note.* The patients to whom it was given were cured, and application was made for a farther supply of the peroxide. The mode of preparing this remedy (Mundarium) varies, but the products of the different methods probably do not materially differ. In that given by Messrs. Geddes and Macdonell, the scales from a blacksmith's forge are rubbed up with urine, instead of oil, the mythological opinions of the Hindoos, leading them to ascribe medicinal virtues to the excretions of the cow, and other animals. "A tola or about a rupee weight of gall powder is mix-" ed with 4 oz. of cow's urine, and this is given daily for the first five days. " It is stated to operate as a diuretic and purgative, and by its influence the " dropsical effusion is removed. When this is the case, and the swelling has " subsided, the mundarium which appears to be a peroxide of iron is exhibit-" ed, and this is likewise continued for five days, when the necessity for medi-" cine is considered to be at an end. At the same time the diet consists of " goat's milk and rice without salt. Among the more wealthy, particularly the " Mussulmauns, the treeak farook is had recourse to, along with good stimulat-" ing diet, and when the swelling disappears, this is also followed by the mun-" darium, each being continued for five days. * * * When medicine is dis-" continued, the richer classes continue a milk diet for upwards of forty days." The gall used in the strange combination mentioned in the above extract, is one of the myrobalans, which possess all the qualities of Aleppo galls. Mr. Burrell of the 11th regiment N. I. employed a similar preparation in beriberi, and from the cases he communicated to me, it appears to possess some virtues. Professor H. H. Wilson gives several formulas, in use amongst the Hindoos as purgatives in leprosy, in which the myrobalans are the principal ingredients. (*Transactions of the Medical and Physical Society of Calcutta, Vol.* 1.)

quently connected with internal disease, much caution is necessary, and it has often been found useless, and sometimes hurtful. Both it, and cheyretta have been of advantage as general tonics.[138]

Counter-irritation. A very important part of the treatment, consists in counter-irritation and external stimulants. Blisters to the chest, when the pericardium is affected, have been useful, both by the discharge and counter-irritation they cause, but on the whole, their effects are not very evident. When the lungs or pleura were affected, they did good, but did not protect the patient from death by effusion or syncope. They were of decided benefit when the stomach was tender or irritable, but, as might be expected, often failed in overcoming the vomiting.

Blisters, sinapisms, tartrate of antimony frictions, caustic issues, moxas, setons and stimulating frictions, have been used to the spine. It has already been mentioned, that blisters to the loins were more effectual in removing pain fixed within the canal, than leeches and cupping. The power of the limbs has sometimes been increased and the numbness diminished, by blisters to the lower part of the spine. They seem to act merely as stimulants and counter-irritants, as the effect on the limbs was produced as soon as they acted on the skin, or even before the patient was sensible of their acting, and sinapisms were often equally and sometimes more powerful. In one patient, the limbs which had been below the natural temperature became warmer, the motions more free, the numbness less, and the feeling of stiffness and weight in

[138] Mr. Flockton of the 22d regiment N. I. has communicated two cases, in which the arsenical solution was employed without advantage. Messrs. Geddes and Macdonell also state that, "the arsenias potassæ has been given "to the extent of fifteen drops three times a day, but with doubtful benefit."

the back diminished: in another very bad case, a blister from the 10th dorsal to the 3rd lumbar vertebræ, caused involuntary extension of the legs. The improvement is often only temporary. The country mustard is always of very uncertain powers, and should never be used in medicine, when the European article can be obtained; the former has been on the back for a whole day without inflaming the skin, when the latter was applied, and before it had been on an hour, was torn off by the patient who was unable longer to bear its action. In the few cases in which moxas were employed, they were not found to be of very certain advantage. I have not used setons, and where I saw them employed, they did not seem beneficial. One or two issues have been inserted on each side of the spine, and have removed the remains of numbness of the legs and feet, and of pain about the lumbar vertebræ; they have also been beneficial in the irritable state of the kidney and bladder in the phosphatic stage, in some degree fulfilling the intention of blisters, which are apt to increase the pain, and the irregular actions of the latter. A friend employed the unguent. antimon. tartarisat. as a counter-irritant to the spine, but in none of the cases I saw or read the history of, did it appear to do any good. Liniments of turpentine, &c. are ineffectual.[139] In Ceylon, blisters to the back of the neck have been used with advantage, when the throat was affected, and in the circars where the symptom is not very common, benefit has been in a few instances derived from them. Local applications to the affected limbs are often of great use, and should be diligently employed, as they are always safe and agreeable to the patient. Fomen-

[139] Dr. Rogers states that they are used with advantage, by the Dutch in Ceylon.

tations are frequently grateful, but they have not been much employed in the circars. Pouring cold water on the limbs has been practised by several, but I believe without benefit, and is said, by Dr. Herklots, to be dangerous.[140] Bandages to the legs have removed œdema which resisted other means, and warm clothing is necessary in all stages.[141] The nitro-muriatic acid bath was useless. Frictions relieve the spasmodic affections and pain, in the very worst cases; and have even restored the power of the limbs, removed numbness, pricking sensations, &c., and with blisters and more frequently sinapisms to the calves and to the soles of the feet, have been effectual in removing the torpor of the nerves which, as in common palsy, has sometimes remained after the diseased condition by which it was caused, has been removed.[142] One or two successful cases, where sinapisms and liniments were the only remedies employed, have been communicated to me, and in one, the partial palsy below the waist had been coming on for two years; but such results are rare, and only occur in mild and neglected cases. In general, the treatment to be successful must be commenced early.

Exercise and change of air. Walking or immersion of the feet in the hot sand at noon, is a favorite remedy of the natives, and from the confidence they put in it, may be employed with benefit, as it induces con-

[140] Pouring a stream of hot water on the affected limbs, has been found a safe and beneficial measure in Mr. Davidson's practice.

[141] "As tending much to strengthen the nervous system of the limb, to support its warmth, and to keep up a gentle perspiration, a flannel bandage "should be rolled rather firmly round the leg after each use of the frictions." Messrs. Geddes and Macdonell.

[142] Dr. Pearse used fomentations containing the Moringa root, with much benefit. Dr. Herklots employed, occasionally, a poultice composed of aloes and black hellebore, which is in use with the native practitioners. It is important to be aware of these easy and effectual means, which can be prescribed to convalescents, and which will be the more diligently used by them, as being consistent with their own notions and easily procurable.

valescents to use their enfeebled limbs, and is itself a powerful stimulant to the parts, and excites free perspiration which is also useful. Frictions with the sand is employed at the same time. When it is doing good, the feet become more sensible, and the heat to which they were before unconscious can be borne only for a short time. This practice was pursued on a large scale at Chicacole, by the formation of a temporary convalescent hospital near the sea, six miles from the station, to which convalescents were sent. The place was surrounded by sand hills, on which the men were fond of sitting or walking, they were removed from temptation to excess, and could be narrowly watched by the dresser, (who resided in the building with them), without the confinement of a regimental hospital; and hadthe benefit of a change of climate by no means inconsiderable. They were also saved from the necessity of returning to duty too soon, a very fatal measure in all Indian diseases, but especially in this, in which so much disease of the vital organs may exist in a latent state.[141] Rest alone relieves

[143] The spinal disease must be aggravated by exercise and fatigue; and very little exertion is sufficient to bring back the pain of the loins. Standing increases it, but in a less degree than *turning* in bed frequently and quickly, hence the pain has been much aggravated by a restless night. *Original note.* Exercise is considered to be one of the most important and unobjectionable means of cure in beriberi, and has been enjoined, whenever the patient could be got to move from his cot with the assistance of his comrades; and as a remedy for the palsy and torpor of the limbs and general hebetude of body, it cannot be valued too highly. There is, however, great danger of aggravating many of the symptoms, by its indiscriminate use. The remark made on this subject, in the text at page 114, is confirmed by the following extract from the detailed history of the first of Mr. Davidson's patients, whose cases are referred to in note 47. "The pain in the spine is always less the less "exercise is taken, and entire relief is obtained from lying horizontally. "It is brought back by sitting long." In another of the same gentleman's cases also, the following symptoms are recorded. "October 12th. Has pain "in the groins and about the thighs, and also in the sacrum or termination of "the spine, *when he moves*. 14th. Has no pain at present in the sacrum as "he is not moving, but on the least motion or pressure, gets pain there and "also in the groin."

The aggravation of the cardiac symptoms by the slightest exertion, has been frequently noticed in the preceding pages, and instances of sudden death from eating, speaking, and other slight causes of excitement, have occurred

many of the most alarming symptoms, in the severe cases often received, after the dissipation of the Mohurrum. The success of this establishment was very satisfactory, and I had great reason to thank my predecessor, Mr. Price, for commencing it; and had much pleasure in observing the improvement in most of the patients, after the intervals of 3 or 4 days between my visits. Many patients were sent to neighbouring stations, where the disease was thought to be less prevalent, but the success was far less than in our convalescent hospital; which was accounted for, by the sepoys on leave, concealing themselves in their houses without leaving the neighbourhood, by their living a dissolute life, or never moving from their huts in the station to which they went; by the want of medical inspection and aid on the return of any of the symptoms, and to their practice of taking mercury to excess. There was reason to believe, that a change after a few weeks, by a return to their own station, was beneficial; but the experience of a native practitioner, that a change within the districts where the disease prevails, is of little use, was on the whole confirmed. He assured me, that he had known men cured by change of climate, after being ill more than a year; a fact of great importance, but stated with too great latitude, as I have seen the disease get rapid-

to various practitioners; it is therefore evident that while these symptoms last, and it is astonishing how long they often continue, rest is essential to the cure; and that to force patients labouring under them, to take exercise, must often be the cause of their destruction. The following statement by Mr. Colhoun Stirling, will impress these observations more, than any appeal to the analogy of similar affections. " I have not a doubt on my mind with respect to the " good effects resulting from a nourishing diet and general tonic plan in ob- " viating the fatal tendency of beriberi, and I am convinced that the use of " regular exercise is the most effectual mean of preventing the paralytic symp- " toms though it may be proper to mention, that an instance or two occurred " where the patient dropt down and died while walking out under a guard, " which was the only mode in which this part of the cure could be carried " into effect." (*Hunter op. citat. p.* 137.)

ly worse, after marching far from the endemic influence. Except carriage and attendance were granted by government, it would not be safe to send men ill of this disease to a distance, as many would die in the road, as I have known to happen several times, from the fatigue of a short journey.

Galvanism. From the want or imperfection of instruments, I have never given galvanism a trial worth describing, but a friend* whose judgement is of more value than mine, has communicated to me the following important facts. A man who had lost the use of his lower extremities, and had œdema, swollen face, pains, &c. had used treeak farook and other remedies, without benefit. Galvanism from fifty small plates was sent through the spine, by small blistered surfaces on the neck, sacrum and feet, for ten minutes: after the first application he was able to walk between two men, after the second with the assistance of one, and gradually recovered. He used at the time and afterwards, nothing but bark. Another man had the peculiar pains of beriberi, and loss of power of the lower limbs; the former were removed by galvanism, but it lost its power and a stronger battery could not be procured. Another patient derived benefit from it, but he passed into other hands and the galvanism was not continued. It had much more effect when directed through the spinal cord, than along the nerves of the extremities. In one case it induced spasms of the chest, and dyspnœa. From these facts there is reason to expect, that galvanism will be of use in the removal of the paralytic symptoms, and probably of some others; and as it is known to be beneficial, only when loss of motion and sensation depend on defective ener-

* Assistant Surgeon Geo. Thomson of the civil station of Masulipatam.

gy of the nervous system without organic defect or pressure, we may conclude, that these are not present in *ordinary* examples of beriberi.

Nux vomica. I have been disappointed in my expectations of advantage from nux vomica, which has been administered in considerable doses, and the constitutional effects of the drug induced, without other effect than some aggravation of the spasmodic affections of the paralytic limbs. I only used it in old cases where the palsy was the prominent symptom, but the same friend who employed galvanism successfully, used nux vomica in recent examples, and to the extent, in one instance, of sixty-four grains in twenty-four hours, and until the specific effects of the poison began to show themselves; but he saw no advantage result from the practice. As the strychnine is a peculiar stimulant to the nervous system, and useful only in its torpid state, inducing irregular actions in the muscles, there are no doubt cases for which it will be found an appropriate remedy, but it will probably have no power over the confirmed disease when the structure of the nerves are injured; nor is it likely to be beneficial in the early stage, when all the muscular and nervous powers are in an irregular, and often, in an excited state. The action of nux vomica in exciting the palsied muscles only, deemed so mysterious, is not of difficult explanation by attending to the fact, that if the medicine is continued, the other muscles also become affected, and that all parts whose nervous power is diminished, are more easily excited to spasmodic actions. Four grains of the dry nut four times a day, is as much as I have administered.

Of the Phosphatic Symptoms. With regard to the treatment of the symptoms dependant on the phosphatic diathesis, little remains to be added to the remarks previously made. The common principles of medical science must be applied, for the relief of the various distressing symptoms which will frequently harass the patient, and he may be preserved in some degree of comfortable existence, when a permanent cure is hopeless. If the spinal affection can be removed, hopes may be entertained of the kidneys resuming their natural actions, and this should make us diligently employ every measure, which may remove pain and tenderness from the region of the kidney and bladder. Nitre, gum, and similar remedies have not been of use, when the urine was of natural or increased quantity; and when dropsy has continued in these circumstances, diuretics have failed to remove it. When the urine is diminished, the secretion is not, in this stage, difficult to restore. To change the quality of the secretion would be of great importance, had we the means of effecting it, but this I fear we do not possess. Prout has denied the efficacy of acid medicine in the phosphatic diathesis, which Brande and many other chemists and practitioners recommend. Mr. Brodie in a lecture delivered last year, says he has only found the mineral acids useful in medicine, in altering the alkaline quality of the urine, for which he states fourteen drops of the muriatic, three or four times a day, to be sufficient. I have found the muriatic acid taken in as large quantity as the stomach would bear, which is seldom more than two drachms of the strong acid in the course of the day, to have no apparent effect in altering the quality of the urine or lessening the quantity of deposit, nor is it to be expected on chemical principles. In an European in whom the paralytic symptoms had disappeared, the urine continued alkaline and the deposit copious, notwithstanding the daily use of a drachm of muriatic acid, and the kidneys and bladder gave him no uneasiness, except when they were firmly pressed on. Twenty ounces of urine voided by him in the night, were examined in the morning, and it was found, that to neutralize the ammonia in each ounce, 12 minims of strong muriatic acid were required; and to neutralize the last 6 ounces and to dissolve the phosphate at the bottom of the vessel, ʒijss; so that five drachms and a half of acid were required, to alter the quality of the urine and to dissolve the sediment. Hardly more than a drachm was requisite for the solution of the phosphate of lime, a slight excess of acid only being necessary, and hence it is to the urine itself that the principal attention must be directed. In other experiments less was required, but in none so little, as to afford a hope, of our being able to administer enough to the patient, even could we secure the passage of the whole through the kidney unchanged. Another circumstance also, which will lead us to expect little from this method, is the fact of the urine containing an unusual quantity of lime, even when it has become acid, the presence of which muriatic acid could only conceal, so long as its use was continued.[144]

The great enlargement and thickening of the bladder, ureters, and internal membrane of the kidneys,

[144] Mr. Davidson has found the muriatic acid effectual in removing the deposit, and in rendering the urine clear. The cases in which he employed it, were not of the same confirmed character as those referred to in the text, (see note 68) and even in some of his cases, the apparent effect probably depended, on the tendency to alternation of acid and alkaline qualities in the secretion itself, or on its being neutral or nearly so when voided. In some instances, the sediment reappeared in the urine while the patient was using the acid, and in others its repetition did not restore the natural appearance of the secretion, as it had appeared to do before. In many of the cases, however, the appearance of the urine was certainly altered, and the passages protected, for the time, from irritation. Messrs. Geddes and Macdonell also, found vegetable acids useful, in restoring the natural appearance of the urine.

suggested the employment of iodine, in two cases. The hydriodate of potassa was prescribed, but two grains caused irritability of stomach and vomiting. The researches of Lugol have shown, that the tincture of iodine is liable to be decomposed and rendered inert, by dilution in the fluids of the stomach, and that the best preparation is pure iodine dissolved in a solution of the hydriodate of potassa. The former could not be procured, I therefore instituted some experiments by which it was found, that the tincture of iodine added to a solution of the hydriodate in distilled water, was a preparation of the same qualities as that recommended by Lugol, and it was used for a long time, but I regret to say, without advantage.

Notwithstanding the benefit derived from the various remedies we have been considering, it must appear but too evident, that none of them are of certain efficacy, or act directly on the most important part of the disease; and that there are few disorders, in which it is more necessary to investigate with care, the powers of all those substances which have obtained the confidence of the inhabitants or practitioners of the districts, in which the complaint is of constant occurrence. Some of these have already been considered, and have received but little praise; but the two we are now to notice, will be shown to possess high claims to our confidence; and the distrust and even ridicule with which the accounts first communicated, were received by the majority of this establishment, including the present writer, will afford an additional illustration of the injury done to truth and medical science, by that supercilious scepticism and indolence, which will receive or examine nothing it cannot explain. As my testimony to the powers of the treeak farook and oleum nigrum has been forced from me, by witnessing their superior efficacy, I may be allowed to claim some degree of confidence, even should the cases I am able to communicate be insufficient; most of my histories of cases treated with these remedies, not being accessible.

Treeak Farook. The treeak farook was brought to the notice of the Medical Board, some years ago, by Mr. W. Geddes; and Dr. Wight extracted from his report some account of its employment, which was circulated to the members of the Medical Society, and thus became more extensively known; but being, in general, only to be procured at Masulipatam, it was not much in use till 1828. Nor do the Hindoo practitioners appear to have been long acquainted with it, as I was informed by one of them, that the dyspnœa of beriberi proved very fatal until it was introduced; and it is not yet *popularly* known at a distance from Masulipatam, where it is procured from the Moghul merchants. The Hindoos have adopted the name from the Arabs, and the most celebrated practitioner in beriberi, in the circars, is a Mussulmaun hukeem, who administered a remedy, which from the account of his patients is undoubtedly the treeak, and with which he is said to have cured many, who had been unsuccessfully treated by European surgeons. I can find no account of the treeak or teriak farook, in Persian or Hindoostanee dictionaries. The first word is borrowed from the Greek, and is used both for a particular composition celebrated over the east as the theriak of Bagdad, and for any antidote. "Farouk" marks its difference and superiority to other treeaks, as would appear from the account of the word in D'Herbelot. "Farouk epi-"thetè d'honneur qui fut donné par Mahomet a Omar,

" qui signifiè celui qui separé."[145] *(Bibliotheque Oriental.)*

The treeak is a thick extract, sold in small lead canisters containing ten or fifteen tolas, and in others of only one tola weight. The small ones are packed in dozens, well rolled up in paper, and cost a rupee each, and the second size is sold for five or six rupees. They are only to be procured from the Moghuls, and in those towns which still keep up some communication with the Arabian seas. Besides its use in beriberi, it is employed in Hyderabad and the circars in numbness, rheumatism, and as usual amongst them with unknown remedies, as an aphrodisiac. Mr. Geddes was very unsuccessful in treating beriberi till he met with the treeak farook, which removed the œdema rapidly, and had more power in lowering the pulse than any other remedy he was acquainted with.[146] In some in-

[145] " تریاق فاروق *tirjāky fārūk*, and تریاک فاروق *tirjakī farook. Ah.* تریاق کبیر *tirjāky kébīr.* Theriaca optima, præstantissima." *(Thesaurus Meninski.)*

[146] The following history of the circumstances which first led to the employment of the medicine, is valuable on several accounts.

" In the treatment of the earlier cases of beriberi which appeared, the bad " success which I met with obliged me to shift from one plan to another, un- " til at last I had exhausted every resource to which I could apply, with any " prospect of a favourable result. I commenced with a plan which had been " brought to my notice by the superintending surgeon, Dr. C. Rogers, as be- " ing found very efficient by Dr. Wight, viz. calomel in scruple doses with " opium and continued until profuse salivation took place, without having any " effect either on the paralysis or frequency of the pulse. I afterwards super- " added blood-letting, blisters to the loins, along with occasional purgatives of " jalap. On this failing, I had recourse to squills and other diuretics, the " warm bath, bleeding followed by daily purgation, scruple doses of calomel " followed by castor oil in the morning, and antimonials, notwithstanding how- " ever all that I could do, the fatal dropsy supervened and killed my pati- " ents. The only plan which appeared to have any effect in keeping off the " dropsical symptoms was blood-letting, followed by daily purgatives; the dis- " ease however was not removed by them, for after a while, the œdema be- " gan to make its appearance, and being completely at a stand, I consented " to the request of my patients, to be allowed to try a native medicine, which " they stated had cured some of them, when affected on a previous occasi- " on." * * * " The patients in whom the bleeding and purging had been used, " but where œdema had begun to make its appearance, had the medicine " exhibited to them, and in a few days the dropsical effusion had completely " disappeared, and the pulse was considerably lowered. In the next case " there was total paralysis in the legs and arms, the feet had been swelled

stances the pulse fell in four days from 108 to 84, and it was also useful in dropsy succeeding remittent fever. He did not find it remove the palsy. Another gentleman informed me, that he found it produce rapid absorption of the effused fluid but did not observe that the pulse was affected, nor in the few cases he employed it in, that the palsy was much benefited. In the experience of others its influence over the palsy has been clearly ascertained, and in differing in some degree from the opinions of Mr. Geddes, I hope I shall not be supposed to do so, with any view to lessen the gratitude the medical men of the circars owe him, for adding what appears to be so valuable a medicine to the materia medica; and saving them the mortification and discredit, of seeing their patients whom they had in vain attempted to cure, recover under the empirical treatment of natives. The prescription employed by Mr. Geddes, was treeak ʒiij, rhubarb ℥ij ʒv, cinnamon ℈ij, cloves gr. xxi, made into a mass with honey, of which four scruples and a half are taken every morning with honey, and is said to procure four or five stools daily. The patient is di-

" for several days, and the pulse when the treeak farook was commenced was " 108, next day it was at the same rate and on each successive day it was " found lowered to 100, 88, and 84, by which time the œdema had disappear- " ed, and the patient had no complaint but of the paralytic affection. In the " next person to whom the medicine was given, there was not much paraly- " sis, as he could walk, although not steadily, without assistance, his limbs " however were œdematous and his pulse on the day of commencing the " treatment was 116, next day it got up to 124, after which it fell daily as fol- " lows: 106, 94, 100, 84, 84, 76, 72; the œdema was by this time removed " and the patient continued to improve daily." *Mr. W Geddes' report for the 2nd half of* 1822.

Mr. Stevenson employed it soon after, and observes that, " the treatment " of this disease having hitherto proved so unsuccessful, I was led to put into " practice a mode of cure suggested to me by Mr. assistant surgeon Geddes, " 1st. batt. 11th regt. Native Infantry, who has lately used a native me- " dicine of the name of ' teriac farook'; in two cases solely treated by that " medicine, I entirely coincide in opinion with that gentleman, regarding " its singular power on the state of the pulse and in removing œdema; the " pulse in one case being reduced from 100, and in the other from 90 to the " healthy standard in two days, and in the course of four days the œdema " had entirely disappeared, and the patients are now convalescent; consi- " dering the repeated disappointment in the treatment of beriberi, I am of " opinion that the medicine in question merits a further trial."

rected to eat animal food, wheaten cakes and milk, and to drink warm water (of which as common drink the natives are fond). As the quantities of these ingredients are reduced from native weights, the minute proportions given, neither justify distrust or demand observance. I have therefore sometimes employed the following, which I received from an experienced native practitioner, who administered it to several patients under my inspection. One rupee weight of treeak, six of rhubarb and of honey, made into a mass and divided into fourteen large boluses, of which one is taken in the morning and at noon. The general effect of this on the bowels was stated to be two or three stools a day, which I have found correct, and six if there were anasarca, which is probably a just observation. But as this was inconvenient in prescription, and such large pills could not be swollowed by Europeans, and as there was no danger of mistake, I substituted the following: pulv. rhei ℥ijss, treeak farook ℥ss, confect. aromat. ʒss, mel. q. s. Fiat mass. et divide in bol. xviii; which were divided into pills, of the size the patient could most easily swallow, and were found to answer very well.

The treeak was sometimes prescribed alone, but in doses of from four grains to fifteen had no sensible effect, unless perhaps in a slight degree constipating the bowels. The urine did not appear to be increased by it, even when all the symptoms had yielded to it or to other remedies. When the case was of long standing, the palsy confirmed, and the urine either scanty, or copious and alkaline, the treeak was equally useless as a remedy for the anasarca as for the paralytic symptoms; and when it was only had recourse to as a last resource, after other means had failed, the patient frequently died the first day or two after commencing its use. It is therefore necessary to employ it early, and to this, is in a great measure to be ascribed, the greater success of this remedy in the hands of Mr. Geddes and others who were fovourably impressed with its usefulness, than in those of gentlemen who were of a different opinion, and by whom I observed the remedy to be given, when success could not be expected from it. Its power over the anasarca is well illustrated, in the case of which the following is an abstract.

Case 45th. Appadoo, sepoy, ætat. 30. Admitted 13th October, complaining of numbness and want of power of the lower limbs, which are œdematous. Face a little swollen, pulse quick and rather full, stools from a dose of jalap green, urine scanty and dark. Ill ten days. Had purgatives, calomel and squills for eight days, and several doses of tincture of squills and of digitalis without benefit, and the face had become more puffy. Dyspnœa not complained of. On the 23rd, the treeak was given in pills with rhubarb. 24th. No change. 25.th Swellings less, but numbness continues. 26th. Very little swelling, but numbness continues. 28th. Swelling gone. 31st. Numbness less. This symptom yielded slowly, as well as the rare symptom of burning in the feet, at night, which came on the beginning of November; and pains succeeded. Great benefit was derived from frictions and sinapisms and the cure was completed, but he was attacked with fever, to which the debility made him more liable, and was easily cured by purgatives and bark. Fever is apt to bring back the beriberi, but it did not do so in this case, and the patient was discharged, well.

It is of great importance to neglect no means, by

which we may assist the efficacy of the remedy, and more especially those of a local nature as frictions, which are in most instances essential to restoring the functions of the nerves: and the habit of trusting to specifics common to the natives, has been injurious with regard to the treeak, along with which they seldom employ any thing else. The hukeem to whom I formerly alluded, was an exception to this remark.

When the treeak relieves the numbness, it does so more slowly than the effusion either into the chest or cellular membrane.

Case 46th. A stout muscular sepoy, aged 30. Was admitted November 22d, on the 10th day of beriberi, with considerable œdema and pitting of the lower extremities which were numb; some dyspnœa, four times purged by pulv. jalap. comp. On the 23d commenced the treeak. 25th. Less swelling, numbness and dyspnœa the same. 27th. Dyspnœa gone. December 2d. Œdema gone, numbness continues in calves and feet. 3d. Less numbness. On the 4th he used sinapisms and frictions also. 18th. Very little numbness, in soles of feet only. Omitt. treeak. 26th. Slight numbness in toes only, and he was soon after discharged cured. Two cases of a milder character admitted at the same time, were treated by ordinary remedies and were not cured.

Case 47th. December 14th. Rownapah, aetat. 47. Had been ill of fever a few days before, numbness and deficient power below the knees since yesterday, with slight hard swelling, no pitting; slight dyspnœa on exertion. Pulv. jalap comp. ℨss. 15th. Treeak. 18th. Numbness less. January 1st. Swelling gone, walks well but there is still some numbness of feet. February 3d. Quite well.

The native practitioners justly observe, that when the face is swollen the disease is most dangerous, and that the treeak must be given without delay; and the following abstract will show, that it will then effect a rapid cure, when the combination of pectoral symptoms with a languid pulse, and the known uncertain or ill effects of mercury, would make it difficult to find any medicine in which we could place confidence.

Case 48th. Tatiah, aetat. 20, November 24th. Suffered from fever and some beriberi symptoms last year, and now complains of numbness, weight and pain in the lower extremities, which are œdematous, as well as the body, arms, and face, which last is bloated and of a glassy appearance; weight and oppression of chest, increased on exertion. Cough and dyspnœa easiest in the recumbent posture. Pulse languid and irregular, bowels slow, eyes yellow, tongue fiery red, moist and clean. Pulv. jalap. comp. ʒj. 6th. Purged, less œdema, dyspnœa worse. To take the treeak. 8th. Less œdema and dyspnœa. 10th. No dyspnœa and œdema nearly gone. 12th. Numbness, dyspnœa, and œdema all gone. 14th. Omitt. medicament. 18th. Weak. Infus. cheyrettæ. 27th. Discharged. But success is not generally to be expected in so dreadful a malady, and there is reason to believe, that the paralytic affections are less certainly cured than any of the others.

Case 49th. Somanah, a stout young sepoy. Was admitted November 27th, with numbness over the body, legs and hands slightly swollen, unable to walk without assistance. Complaint of four days standing; he says he has had dyspnœa only since last night. Pulse quick and rather full, eyes yellow. Pulv. jalap. comp. ℥j. 28th. Swelling less. Dyspnœa, numbness, and weight in thorax. To commence with the treeak. 29th. Very little swelling. December 2nd. Swelling gone. Breathing free, numbness and weakness of lower limbs, and knees feel weak. It was continued along with frictions with some advantage, but he was lost sight of in January, not having recovered the full use of his limbs.

The experience of the natives has convinced them, that the treeak removes the spasmodic and other nervous symptoms, but they say, that if there is no œdema the cure is usually slow, and that the same is the case when there are sensations of biting of ants. Whether any of the cases they spoke of, were of old disease in which the œdema had been cured, I could not ascertain. In some examples, the numbness and peculiar unsteady walk of beriberi are benefited earlier and to a greater degree that the anasarcous symptoms, especially when these had resisted other means. The affection of the *pericardium* and *œdema of the face and hands depending on it*, are removed *simultaneously* and earlier than the œdema, numbness, &c. of the lower extremities; and the same remark applies to the numbness over the chest and body. It is occasionally necessary and generally expedient to give cream of tartar at the same time as the treeak, when the urine is scanty or the œdema extensive. Purgatives will frequently be necessary in the course of treatment, and when the stools are disordered, and the œdema does not rapidly yield, they should be repeated; it is also advantageous to commence the treatment with a smart purge; and jalap is the best. The treeak has been found most useful in that form of the disorder in which there was little excitement, the pulse being usually, though not always, feeble and small.[147]

[147] Dr. Pearse observes, that "having employed the native remedies oleum "nigrum and treeak farook, in several cases of beriberi during the latter "part of last year, I am induced to make a favourable report of their effects "in cases of the chronic form of beriberi, and am inclined to believe, that "they may be used not only with safety but with much benefit, *after the re-* "*moval of the stage of excitement* by the means before advised. The treeak "farook usually acts as a purgative or laxative, and some patients also com- "plained of a feeling of internal heat in the chest and abdomen, and after "continuing its use for 3 or 4 days, it caused a good deal of irritability with "increase of the pulse, and a feverish heat of skin."

Holding in view this observation and the remarks made at page 268 regarding the efficacy of purgatives, we may perhaps be justified in thinking, that the combination of the treeak with rhubarb and aromatics, will fulfil the conditions which Dr. Herklots considers to be essential, in a medicine to be employed in this disease: "having premised a suitable purgative, we must "commence upon a course of medicines; and that should possess the com- "bined properties of being purgative, diuretic, diaphoretic, stimulant, and "antispasmodic; or different medicines having these virtues individually, "united together into one or more formulæ." The enquiries alluded to in note 126 have convinced me, that much is to be ascribed to the gentle purgative effect produced, but the following observations by Mr. Davidson, seems to show that its operation does not depend on this alone. "With regard to "the treatment, it appeared to be sufficiently simple. In cases of *short* stand- "ing though there be œdema, heaviness, or anasarca, with a tense fulness of "some parts (as the arms), numbness, frequent pulse, puffiness of the face, "high coloured and scanty urine, &c. purgation aided by diuresis, in the "course of ten or fifteen days has effected a cure. The medicines used were "a drachm of compound powder of jalap early every morning, having its ten- "dency to act on the kidneys assisted by a diuretic powder (composed of "squill gr. ij, nitre gr. x, &c.), given twice during the afternoon; which was "found speedily to remove all the symptoms. During the copious purgation "so produced, the urine became daily less scanty and less high coloured, the "feeling of heaviness, numbness, and œdema decreased, beginning at the "right side. The rhythm of the heart was gradually recovered, that is, the "contraction of the auricle took up less time, the pulse became less frequent "and less strong; in short, this went on till the last trace of the disease dis- "appeared from the left side; leaving the patient not much reduced in flesh, "if not so on admission. There seems to be little in the shape of disease "during this time in the abdomen, the tongue clean, appetite good, the stools "composed of indigested food and water. Besides the above, was given ge- "nerally and apparently with good effect every night, ten or fifteen grains "of one of the preparations of aloes, the compound pill seemed to be the best, "producing stools more feculent and consistent. Indeed the compound ja- "lap powder seems to be well fitted for this disease, for there are several "persons here now, who have had the first symptoms of the disease for some "time but are going about, and who find that by taking a dose of compound "jalap, they can remove for a time the heaviness, numbness, &c. and when "they feel these returning, they repeat this dose and so keep the disease in "check."

"However in cases of *long* standing, where perhaps some organic change "had already taken place, the above means were found ineffectual and so "was also the infusion of digitalis, tried after them, to the extent of ℥iij in the "day. The pulse, numbness, general swelling, scanty and high coloured "urine, &c. continuing all unchanged notwithstanding copious purgation dur- "ing ten days; the only effect produced was merely a diminution in the feel- "ing of heaviness, but very soon after treeak in combination with rhubarb "began to be used all the symptoms began to disappear. The pulse which "had kept invariably near 100 was, on the third day of the use of this medi-

It is not without efficacy in other circumstances, but I am not able to point out the limits where its virtues are counteracted by inflammatory actions, in which the stimulating diet combined with it must act injuriously. Mr. Geddes ascribes to the treeak very extraordinary virtues as a direct sedative to the vascular system, and states, that in four days it has lowered the pulse from 108 to 84. My experience did not justify this opinion as a general fact, although striking instances of rapid lowering of the pulse under its use occurred, and the circumstances on which the difference depended, therefore demanded enquiry

" cine, reduced to 72, swelling much less, tongue moist. On the fourth day " the pulse was reduced to 42 beats in a minute, and other symptoms also less. " On the fifth day of its use pulse was 37 in a minute, all the other symp- " toms disappearing, the urine becoming more copious and less high colour- " ed, stools copious, semifluid and feculent. On the sixth day the pulse was " only 36, all the other symptoms dissappearing. The pulse kept equally low " for the next two days; at the end of which the medicine was discontinued, " all the symptoms having nearly disappeared; immediately after which the " pulse began to rise and continued gradually rising to its natural standard. " The combination in which the treeak was used in this case was that given " by the natives, namely a bolus morning and evening containing, grains vijss " of treeak, ϶ijss of rhubarb, and one clove."

" Indeed it seems probable, as a general rule, that the above bolus morning " and evening is adequate to the cure of the disease in any remediable stage; " it has been found to purge very copiously, producing stools not at all wate- " ry but semifluid and about ℔ v every twenty-four hours, restoring the ap- " petite and digestion, should these have been impaired."

The following remarks however by Messrs. Geddes and Macdonell are to be carefully attended to, in observing its effects, although the importance assigned to the diet used along with it, is perhaps exaggerated.

" It is right however to state, that the treeak farook has been considered " by several medical men who have used it, as devoid of those effects in be- " riberi which have been ascribed to it, and it has been supposed that the " diet attending its exhibition has had the chief share in producing those " advantages, which seem at first to be the result of the medicine. It is cer- " tain, that without the aid of a nourishing diet, little permanent relief has " been shown to have been obtained by the use of the treeak, but when ge- " nuine and fresh, the cordial and stomachic properties admitted to belong " to the theriaca venetiana, combined with the gentle laxative effect of " those medicines with which it is given, must tend to assist digestion and " assimilation, and to aid in improving generally the tone and energy of the " whole body. In producing this effect however, generally, it must be ad- " mitted that medicines can only act as auxiliary means of cure. Nourish- " ing diet particularly the use of milk, exercise where practicable, or fricti- " ons if the patient cannot walk, change of place involving as it does a re- " moval from the atmosphere in which the patient has been seized, with its " concurring consequences of mental excitement and exercise will do more " of themselves, it is believed, for the recovery of the patient, than any re- " medies which could be given without their assistance."

and some of them have been ascertained. If the pulse were natural or raised above the common standard by general irritation only, no change was caused by the medicine; but when it was rapid, small and otherwise disordered in connection with cardiac affection, especially dropsy of the pericardium, the pulse was restored rapidly to a more natural state, but as far as I have observed, only in proportion to the removal of the thoracic affection, and when this took place slowly, the pulse remained long very quick. The general fact is established by a sufficient number of examples, but the observations tracing the correspondence in the degree of alteration in the pulse and in the quantity of effusion and of disorder of the heart, have been few, although satisfactory to my mind. The following abstract will illustrate these observations.

Case 50th. A native woman who had laboured under rheumatism in the joints and shoulder-blades for sometime, got numbness and sense of weight from the middle of the thighs downwards, and of the abdomen, forearms, hands, and lower lip. The walk was unsteady, and the legs and feet œdematous. There was extensive pulsation felt by the hand over the chest, the sound of the heart loud, and there was oppression at præcordia. Pulse upwards of 100 and weak, as was the action of the heart. Had used the juice of the leaves of the sikiserum chettoo (Acacia frondosa) and purgatives, without much benefit. The treeak was commenced, and in two days the numbness was lessened and the opppression diminished. In three days more, the numbness, difficulty of motion, and oppression at præcordia had nearly left; there was still some œdema; the bowels were five times opened daily, and the urine remained scanty and red: the respiratory murmur could be heard distinct and natural round the cardiac region, where it could not previously be distinguished; the impulse could not be felt *much* beyond the cardiac region, although its sound could be heard rather loud, some way over the right side. Pulse still quick. When she had taken twelve boluses there was no dyspnœa or oppression, the impulse, and respiratory murmur were natural, the pulse 70 and soft; the sounds of the heart, especially the auricles, were loud, and there was numbness of the hands and feet only. Six more of the boluses removed every symptom of beriberi, but the rheumatism was not relieved. In the following case the medicine acted powerfully on the nervous and absorbent system, and had little effect on the pulse, the strength of which was increased before its frequency was at all diminished.

Case 51st. A woman who had used the dursan chettoo, jalap, and diet of wheaten bread and milk with some little benefit, had on the 25th May, numbness downwards from the middle of thighs, and sensations of biting of ants and œdema of the legs, with difficulty and staggering in walking. Lower lip numb, as were also the forearms from one-third above the wrist, the power of directing the motions of the fingers nearly lost, they move over each other involuntarily, and although she has power to grasp objects, they fall from her hands apparently from want of sensation in the fingers. Respiration hurried by slight exertion, is easy in the recumbent posture. There is tightness, weight, and oppression in præcordia and pit of stomach, action of heart communicated to the hand over the whole front of the chest and epigastrium, but is weak, its sounds rather loud as heard with the stethoscope; respiratory murmur cannot be heard below the third rib for a considerable extent round the cardiac region, but is perfectly natural every where else. Pulse 116, feeble, small and regular, (has been observed slightly to intermit once or twice). Menses regular, urine scanty and red, bowels costive, tongue white, pale and clean, no thirst, slight swelling of the face. The hands are smooth and moist like soaked leather, and several degrees below the temperature of the body. Her husband says she is worse in the evening, and that she is indolent and the mind weak. A dose of jalap purged her well, and on the 26th the treeak was given with rhubarb only, and meat, wheat and milk were ordered for diet. On the 28th felt herself better about the chest. Pulse more rapid (130), two stools daily, numbness did not extend so high up the legs and hands. On the 31st pulse was stronger but frequent, numbness and biting sensation only from the middle of hands and diminishes in the legs. Less weight at epigastrium. June 3rd. Feeling and temperature nearly restored, but there are sensations of sleeping from the middle of the legs and of the hands, walks about pretty well and is able to attend to house affairs, no weight or tightness at præcordia or epigastrium, the extensive pulsation cannot be felt and respiration is natural. Pulse 100, of better strength. On 3rd and 4th took no medicine. On the 5th was in the same state. The treeak was repeated, and a perfect cure effected. The combination of the rhubarb was very useful.

It is probable from some facts, that the treeak by removing the irritable mobility of the system, by its powers over the nerves, will restore the pulse to a healthy standard, but this is not often to be expected. The virtues this remedy appeared to possess, naturally excited a desire to learn something of its history and nature, but it was long before I could obtain any information. Some roman characters stampt on the boxes increased the curiosity, but the native doctors knowing only that they were brought to Bombay by the Arabian traders, it was uncertain whether they were imported through Persia, the red sea or the Portuguese settlements in Africa. To obtain more accurate information and in hopes of finding some intelligible inscriptions, I visited the Moghul merchants at Masulipatam, and was informed that the treeak farook was brought from beyond Istamboul (Constantinople) by way of the red sea; and I purchased some cannisters with distinct characters stampt on their lids, and procured a number of papers in which they were packed. The larger cannisters had on the lids, a head well executed and surrounded with a wreath of laurel, and on one of them the following legend in fine roman capitals; TERIACA. F. ALI. A. TESTA. DORO. IN. TRIESTE. Two half sheets of paper, ornamented with a gilded head, containing a long account of the medicine well printed, the one in Turkish and the other in modern greek, are wrapped round each packet, and to many the signature of Eredi L. B. Silvestrini is attached, who appears, from the inscription around the head, to be an apothecary on the Rialto at Venice. Some of the papers bear the words " Ponte de Rialto" and others " Strazzo d'oro" " in Venezia", and common Italian notes and printed lists of drugs, some of which are curious,[148] are wrapped round the packet, within the

[148] The following is a specimen. Liquor. Corn. Cerv; Lignum Nefriticum; Liquor. Nitri fixi; Magisterium Antimon; Magisterium Jovis; Lima Caustica. *Original note.*

others papers. (Having procured, through Mr. Thacker of Calcutta, a translation of one of these papers, the following extract from it will leave no doubt of the medicine being procured from Venice, of whose commerce with India it is one of the last remnants.

"Theriakh of Andromachi. An invention of Theron, "the Prebyster. It is prepared, measured and made "public by me, John Baptist Sylvestrius, in the Rial- "to, by the authority of the excellent Governments' "physicians, of ancient righteousness, and of the "council of the apothecaries and learned physicians."

"The within mentioned treacle is prepared in Ve- "nice with every care and faithfulness by me, John "Baptist Sylvestrius, Apothecary in the Signal *Tes-* "*ta d'oro* in St. Bartholomy, in the presence of ex- "cellent and superior physicians of ancient righte- "ousness, and of the assembly of apothecaries and "others connected with the medical institution. The "virtues and properties of the treacle are particula- "rized below, in common benevolence and for the "good of the public." A long list of diseases for which it is an infallible remedy follows, and the paper concludes by informing its readers, that other diseases are omitted as the name of this medicine "is universally known throughout the world;" and that the young and strong should use it in small doses, and that the old and those accustomed to the use of opiates may take it more freely, but still in small quantity.

The treeak farook being thus identified with this celebrated compound, we can more easily appreciate the effects which it appears to produce in this disease; and while we are not to expect it to exert any specific powers over the heart, the known composition of the drug itself, and the combination in which it is given, are such as to confirm the inferences as to its virtues suggested by the whole mass of evidence for and against it, and cannot fail to suggest important improvements in the combinations employed by those, who may not chuse to adopt the empirical and expensive remedy itself. Nor will it be difficult to compose a formula containing the more important purgative, diuretic, stimulating and anodyne medicines which enter into its composition.)[149]

When of good quality, the taste of the treeak is at first sweetish, then nauseous, hot and acrid; its smell is aromatic and resembles spruce, which, and it is alleged, the information obtained from some traders from the Persian gulf, has led to the occasional substitution of that article for the genuine; and its comparative cheapness will probably lead to frauds fatal to the character of the remedy.[150] The small cannisters should also be avoided, as they do not appear to be of equal quality and are sometimes half empty.

Oleum Nigrum. It remains to communicate such

[149] Some additional information on this subject will be found in the appendix. The paragraph within brackets has been substituted, for a few sentences of the original paper which have been omitted, as the translation of the envelopes obtained soon after, superseded the incorrect speculations on the nature of the compound, contained in them.

[150] Dr. Herklots was iuduced by this similarity in appearance and smell to employ the extract of spruce in beriberi, but he found it to have no effect. The following observations on the treeak are extracted from his second half yearly report for 1823.

" Instead of commencing with the oleum nigrum, you may begin with ano-" ther remedy which I shall term here *bolus ex teereeaq farooq*, since the " chief ingredient in its composition is a medicine called teereeaq farooq used " by natives all over the country, and considered by them as a most sovereign " remedy: though according to my experience on the subject, after trying " it in a variety of cases, I must confess it falls far short of the oleum nigrum; " however it deserves the second rank; it possesses the same virtues with its " predecessor, but in a weaker degree; it removes œdema in a few days, but " not in quite so short a time as the oil. As rhubarb enters into the compo-" sition of its boluses (which will procure three or four evacuations daily) there " is no occasion to interpose cathartics as in the former case, but the boluses " (fourteen in number) are to be taken morning and evening for seven days, " during which time as well as throughout the whole complaint, the patient " is to adhere to the full diet mentioned before."

observations as I have made, regarding another native remedy of great value, styled by Dr. Herklots, to whom we owe its first introduction to the notice of Europeans, the oleum nigrum. It is prepared in the following manner. Into an earthen pot whose bottom is perforated by a number of small holes are put, malkungnee seeds ℔ijss, benzoin, cloves, nutmegs, mace, of each ℥ss; the mouth is closed and the pot placed over another and luted to it. They are then placed in a pit three feet deep and nearly as wide, and surrounded by cakes of dry cow dung which are set on fire, and when they are consumed about six ounces of the oil is found in the under vessel ready for use. It should be kept in well closed bottles. As we would expect from the nature of the process, the appearance and sensible qualities of the product resemble those of an empyreumatic oil, possessing the peculiar powers of the principal ingredient, the malkungnee seeds. These do not appear to be the produce of the circars, or as far as I can learn, of the Deccan, but Mr. Royle has included them in a list of Indian materia medica, and states that the plant is the Celastrus nutans.[151] It is stated by Hukeem Mahomed Hussein Khan to be a native of Hindoostan, and the seeds are imported from Calcutta or brought to the circars from Hyderabad, and are only found in the princi-

[151] I have since found the plant, growing in the jungles which cover the primitive hills of Ramteak north of Nagpore, and in similar situations in the neighbourhood of Hyderabad. Roxburgh, also, obtained living plants from the Mysore and introduced them into the botanic garden of Calcutta, where Dr. Wallich found six plants, of which only one is hermaphrodite and fertile, all the rest are male-hermaphrodites and barren. Two varieties were pointed out to me in the Hyderabad jungles, the leaves of one of which were smaller, and it in no instance bore fruit. The other plants were in fruit in October and November. Dr. Wight is of opinion, that the Celastrus paniculata of Roxburgh, who had only seen dried specimens obtained from the circar moundains, is the same with his C. nutans. The malkungnee must be rare in the circars, as neither Dr. Wight or myself could obtain any specimens in these districts; it is, however, always a scarce plant.

pal towns, where they are kept in bags containing the seeds, seed vessels and stalks, from which the genus can be ascertained, as was done by Dr. Wight some years before the publication of Mr. Royle's catalogue. The name used in Hindoostan has been introduced into Arabic, Persian, Teloogoo, and Tamul. A tree called by the Mahrattas "malkanee," the seeds of which afford an oil, grows in the forest of Dongatal north of Nagpore, but I did not see the tree nor am I sure that it is the same.[151] The seeds differ in quality, sometimes from age, but I have seen very fresh ones of inferior quality, apparently from their being pulled too soon. When new, the seeds are partially surrounded by a yellow unctuous tasteless farina, and when they are reduced to powder they form a paste from which a yellow oil, having in some degree the qualities of the seeds, may be expressed. These have a hot biting taste, permanent in the palate, and if many of them are masticated, a sense of giddiness and a peculiar slight sensation extending over the face and brow are felt. A very slight taste and no acrimony is given to water distilled from them, and the oil on the surface of the residuum is bland. The seeds retain their taste. It was evident from this, that their virtues did not reside either in a fixed or volatile oil. Some of the seeds were coarsely powdered, and alcohol rubbed up with them and afterwards filtered; it had acquired a light yellow tinge. On this being dropped into water, an immediate separation of the resin it held in solution took place, in a white flake, which had a strong biting acrid taste exactly like that of the seeds but much more powerful, and in which it appears the virtues of the plant reside. The alcoholic solution evaporated, leaves a beautiful yellow resinous paste which also possesses the qualities of the seeds. The black oil itself is a thick deep brown fluid, burning with a white flame and not acted on by acids. Its specific gravity is, at ninety, 0975. which is higher than any of the fixed oils; its taste is rough, bitterish and acrid, its smell empyreumatic and peculiar. Water distilled from it is limpid, but has a good deal of the taste of the seeds, and the oil floating on the water in the retort is tasteless. The oil when rubbed up with alcohol forms a deep olive brown partial solution, and there is only a little thick oily matter left on the filter, which has much less taste than the oil itself or the oily tincture. This last, on being dropped into water, separates into a white flake sinking in the water and of the same quality as that obtained from the alcoholic solution of the seeds, and a fixed black oil having a slight bitter oily taste. On the mixture of the oil and alcohol standing for some time, the fixed oil partly separates from the tincture; and seems to pass through the filter with, butnot dissolved by it. From these observations it appears, that the resin is combined with the oils existing in the ingredients employed, which are partly converted into an empyreumatic compound, and thus acquire the property of partially dissolving the resin.

The black oil is administered to natives in betel leaf, but as Europeans cannot take it in this form it is made into pills, which are inconvenient from their size; it is therefore desirable that a form of administering it may be founded on the above experiments, which will be more convenient, and avoid the uncertainty which must attend all processes like that described; but as the empyreumatic oils possess powerful stimulating properties and the combination seems so far judicious, it will be necessary to be very cautious in rejecting it, or substituting another, without extensive observations of their effects in disease. The genus Celastrus belongs to the natural family of Rhamneæ of Jussieu and the frangulaceous plants of Decandolle, the berries and inner bark of many of which are stated by that eminent naturalist to have virtues but little known, offering curious subjects of investigation. The Cassina, nearly related to the Celastrus, exerts an influence over the nervous system causing drunkenness, and the Celastrus maytenus affords a wash, useful in removing the swellings caused by a poisonous tree in America. It is therefore interesting to find, that great powers over the nervous system and digestive organs are ascribed to the seeds of the Celastrus nutans, in the "Mukhzun ool adrea" or treasury of medicine, a compilation in Persian, from Hindee, Persian and Arabic works composed by Hukeem Mahomed Hussien Khan of Calcutta; and that besides its supposed effects when taken internally, frictions with preparations of the seeds are said to be efficacious in cases of palsy, spasmodic distortion of the face, cramp, &c. It has already been observed, that the proportion of deaths in cases of beriberi was remarkably diminished throughout the division, at the time the black oil came into general use, which I had the best means of knowing, having supplied a large portion of the corps with the oil or directions for its manufacture. But it has been in Dr. Herklots' experience that it had the most astonishing effects, that gentleman having lost only one patient in fifty cases of beriberi treated by it, while he had eleven deaths out of fifteen, before he adopted the native treatment.[152] Al-

[152] More than one half of the admissions with beriberi, died in the jail of Masulipatam, in ten years, during which it was in charge of a succession of the most skilful and experienced surgeons in India. Bleeding was used freely and judiciously. *Original note.*

though unacquainted with Dr. Herklots, I have had opportunity of knowing, that his intimate knowledge of the language and opinions of the natives had acquired him their confidence, which was increased by his use in practice of their own remedies and diet: hence he saw his patients earlier and before the dangerous thoracic symptoms developed themselves, and therefore it is not to be expected, that in other hands it will prove nearly so certain a cure. Unfortunately Dr. Herklots weakened the force of the evidence of this astonishing success, by ascribing part of it to remedies in their nature evidently absurd, although they may have been useful in inducing a zealous employment of frictions. But the testimony of this gentleman having been received with general indifference and even ridicule, and my experience affording nothing approaching to similar success, I shall present the result of my enquiries in detail; as the efficacy of a medicine can only be appreciated when the circumstances in which it has been administered are faithfully stated.

The diet directed by Dr. Herklots, viz. water and wheaten cakes has generally been followed, and although not essential to its success, I did not consider myself justified in making any change, till I knew more of the power of the remedy; and there is reason to believe, that its stimulating qualities are prevented from being injurious and the absorption of the fluid hastened by the low regimen.[153]

Dr. Herklots gave fifteen drops of the oil twice a day, which, he states, mitigate the symptoms the se-

[153] The propriety of confining the patient to a wheaten diet, will be strengthened by the fact of the exemption from the disease, enjoyed by those who live on it. (See page 48.) Although this diet is low even to a native, it is sufficiently nourishing, and is more easy of digestion than rice and the other grains in common use.

cond day, and the œdema begins to lessen; on the fourth it is gone and the patient is much better; on the sixth or seventh day the medicine may be omitted, and is never to be continued more than fifteen. If it prove too heating the number of drops may be diminished. The diet is to be continued twice the time of the medicine, frictions are to be diligently employed, and blisters and tonics will often prove useful. He considers the treeak to have similiar but weaker virtues.

A purgative should be given at the commencement; I then order the oil in doses of from eight to fifteen drops twice or thrice a day. I took a number of notes regarding its effects on the pulse, but having lost them, I shall not venture to state the results from memory, but they were not uniform. Above twenty drops have caused abdominal uneasiness and dysenteric stools. The effect of the medicine first perceived, is a sense of heat in the stomach extending up the throat, and an extrication of flatus compared to that produced by peppermint. In many instances no other sensible effect follows, but frequently a general sense of heat is experienced, and a free perspiration breaks out some hours after and is not followed by exhaustion.[154] If there is, or even has been, ten-

[154] Dr. Herklots thus describes the sensible effects of the medicine, in two cases of hemiplegia of upwards of six months standing, in sepoys of the 14th regiment N. I who had been discharged the hospital as incurable. "In one "case there was *numbness* in both the affected upper and lower extremities, "with diminution of power of motion of the left half of the body, *but no œdema*; "while in the other, *there was œdema*, with diminished nervous energy, but "*no numbness*. By the use of the above remedy for ten or twelve days, the "one patient had completely got rid of all his insensibility; the other of his "œdema, though neither had improved in the more effectual use of their "limbs. During the exhibition of the medicine both complained of excessive "internal heat, (which one of the patients could latterly suffer no longer); "and they perspired constantly, though not freely. After the employment "of the above medicine for the before mentioned period it was omitted, and "agreeably to the native system, the very low diet of wheat cakes and water "continued for as many days, together with the use of the very powerfully "stimulating liniment denominated, in my report above alluded to, liniment. "ex resin. chloroxylon. dupad., but without benefit."

derness at the epigastrium it is inadmissible, and I have seen eight drops three times a day, bring back pain of stomach, a red fiery tongue and other symptoms of gastric irritability; and when there is a tendency to this affection, the medicine has little effect on the other symptoms.

Mr. Macdonell has found the black oil increase the action of the kidneys, which he ascribes to its direct effect on these organs, having detected the peculiar smell of the medicine in the fresh urine. He thus reports the result of his experience with it in mild cases. "After a purgative the oleum nigrum is given from five to six days, in which period the swelling is generally removed, leaving the limbs relaxed and flabby. As the swelling disappears the pulse comes down to the natural standard, or even below, and instead of being full, soft and round, it becomes weak, soft and feeble. In the graver forms of the disease, however, with a very frequent pulse, throbbing heart, &c. the black oil is a medicine not of sufficient power to be trusted; at the first I was inclined to give it a direct controling power over the heart's action, but in doing so, I am afraid I overrated its qualities. It is true that under its action the pulse is lowered, but this may be more correctly attributed to the stimulus of the effusion being removed. I may add that the diuretic effect of the black oil appears to be confined to cases of an asthenic diathesis, for I have given it in dropsical affections of prisoners in the Rajahmundry jall connected with organic obstructions, but without its showing its characteristic effects, as in beriberi. The direct diuretic effects will be seen in the following cases."

"Dandy Hommet, naigue, 41st regiment, admitted 17th November, 1831. Had fever for two days, but it has subsided, his legs and the anterior part of the abdomen are now numbed, but his thighs and hands are exempt, legs swelled and tense, with pain; tongue clean, urine high coloured, bowels irregular. Let him have an emetic immediately and afterwards two purgative pills. 18th. Vomited and purged yesterday. Pulse 80 and full. ℞ Ol. nigri gtt. x bis in die. 19th. The œdema less, urine increased. Cont. 20th. Urine much increased and the swelling diminished. Numbness the same. Cont. 22d. Swelling gone and his urine is less in quantity. Pains in the muscles the same. Omitt. ol. nigrum. Frictions with stimulating liniment, and to have five grains of sulphate of iron, morning and evening. 26th. Pains less. Pulse a little frequent, otherwise feels well. Cont. medicament. A flannel bandage to his legs. 4th December. The state of his limbs from his knees downwards continue the same, the pains are however gone, has a peculiar sensation at the heel of pricking but none at the toes, health good, but his tongue is white. Pulse firm. Cont. ferri sulphat. et pil. hydrarg. gr. x ommi nocte. On the 7th, took a dose of jalap. On the 14th, gums touched, tongue white, state of his limbs improving, pulse of a moderate strength. Repeat the jalap and omit the pill. 19th. Feels quite well, save a slight pricking at the soles of his feet, and he is discharged."

"Gooriah, naigue, 41st regiment, admitted 22d November, 1831. Has swelling and numbness of the legs, the latter also extends to the abdomen and hips, no fever or heat of skin, has been six days ill. Pulse feeble, urine high coloured and bowels irregular. Had a purgative of jalap and calomel with a few grains of ginger. 23rd. There is no pain in the limbs and the swelling is moderate, there is fulness of the epigastrium and a sense of weight. Pulse 96, had four stools. ℞ Ol. nigri gtt. x, bis in die sumend. 24th. Puffing less. Pulse 66 and feeble. Cont. 25th. Much better. 26th. Repeat the jalap and omit the oil. 27th. Bowels not well moved. Repeat the purgative. 28th. The puffy state of the stomach less and had eight stools. A little swelling observable to day over the shin bones. Rept. ol. nigrum. 1st December. Swelling gone and feels better, numbness less. Pulse good. Omit the oil. Frictions of volatile liniment. On the 4th the puffiness of the abdomen was felt during the night and his bowels are not regular. Urine high coloured and deposits a sediment. Pulse feeble. ℞ Pil.

Case 52nd. Tantiah, ætat. 35, a stout sepoy, had rigidity and total loss of power of the lower extremities without œdema. Pulse 76, small and weak; could not sit up in bed. Purgatives and oleum nigrum did no good, and *vomiting* with dyspnœa and loss of power of the upper extremities came on. The dyspnœa increased, œdema of shoulders, arms, and face supervened, and he died in a few days. The pulse was latterly only 64.

In comparing the oleum nigrum with the treeak farook, the former appears to me to have less power over the œdema and perhaps more over the nervous affections, and that it is through the latter effect only, that it removes the hydropic symptoms. In the following case, the œdema was not diminished till the palsy was relieved at the end of two months.

Case 53rd. Gooranah, a weakly man, ætat. 50, ad-

" hydrarg. gr. x ommi nocte. 5th and 6th. Continue the pill. 7th. Bowels " regular. Took the pill up to the 14th when his gums were touched. Puffi- " ness daily subsiding and numbness much better. Pulse feeble. ℞ Ferri " carbon. ℈j, pulv. rhei gr. vi, syrup. simplic. q. s. misce, bis in die sumend. " 23rd. Improving slowly and took a dose of oil. 1st January. Pains and " numbness entirely subsided and he feels well and went to his duty."

The failure of the black oil to increase the urine in cases of ordinary dropsy, and the apparent effect on the kidneys ceasing in the first of these cases as soon as the œdema had disappeared, confirm the more common opinion, that the black oil possesses no decided *direct* diuretic virtues. Mr. Macdonell seems to have been led by this opinion, to omit it as soon as the œdema was removed, and before its more important effects could be expected to have been produced. In regard to the effect on the pulse see note 93. It is also necessary to observe that Mr. Macdonell considers beriberi to be an asthenic disease, caused " by a long course of poor diet insufficient to sup- " port the energies of the nervous system and deteriorating the whole frame." The diet used by him along with the black oil differed from that recommended by Dr. Herklots, by the addition of a liberal allowance of milk. He also insisted on his patients generally, adopting a more nutritive plan of living than they had previously allowed themselves. " It is most fortunate for them, " that their appetite seldom fails. In the severe forms of the disease I di- " rect each man to be put on milk diet, two pints in the day, with a pint of " good arrow root congee at night, and for the less severe forms a pint of milk " for breakfast with the unleavened bread of the country, a good curry with " meat, and the alliaceous vegetables for dinner and a little more of this for " their evening meal, if so inclined. It is to this, that we must look for a per- " manent restoration to health. In the diet of sepoys the medical officer has " no control, and they are but too apt to neglect his advice on this very im- " portant subject, some from their necessities, and others from inveterate " habits, are disinclined to a full meal, on the plea that it heats them, but I " had to overrule this, knowing it to be a futile argument."

mitted March 1st. Has been long ill; was carried yesterday morning to the hospital, having lost the use of his legs which are stiff and numb. Weight at lower part of sternum and slight oppression at præcordia. Says he has no dyspnœa, but respiration is hurried on the least exertion. Pulse 80, weak; tongue clean, appetite slightly impaired. Had a purgative. Habeat olei nigri gtt. xv bis die. To use the dammer liniment (Liniment. resin. chloroxylon. dupad). 4th. No better; increased weight at chest, rested ill, slight œdema of feet. Pulse 88, stronger. Cont. medicament Emplast. vesicator. pectori. Habeat statim pulv. jalap comp. ʒj. 5th. Physic operated; the same. 6th. Œdema of feet increased, paralysis the same, pectoral symptoms relieved. 8th. Paralysis and œdema rather increased, slept badly from pain in the legs. Pulse 90, small; slight dyspnœa on exertion. Rept. pulv. jalap. Cont. alia. 12th. Much pain in the legs, no dyspnœa. Pulse 80; œdema the same, feet pit deeply. 16th. Chest well; pulse fuller. 20th. Numbness a little better, œdema the same. Omitt. ol. nigrum. 25th. Œdema rather less. Pulse pretty good. Has taken tincture of squills and digitalis with a little benefit to the swellings, and they are now omitted. Habeat ol. nigri gtt. viij bis die. 28th. Palsy and numbness the same, abdomen a little swollen. Pulse 70, small and irregular, sleeps ill. Habeat ol. nigri gtt. xv bis die. April 1st. Œdema gradually subsiding, the numbness is relieved and he sleeps very well. Ol. nigri gtt x. Pulv. jalap. c. m. 8th. Œdema has left the right foot, a very little still of left. 15th. Œdema not yet quite gone. Omitt. ol. nigrum. 24th. Not so well. Rept. ol. nigri gtt. viij. 29th. Is now able to walk and œdema entirely gone. May 2nd. Walks well. 10th. Discharged cured.

In an old case, where repeated relapses had left great emaciation, distressing pains, with partial loss of power of the limbs, the oleum nigrum did no good;[155] œdema continued until a flannel bandage was applied, when it disappeared. This patient took mercury when on the convalescent list, and was much the worse for it. The œdema has occasionally been observed to diminish a day or two before the numbness, pains, or palsy, and its diminition under the use of the oil *alone* may be considered a favourable sign as to these symp-

[155] The length of time during which the disease has existed, is not, of itself, sufficient to discourage us in the diligent use of this and other remedies, as will appear from the following case. It also impresses a most useful lesson; viz. that formidable trains of symptoms of long standing often depend on slight causes, admitting of alleviation or removal by appropriate remedies.

"Thomas Clynch, 14 February; his disease is of six years and four months "standing. On admission complained of the following symptoms, œdema of "both legs and feet, numbness from the groins down to the extremities of "the toes, of forearms and hands, and all over the head, with pain in all the "joints of the affected parts, feels his lower extremities rather weighty. Urg "seeah (oleum nigrum) bis in die. 16th. Numbness of head somewhat less. "Affrict. rowg. bulsan, (the dammer liniment). 19th. Some degree of sen-"sation in the scalp returned, œdema rather less, feels his right thigh some-"what lighter. 21st. Right thigh much lighter, some degree of feeling re-"turned in it, pain, œdema and numbness of other parts all diminished, "numbness of head nearly gone. 24th. Numbness of lower extremities des-"cended from the groin to above the knee; œdema quite gone, occasionally "returning however of an evening, but on assuming a recumbent posture dis-"appearing again; numbness of head completely removed. 28th Every "symptom relieved, but complains of great heat in the knees and legs. Omitt. "urg seeah. Cont. liniment. 10th March. Both legs lighter and numbness "less, left toe completely benumbed; not the slightest feeling in it, some de-"gree of sensation returned in the toes of right foot as well as in both soles "of feet and in the forearms; for the first time to-day is sensible of some de-"gree of feeling at the extremities of some of the fingers. Cont. liniment. "12th Can close his fists to-day, which he could not do before. 14th Has a "very slight degree of numbness above the outer angle of the right eye. In "other respects much about the same. Sumat pilul. ex acid. benzoic., croc. "sativ., et piper. nigri mane et vespere. 17th No numbness whatever of "thighs, legs easier, fingers much more flexible, numbness over the eye gone, "numbness of forearms has descended from the elbows to middle of forearm. "Cont. liniment. et pilul. 21st. Numbness descended to below the knees. "29th. Since the last four days some degree of œdema is visible every morn-"ing but disappears towards evening, chiefly about the ancles. Seven leech-"es to be applied round each ancle. 1st April. Pain of leg better, numb-"ness and œdema much the same. Habeat decoct. smilac. chinæ. Omitt. "pilul. et liniment. 5th. A couple of sinuses have formed on his leg which "discharge a small quantity of water, and are considerably swelled. Utat. "pediluv. cum decoct. ex smilac. chinæ, curcum. long., et folior. meliæ "azadiracht. bis in die." *Dr. Herklots' 1st half yearly report*, 1823.

Dr. Herklots left Chicacole at this time, but it appears from a subsequent report that the patient ultimately recovered.

toms; but if the absorption is caused by other means, the palsy may be obstinate, as in the following case.

Case 54th. Veerasoo, a stout man walked to the hospitalw ith difficulty in the 10th day of the disease; the next day he could not move his legs, and there were great numbness and loss of power of the upper extremities. Œdema was at once removed by a purgative, but his recovery was only partial after using the oleum nigrum a month. The numbness first diminished, then the palsy in the hands and lastly in the feet, so that he was able to walk about with crutches. In this case as in others, it was found, that the numbness and palsy had no fixed relation to each other, as might be inferred from these depending on affection of different parts. On the other hand, the lower extremities are always the first disordered and last cured, and the disease is most severe when the upper extremities are affected, being a proof of the disease being usually seated low in the spine and having a tendency to ascend. In many old cases, the œdema was not in the least diminished by the use of the oil, and often, in examples of this kind, no benefit was derived to the other symptoms; and in many it was necessary to continue the remedy for a long time, before its effects were obtained, as in the case of Gooranah page 319: and notwithstanding that Dr. Herklots says, that it should not be continued more than two weeks, I can state that it has not been found to do harm when taken for a much longer time. The early omission of the remedy in deferrence to his authority, has been often injurious and disappointed the hopes entertained of a cure.

Case 55th. Syed Budday. When convalescent from fever got beriberi, and lost the use of his legs. He was admitted 9th December and derived no benefit from remedies. On the 4th January was in a helpless state, hardly able to sit up in bed, limbs contracted, the legs being bent on the thighs and powerless, numb and painful; commenced with ten drops of the oleum nigrum twice a day. On the 13th numbness and pain had left him, and the limbs could be extended further. The oil was omitted, the improvement ceased and the symptoms were aggravated under the use of the black or dammer liniment, sinapisms, cajuput oil internally, and he returned to his village in a miserable state of emaciation and disease. The following case is still more instructive.

Case 56th. Shaik Ally was admitted 27th December having been in good health previously, except that he had pains of the lower extremities for some days before. His knees suddenly gave way under him when on guard, and numbness, palsy, and pains of the calves were complained of. The pains had left him, but the numbness was little diminished and he had a creeping sensation in his legs as if a worm were crawling up them on the 9th January, when the black oil was given him in *baugra juice.* 13th. Pain and numbness gone, no œdema, only complains of weakness. Omitt. ol. nigrum. Frictions and low diet to be continued. On 20th got full diet. On 2nd February had no power whatever of his legs. Went on leave and used treeak farook, and in July, when he was lost sight of, he was emaciated, weak, and complained of deficient power of the limbs but no numbness. The following cases illustrate several other points in the history of the disease, besides the success of the black oil in the paralytic rigidity of the limbs.

Case 57th. Shaik Abdul Hussain, sepoy, ætat. 50,

admitted 9th December, 1827. 10th. Has for some days complained of stiffness of the legs and thighs, with numbness of the former, accompanied with slight œdema of the ancles; skin rather hot, pulse 88. Five stools from a dose of jalap. Habeat calomel. gr. viij. Pulv. jalap. gr. xl. Habeat ol. nigri gtt. xv bis die et infricet. liniment. resin. chloroxyl. 11th. Is slightly worse the œdma having increased, and the numbness prevented him from sleeping well last night; pulse 86. Rept. pulv. purgans. Cont ol. nigrum. 12th. Had five stools from the purgative, thinks the numbness slightly less; the œdema is the same as yesterday, slept badly, pulse 86. Cont. ol. nigrum et liniment. 13th. The œdema is subsiding and the numbness is less, slept better, no heat of skin, complains of rigidity of the extremities. 16th. The numbness and œdema are gradually diminishing but the stiffness continues. Cont. 18th. The œdema has entirely subsided and he now only feels a slight numbness in his feet, had four stools from a purgative. Cont. ol. nigri min. viii bis die, et liniment. 20th. Complains only of slight stiffness and debility in his legs. Cont. 22d. Convalescent. Omitt. medicament. 23rd. Discharged.

Case 58th. Royapah, fifer, ætat. 40. Has anasarca of the face and body. Pains and numbness of legs of three days standing; pulse quick and strong, increased action of the heart. Bowels regular. Has a purgative and oleum nigrum. In three days *action of heart was natural,* and *œdema of face gone.* Pulse was still quick. On the 6th day numbness was diminished but belly and thighs were much swollen. On the 14th day there was only a little numbness remaining, and he was soon after discharged.

It is observed by Dr. Herklots that relapses are

rare when the oil is employed, and there is no doubt that the observation is for the most part correct; this patient however had another attack three months after, and again suffered from dyspnœa, increased action of the heart, œdema of the face, tumid belly; and as often happens in relapses, the œdema was great compared with the numbness and loss of power, probably from incipient organic disease and general debility. He was again relieved by purgatives and oleum nigrum. A relapse has been brought on by ague, and bark was then useful along with the oil. In the following example the same fact is illustrated, as well as the connection of the cardiac affection and œdema of the face, and the necessity of using frictions to the benumbed parts.

Case 59th. Roodray, ætat 40. Admitted 3rd December with œdema of the face and legs, lower extremities heavy and numb but power undiminished; increased and irregular action of the heart, pulse quick and full. Takes a purgative and fifteen drops of oleum nigrum twice a day. On the 9th, action of heart was regular and œdema of face gone, other symptoms the same. On the 18th, œdema of legs gone but numbness continued. In a few days under the use of frictions the numbness descended to the feet, and afterwards a heaviness of the feet only remained and he was soon after discharged.[156] In a man of the name of Shaik Hussein it removed anasarca, swelling of the neck, and œdema of the face with weight in chest and quick pulse; and at the time these patients were under treatment, a lad of 17, Shaik Madinah, was ad-

[156] In reviewing the rapid cures often performed by this remedy, it will be evident that the cause of the symptoms is neither effusion on the spine, inflammation, nor extreme venous congestion, over none of which is it likely, that it possesses direct powers of such sudden operation. It certainly may cure functional disorder preceding or following these. *Original note.*

mitted with beriberi; there were severe pains in the calves and down to the ancles with stiffness and numbness, evening exacerbations of fever and pain, violent action of the heart, weak hurried pulse, bad rest and emaciation. Rest and purgatives relieved the affection of the heart, but European medicines could do no more, and he remained long in hospital in the same state. The following case is remarkable in the nervous affection being evidenced only by the muscular pains, in the slow supervention of thoracic symptoms, their cure by diuretics, and the wonderful effect of the black oil, which induced the gentleman by whom it was given and little experienced in its effects, to doubt that it had any influence in the rapid cure after other remedies had failed.

Case 60th. Apanah, ætat. 24. Admitted July 12th, complaining of œdema of legs without numbness or palsy, no dyspnœa. Has taken medicine, supposed to be mercury, for the cure of pains of the lower extremities. Treated with purgatives, nitric acid, iron, &c. August 3rd. Swelling extends towards the pelvis with pains in muscles of thighs. Belly a little tumefied, urine scanty. Calomel and squills prescribed. 5th. Œdema increased, pain all over him, weight in chest and slight dyspnœa. Face bloated. Pulse quick and full, bowels costive, made no urine last night. Pulv. jalap comp. ℥j. 6th. Swelling has extended up the thorax, dyspnœa on any exertion. Face swollen, urine scanty. Calomel. gr. j cum pulv. scillæ ter die. To have a little gin. 8th. Breathing much impeded, œdema of abdomen and chest the same. 9th Better. 11th. Urine increased, œdema less and chest better. Uses cream of tartar. 22d. Has got rid of the *pectoral symptoms* and *œdema of face*. Pulse natural, urine more copious, but œdema is increased in lower limbs. Omitt. calomel. et pulv. scillæ. Gamboge four grains, with calomel. 24th. Less œdema, more urine. Tinct. scillæ gtt. xx, spt. æther. nitric. ʒss ter die. 29th. Same; œdema considerable. The oleum nigrum having been received, fifteen drops are given three times a day, and on the 1st September he is free from complaint, and is discharged on the 10th.

The oleum nigrum is useful in beriberi with low action, and we have seen it successful where the pulse was full and the action of the heart unusually strong. In the case of a sepoy (Venketsawmy) in whom the heart was acting violently, the pulse quick and full, with sensation of internal heat, green stools and hard swelling of the extremities, it effected a cure of these symptoms in six days; and in Chinniah, a sepoy, aged 30, suddenly attacked with numbness of upper and lower extremities, œdema of face and other symptoms of beriberi with quick full pulse, and fever taking on an intermittent character, nearly equal success attended it. The low diet so strictly enjoined, is probably with a view to obtain the effects of the medicine on the nervous system, without aggravating or inducing inflammation by its great stimulating powers.

That the most alarming affections in the cardiac region are rapidly removed by it cannot be doubted, but how far it may be safe to trust to it in the circumstances in which general bleeding has been recommended, I am not prepared to say; but believe that the secondary effects of the spinal disorder are not unfrequently of a character demanding the same treatment as if they were primary affections, and that a combination of all those means which experience has taught to be useful, will often be necessary to subdue so terrible a disease.

Many examples of failure of the oleum nigrum have come to my knowledge, and although the majority were old and confirmed cases beyond the reach of any medicine, some were not cured, from adhering to one method of treatment and neglecting the aid of auxiliary means. In a few, which I am not able to class under any general heads, except that in most, the spine was affected high in the back, it did not seem adapted to the state of disease, (see Ramasawmy's case at page 124). The remark of the native doctor regarding the failure of the treeak when there was no œdema, is confirmed by the following case, in which numbness round the lips, which is rare in the circars, was present.

A washerman got pains in the thighs and legs in April, followed by numbness, partial palsy of the lower limbs, tottering gait and pain of the loins; no œdema. In three days numbness of upper extremities and round the mouth supervened. The oleum nigrum had little effect and he was not cured, when lost sight of some time after.

In some of the preceding cases the black or chloroxylon liniment recommended by Dr. Herklots was used. It is formed by distilling nine ounces of dammer or the chloroxylon dupada resin and of benzoin, four ounces of the gardenia nuts, two ounces of white sanders wood and half an ounce of cloves and of camphor, which afford two pounds of the liniment; which is stated to relieve spasms, numbness and pain. I can say nothing as to the advantage of this over other liniments, but it appears to be a good combination, and from its cheapness and the confidence the natives place in it, is likely to be used more efficiently than the officinal combinations, always scantily supplied to hospitals, and to be superior to the common camphor oil, which is an inert preparation.

The oil has sometimes been administered in the juice of the goonta kulga (Tel.) or gulgura ("baugra," Duccanee), the Eclipta prostrata, which belongs to the natural family of the Corymbiferæ; which mostly possess oils both volatile and fixed, but are stated by Decandolle to have been little investigated. These virtues reside in the goonta kulga principally in the leaves and branches, which afford with boiling water a strong bitter decoction (extractive), and the seeds a fixed but no volatile oil, and a little bitter resin. The powers are not great, but they probably are a useful addition to the other medicine. The natives of Telingana ascribe to it virtues in jaundice and dropsy, as stated by Ainslie of the Verbesina calendulacea.

I shall conclude this essay by directing the attention of gentlemen residing in the south of India and the western coast, to a grey powder said to be employed with success by the native doctors in these parts. I procured a very small quantity from a man who bought it at a high price from a Malayalim practitioner, and appeared to have derived some benefit from it, in what appeared hopeless circumstances. It was irritating to the stomach and bowels in the dose of a few grains, was not a metallic oxide and seemed too heavy to be a vegetable powder; but the small paper I obtained did not admit of many experiments, and the doctor had returned to his native country when I was in his neighbourhood.

THE END.

APPENDIX A.

21st Regiment N. I.

The 21st regiment N. I. arrived at Ellore, from Kulladghee in the southern Mahratta country, in April 1830 and marched to Vizagapatam in February 1833. The remarks made in the monthly returns of this corps show, that many sources of error are to be avoided in drawing up tabular statements of sick when beriberi is present. (Note 4, page15.)

Abstract of diseases from which deaths occurred during the years 1830, 1831, 1832, *and* 1833, *respectively.*

DISEASES.	Remained last return.	Admitted in January.	February.	March.	April.	May.	June.	July.	August.	September.	October.	November.	December.	Total.	General Total.	No. of Deaths.	REMARKS.
1830.																	
Beriberi.........	0	0	0	0	0	0	0	0	0	0	1	1	0	2	2	1	
Palsy............	1	0	0	0	0	0	0	0	0	1	0	0	0	1	2	1	
Phthisis.........	0	0	0	0	0	0	0	1	0	0	0	0	0	1	1	1	
Rheumatism......	4	2	6	8	0	1	1	0	0	3	3	3	2	29	33	2	
Syphilis, &c	4	3	4	0	0	0	0	3	1	3	2	3	2	21	25	2	
Total..	9	5	10	8	0	1	1	4	1	7	6	7	4	54	63	7	
1831.																	From remarks made in the
Beriberi	0	0	0	0	1	0	1	0	3	1	10	4	2	22	22	0	monthly returns it appears
Consumption	0	0	0	0	0	0	1	0	0	0	0	0	0	1	1	1	that 3 of the fever cases ter-
Dropsy	0	0	0	0	0	0	0	0	0	2	1	0	0	3	3	3	minated fatally by beriberi;
Fever Intermitt...	5	6	5	4	1	2	3	3	6	13	5	6	40	94	99	4	and that the death of a se-
Do. Remittent...	9	4	0	0	0	3	2	0	3	1	4	7	15	39	48	5	poy which happened on the
Indigestion......	2	2	3	5	3	4	2	5	1	4	2	4	2	37	39	1	march from Condapilly, was
Inflam. External.	4	2	6	10	11	14	5	8	2	4	5	4	1	72	76	1	from the same disease.
Rheumatism.....	1	3	3	3	6	4	4	5	4	4	3	2	3	44	45	1	Six cases of indigestion, 9 of rheumatism, and 2 of fever
Total..	21	17	17	22	22	27	18	21	19	29	30	27	63	312	333	16	turned out to be beriberi.
																	Two deaths of beriberi oc-
1832.																	curred under the head of
Apoplexy........	0	0	0	0	1	0	0	0	0	0	0	0	0	1	1	1	rheumatism, and 2 of fever;
Beriberi	11	2	2	2	2	1	3	1	2	1	3	6	1	26	37	6	and numerous cases of indi-
Cholera	0	0	0	0	0	0	0	3	2	1	2	0	1	9	9	5	gestion, fever, &c. are noted
Cough	1	0	0	0	0	0	1	2	0	0	0	0	0	3	4	3	as having been beriberi, but
Fever Intermitt..	14	35	27	7	2	5	3	8	0	5	4	10	7	113	127	1	the number of these cases
Do. Remittent ..	14	7	3	2	0	4	3	10	22	1	4	7	2	65	79	2	remaining at the end of each
Rheumatism	8	1	2	5	4	6	8	10	4	1	3	5	2	51	59	2	month only being stated, it is impossible to determine
Total..	48	45	34	16	9	16	18	34	30	9	16	28	13	268	316	20	how many were fresh cases.
1833.																	* One man died sudden-
Beriberi.........	9	1	3	0	0	1	0	3	4	0	1	1	1	15	24	*0	ly of beriberi at Cassimcot-
Cholera..........	0	0	2	0	5	1	0	1	1	0	0	0	0	10	10	6	tah, and not having under-
Dysentery	0	0	1	0	1	0	0	0	0	2	2	0	1	7	7	1	gone medical treatment is
Fever Remittent..	7	4	10	6	3	0	3	7	2	28	6	5	1	75	82	†5	not included in the return.
Hepatitis........	0	0	0	0	1	0	0	0	0	0	0	0	0	1	1	1	† One died of beriberi
Insanity.........	0	0	0	0	0	0	1	0	0	0	0	0	0	1	1	1	and two of pulmonary af-
Palsy............	0	0	0	0	0	2	0	0	1	1	0	0	0	4	4	1	fection.
Rheumatism......	11	11	9	2	2	0	4	3	2	4	4	5	4	50	61	‡3	‡ One died of beriberi, one of diarrhœa and hectic,
Total..	27	16	25	8	12	4	8	14	10	35	13	11	7	163	190	18	and one of consumption.

APPENDIX B.

Prevalence of Beriberi in the interior of the Peninsula.

A number of cases of beriberi having been reported to have occurred amongst the troops composing the Nagpore subsidiary force, advantage was taken of the opportunity afforded by my return to Kamptee, immediately after the foregoing paper was transmitted to the Medical Board, to examine the records of several of the hospitals, which were kindly communicated by the medical officers in charge.

The regiments at that station are usually relieved from the northern division; it may therefore be supposed that they will be, for some time, subject to the diseases of the circars. To ascertain how far this was the fact, abstracts were made of the history of every case of beriberi which had occurred for some years previous to November 1833; and wherever it was practicable, the patients were themselves examined as to their former history, and whether they had similar symptoms in the circars, or had been on leave to these districts since the departure of the regiment from them.

The 22d Regiment N. I. arrived at Kamptee from Samulcottah the beginning of 1831, having left some men ill of beriberi in the hospital of that station. Of these, one, who had rejoined the regiment in the following April, relapsed in October and died. The second case occurred in a sepoy who had formerly suffered from beriberi, and was admitted in April 1832 with ulcerated sore throat, which was cured by mercury, acid gargles and blisters. On the 10th of May pains of the limbs were complained of, and were not relieved by sinapisms, guaiac and sulphur. On the 15th slight swelling of the face, hands, and feet supervened and there were slight palpitations. On the 16th the swelling had increased. Small doses of squills, blue pill and powder of digitalis were prescribed but without benefit, and on the evening of the 31st he complained of headach and dyspnœa. The pulse was 90, jerking, the skin cool and clammy, and notwithstanding the employment of sulphuric æther, the dyspnœa and coldness of the extremities increased, the eye became fixed and the pulse imperceptible, and he died on the 1st June. The third case appears rather to have been dropsy following fever, than beriberi. The fourth was a recruit who came to Kamptee from the circars with the 34th regiment N. I. in 1830.

Ramkisnamah, ætat. 23. Admitted 5th October 1832, with œdema of the lower limbs, puffy face, some numbness, appetite bad, sleeps ill. Pulse 76, tongue pale. Had calomel and jalap and infusion of cheyretta 8th. No better. Omit. infus. cheyrett. Rept. pulv. cathartic. Habeat olei nigri gtt. x ter die. 9th. General numbness. Urine not free, some dyspnœa, sleep disturbed. Pulse 80, small. 11th. Much better. 13th. Improves. Urine free. 17th. No complaint but of debility. 31st. Convalescent. He was readmitted with beriberi 17th November, and discharged 12th December. He had been twice in hospital with intermittent fever in July and once in September. I examined this patient in October 1833, when he appeared to be in excellent health. He said he had not suffered from numbness, and ascribed the disease to fever.

The 5th case is still more doubtful. Shashiah, ætat. 25, was admitted 24th November, with swelling of the face and ancles, palpitation of the heart and slight vertigo, no pain. Slight uneasiness of limbs; pulse 65 soft, tongue white. Jalap and calomel were prescribed, followed by five grains of the pil. ferri comp. three times a day. 27th. Much better. December 8th. Swelling nearly gone. Debility. 18th. Stronger, rests ill. 29th. No complaint. Discharged. This man was also examined in October 1833, when he was in good health. The action of the left ventricle seemed rather strong and diffused, but he was agitated. He stated that he had never suffered from numbness or palsy and ascribed his complaint to cholera and purging, of which he was discharged cured on the 15th November. He had suffered from fever once in August and twice in September 1831.

Two other cases having symptoms allied to those of beriberi occurred in November 1833, but although interesting in other respects they do not afford satisfactory evidence on the question now under consideration. The gums of both patients were swollen, of a deep red colour over the roots of the teeth with a pale line above and below. One of them had taken bazaar medicines previous to admission, and the other had had about twenty grains of calomel during the eight days he had been in hospital, before the state of the gums were observed. He had suffered from fever for seven days previous to the appearance of the œdema.

THE 7TH REGIMENT N. I. returned to the coast from Ava in 1826 and from 1827 to 1829 was stationed at Hyderabad, where no case of beriberi occurred. In the beginning of 1829 the corps arrived at Kamptee, having many men in the ranks whose constitutions had not recovered from the effects of the service in Burmah. Eight cases of anasarca having a resemblance in some of their symptoms to beriberi, are recorded in the journals of the regiment for the succeeding four years.

Hoosman Khan, ætat. 50, 11th September, 1830. Pain and sense of pricking in the legs and arms; the former œdematous. Face puffy and bloated, Pulse 120, tongue clean. Little appetite and has nausea after eating. Tremor of the hands. Uses calomel, squills, nitre, &c. 13th. Less œdema. Nausea and frequent vomiting. Urine scanty. Mouth slightly affected. Tinct. digital. min. xx, spt. æther. nitric. ℥j bis. 14th. Pulse *down* to 100. Mouth sore. Œdema increases in the evening. 16th. Action of heart seems violent and irregular, oppression in thorax compared to a rattling; swelling the same. Urine increased. Ptyalism. Omit. hydrarg. Cont. alia. 17th. No dyspnœa, nausea returned. 18th. Action of heart still violent, pulse at wrist less frequent and softer; still sick and vomits. Emplast. vesicator. præcord. 20th. Urine scanty. No swelling, or dyspnœa. 21st. Increase of œdema of feet. Omitt. digital. Ol. terebinthin. gtt. xv. 22d. Rigors followed by heat but no sweating at 1 P. M. 23d. More urine. Œdema the same. Pulse 96. 30th. Little œdema. Pulse 80. Mouth has got better and now takes calomel and opium. By the end of October he was rather better and recommended for change to the coast, but on the 31st, vomiting followed his forenoon meal, with dyspnœa and vertigo; no pain of head, pulse scarcely perceptible at the wrist, quick aud undulating in the carotids. Extremities cold. Two consistent stools. Æther and wine prescribed, but he got worse and died with great dyspnœa at 10 P. M. There was a case in some respects similar during October 1829, in which the anasarca was accompanied with dyspnœa and abdominal pain. The integuments of the chest and arms were much distended with fluid, and for some days before death there was so much swelling of the wrists that the pulse could hardly be felt; it was rapid, and "that of the carotids seemed more equable."

John Mackeen, drummer, A company, ætat. 30. September 29th 1830. Tense œdematous swelling of the lower extremities terminating by a hard margin at the hips. The hands and forearms are also affected. Complaint of two days standing. Functions reported natural. Pulv. cathartic. Vesp. One yellow stool. Tongue clean. No dyspnœa. Says he had a similar affection at Rangoon for which he was bled and purged. Calomel. gr. ij, pulv. antimon. gr. iss, quarta quaque hora. Ol. terebinth. gtt. x ex mist. camphor. ter die. October 1st. Œdema less. 4th. Urine increased. 5th. Pulv. cathartic. 6th. Less œdema. 8th. Rept. pulv. cathartic. 9th. No œdema. Discharged.

Moothoo, a robust sepoy, ætat. 31. Admitted 25th October, 1831, complaining of debility and œdema of the legs. Tremor when in the erect posture and has "loss of power and pain of the thighs." Pulse small and quick, tongue clean, bowels reported regular, urine high coloured and not scanty. Habt. stat. calomel. gr. iv, pulv. jalap. ℈j; postea ol. nigri gtt. xv ter die. 27th. Less œdema, stools scanty. Complains of pain in the lower extremities and also in the abdomen. A saline purgative, frictions, and 30 drops of the black oil prescribed. 29th. Considerable œdema about the chest. No abdominal pain. Pulse 80, weak. Urine does not coagulate by heat; dyspnœa, slept ill. On the 30th his pulse was slow and weak, his bands and feet became suddenly cold, the breathing laborious and irregular, and he died at 7. P. M.

The next patient had anasarca only, which was removed in six days by a purgative and black oil.

Another of these patients was admitted 29th July 1831 with œdema, cold extremities and dyspnœa, and died when talking, with a single struggle. He had no evacuations. Such cases are of frequent occurrence amongst native troops, whose constitutions have suffered from any of the fruitful sources of disease amongst them, such as fatigue and food to which they are not habituated, the effects of a moist climate on men accustomed to the dry atmosphere of the Carnatic, and from febrile influences. The successful illustration of this class of complaints, is of great importance to the Indian practitioner, but the prejudices of the natives to dissection and other causes, oppose almost insuperable obstacles to the investigation. I am not satisfied that any of the above cases are examples of beriberi. The following case is important from the relief afforded to the tingling sensations, by a blister to the loins.

Oomar Sahib, ætat. 33, robust, 21st December, 1831. Œdema of feet and legs. Sense of weight over the body. Pulse full and quick, urine high. Pulv. jalap. et calomel., postea ol. nigri gtt. xv ter. 25th. Less œdema. Pulse still quick. 27th. A little œdema. 30th. No œdema now perceptible. Omitt. ol. nigrum. 1st. January, 1832. Tingling and sense of pricking of the surface. Applict. vesicator. dorso. 4th. The pricking and tingling sensations have been removed by the blister. 5th. Convalescent.

Mr. Butler informs me, that a havildar of the corps who was on leave for recovery of his health in October 1833, was considered to have laboured under beriberi. He had paralysis of the lower extremities and occasional excruciating pain about the sacrum; and another man admitted about the same time was long paralytic, but gradually recovered and has had good health since.

THE 3RD REGIMENT LIGHT CAVALRY arrived at Kamptee from Arcot in 1829. Two cases occur in the journals as beriberi in 1831, two in 1832, and one 1833. In one of these there was numbness of the lower extremities with œdema and dyspnœa, and in another pains and numbness of both upper and lower limbs and, subsequently, slight œdema and tremors of the legs. The other three cases also resembled some forms of beriberi; and from enquiries made by Mr. Stokes who communicated the histories, none of the patients had been in the circars. It is impossible however to draw any positive conclusion on a subject involving so many sources of mistake, from so few cases occurring during so long a period. They all occurred the latter end of the rains, yet certainly want that endemic character so remarkable in beriberi; and even if they are allowed to have been examples of that disease as I am inclined to think they were, the fewness of the exceptions confirm the general truth of the observations made at page 39.

The detailed histories of several well marked and interesting cases of beriberi which occurred in the 11th regiment N. I. at Hyderabad, have been furnished by assistant surgeon Burrell. This corps left the circars 1830, but the liability to the disease does not seem to have been removed by time, as the year in which most of the cases occurred was unusually dry. The gums of one of the patients, I observed to be exceedingly pale with some lividity at the edges, but the patient was otherwise in a cachectic state.

A few examples of dropsical and paralytic affections have been observed in Europeans at Nagpore which have been supposed to be cases of beriberi. An interesting case of this kind occurred to Mr. Geddes in a soldier (James Dooly) who was employed as a clerk. In April 1829 he had anasarca, scanty urine and the gums were red and spongy. He was treated with calomel, squills, cream of tartar, &c. Salivation took place on the 5th day without any immediate effect on the disease. He was then allowed two measures of gin and was discharged on the 10th of May. He was re-admitted on the 13th, with general anasarcous swellings, increasing in his legs on walking about. Pulse 84, strong; urine very scanty, appetite good. He was put on a full diet with six oranges daily, and was purged by calomel and jalap. On the 18th the pulse had come down to 60, the œdema had disappeared, his urine was of natural quantity, and he was discharged. From this time until October 1832 he continued in good health with the exception of a slight attack of indigestion and disordered bowels, which kept him in hospital for ten days. "On the 17th October 1832 he was admitted, having "been affected from last night with pains and feeling of numbness in the "calves and shins of both legs, and partially in the knees, and after sitting "for a little or walking, the legs became considerably swollen assuming a "tense appearance and a bluish hue. The gums were at the same time "evidently swelled, red, and he said they very readily bleed. Had also been "feverish for two days, and his pulse was 100, and skin somewhat heated "on admission. Bowels were regular, and appetite good. From the following "day he was put on a diet of two pints of milk morning and evening, in "addition to the regulated half diet of the hospital, with six oranges daily and "lemonade for drink. For the first two days of being under treatment, "he had sulphate of quinine succeeded by bark, and the pulse gradually "came down in frequency, being by the 23rd at the natural standard. "He had also six doses of jalap in the course of twenty four days, some spirit "of nitrous æther for a few days, the acid. sulphuric. dilut. with the bark; "and on the 2nd of November, ℥ij of lime juice were substituted for the acid "and were given four times a day. Turpentine frictions were also used, "which completed the treatment employed. The following are extracts "from the reports of its effect. On the evening of the 18th pulse was 88, "pretty calm, 'has felt more numbness and loss of power in his hands to-"day.' 20th. Makes no complaint but of the numbness, which is as before. "Appears to walk a little more steadily, and to direct his feet more pointedly "than before. 23rd. Thinks he can walk better, but has darting pains in the "calves of his legs, on stretching them out. 27th. Pulse 64, skin natu-"ral, can walk a good deal more steadily, and with less delay in raising "his feet, the calves of the legs are also not so distended in walking, and do "not put on so turgid an appearance. 31st. Thinks he has more use of his "hands although he could not write with them, and on the 2nd November it "was all he could do to cut his meat, but he had not power to cut the bread. "He walked however pretty steadily; stretches out his leg firmly but had a "pain in the upper part of the calf in doing so. On the 10th continued to "improve, and could walk without assistance excepting of a stick, while for-"merly he required a man to support him either on one or both sides. On "the 18th he could write a little, and on the 26th it is reported that 'he "can now walk steadily and raise himself easily, still a good deal of pain and "tenderness increased by pressure in the calves of the leg and up to the "ham.' On the 28th he was discharged convalescent with instructions to "continue the exercise, &c. as much as possible. He did not however conti-"nue to improve in the same degree as when in hospital, and it was judged "proper in January, to give him the benefit of change of air, &c. by removal "to the coast." In September 1833 Mr. Geddes saw the patient at Masulipatam; he had regained the use of his limbs and was nearly restored to health, but there was still slight redness of the gums. This patient was seen by several other experienced practitioners who acknowledged that his gums were spongy, and the case was considered to require the antiscorbutic treatment which was adopted.

The case is undoubtedly important, but similar symptoms have frequently arisen from very different causes, and much caution is therefore requisite in admitting conclusions derived from individual cases. The following history will show that the spongy gums may have been caused by obstruction to the circulation in the liver. More decided examples might be adduced, but as the case was transferred to my care on the sixth day of treatment as an instance of beriberi occurring in an European at Nagpore, and as the apparent effects of the interrupted circulation in the lungs on the vessels in the spinal canal illustrate the observations made at page 119, it is selected for insertion here. As

I have reason to believe that the case belongs to an important and obscure class of affections not very uncommon in India, the history is extracted at length from the hospital journal, with the omission of a few immaterial daily reports.

Geo. White, Madras European regiment, aetat. 26, in India 9 years. Admitted 10th June 1833 with œdematous swelling of both legs. No fever, tongue clean. Habeat pulv. jalapæ comp. ʒj. 11th. Purged three times, swellings less. Rept. pulv. purgans. Vesp. Swelling extending up to the trunk, no pain, has passed no urine. Pulse 86, rather small. He voided urine frequently in the night which showed some cloudiness on being boiled. A moist exudation was observed on the feet on the 12th. On the 13th numbness of the feet was complained of, the pulse was natural. On the 14th the swelling was less and had become soft, but on the 15th it had again increased. He had used only a very small quantity of the black oil. On the 16th I took charge of the patient. 16th. Swellings increase towards evening, scrotum distended, some abdominal fluctuation, urine said to be pretty natural, some short cough, which he thinks did not precede the swelling. Thinks himself better, gums white and have bled for 8 years on cleaning the teeth. Tongue white, much thirst. Omit. medicament. V. S. ad ℥ xij. Rept. pulv. jalap. comp. Cream of tartar ℥ss. 17th. Blood strongly buffed, hardly any uneasiness or cough since; urine pretty free, of rather deep colour, one pint in the night, sleeps ill and starts out of sleep. Pulse 70, small and a little sharp; otherwise as yesterday, 3 stools. Rept. V. S. ad ℥ vj. Continue the cream of tartar. 18th. Blood slightly buffy, urine coagulated strongly, no difference in the swelling except that the face is puffy. Respiration free, slept better. Pulse 80, small and soft, four stools of good appearance. Continue cream of tartar ℥j. Habeat tinct. digital. gtt. xxx, tinct. scillæ gtt. xv ter die. Has no pain of the back now, but has been subject for a year to pains on each side of the lumbar vertebræ. They came on after a liver complaint, and he thinks they may be caused by sitting or working at his trade of tailor; urine has never been obstructed. 20th. Urine more than a pint in the night, scanty yesterday, and swellings increase in the evening, rested well, feels much better and numbness is diminished. Pulse 84, small, two stools, tongue pretty clean, cough nearly gone. Rept. pulv. jalap. comp. Cont. alia. 21st. Four stools, urine rather freer, pale, and only slightly coagulable. *Face more swollen in the morning and the feet less.* Pulse 96 small, a little sleep. One pint of milk instead of sago at dinner. 24th. Improves, swelling of legs subside and are lax. Face natural, feels better, urine pale and copious. Pulse 70. Thinks the milk binds him. Slight cough, tongue white. Cont. medicament. Habt. pulv. jalap. comp. Chicken broth. Omit the milk. 26th. Urine increased, pale, smelling strongly and not coagulable, œdema the same, cough now slight and only after sleep in the morning, no starting from sleep. Cont. medicament. ℞ Calomel. gr. ss, pulv. scillæ gr. iij. Fiat pil. ter die sumend. 28th. Sweats much. Pulse 70, small and soft. Omitt. haust. Cont. pil. et supertart. potassæ. 29th. The same. Urine 40 oz. pale, ammoniacal with some white deposit, cold sweats over the legs only, swelling goes down slowly. Less thirst. Two stools a day. Pulse 60, small. Cont. med. Rept. pulv. jalap. comp. 30th. Five stools only, 24 oz. of urine, swelling diminishes slowly, numbness confined to the instep and soles, no starting from sleep, abdomen full and fluctuation is pretty distinct. Cont. pilul. et potass. supertartrat. Rept. pulv. jalap. comp. July 1st. Much purged, urine only 14 oz. but made it several times at stool. Cont. pil. et supertartrat. potass. Rept. haust. tinct. digital. ut antea. 4th. Urine 44 ounces, pale. Same. Slept ill, no starting, numbness as it leaves the legs is followed by soreness of the skin. Pulse 72, soft. Gin ℥iij. Rept. pulv. jalap. comp. Cont. alia. Spoon diet. Bread pudding. 5th. Much purged, swelling diminished, urine 30 ounces, ammoniacal with white sediment, slept well, tongue a little white. Cont. medicament. 6th. Urine two pounds, cold sweats in the night, Pulse 68, soft and weak, less thirst. Omitt. haust. Cont. pil. Habeat pulv. jalap. comp. ʒj. Habeat ter die spt. æther. nitric. ʒj. 7th. Several stools yesterday and in the night, urine only one pound, reddish. Face and skin of chest puffy. More swelling of abdomen. Cont. pil. et spt. æther. nitric. et supertartrat. potass. 8th. Urine again increased and reddish, two pounds and ten ounces. Feels better and puffiness of face has disappeared. Cont. 14th. Urine 2℔, red and acid, bowels loose yesterday and swelling in the legs rather larger since yesterday, ascribed to the rains. Tongue pretty clean. Gums felt a little tender yesterday. Omitt. pilul. Cont. alia. 15th. Purged since the rains, stools good, urine 2℔ 10 oz. Cont. 18th. Puffiness in limbs and dropsical effusion in general over the body, bowels moved four times, has voided urine of straw colour. Cont. 25th. Legs perhaps less swollen, arms much more so and the thighs are œdematous, face puffy, slept well. Pulse 80, small, bowels open, urine from 2℔ 12 oz. to 1℔ 10 oz., tongue pretty clean, gums spongy and white, no numbness or indeed any uneasy sensation unless from bulk of limbs. Ol. nigri gtt. viij ter die. Half diet. 26th. Gin one measure instead of the wine. 28th. The urine is now 2℔ 3 oz., ammoniacal with a heavy white deposit. Feels easy. Face puffy, rested rather badly. Cont. medicament. 31st. Urine 2℔ 12 oz. not coagulable, clear and reddish, no change for the better, breathing oppressed in the recumbent posture and on the slightest exertion, tightness round the whole thorax. Pulse 80, feeble; scrotum less swollen, abdomen more so, tongue rather white. Omitt. medicament. Augt. 1st. Same. Urine 2℔, pale and ammoniacal, some short cough, loins œdematous with some aching numbness ascribed to lying in bed, and says it goes off when he is able to move about. V. S. ad ℥viij. 2nd. Slept, but badly in the night, breathing improved, urine as before and pretty copious, says he is much the same, bowels open. Blood buffy in patches. Urine not coagulable although clear. 3rd. Slept better last night than usual, bowels lax, urine as before, sediment white. 4th. Breathing easier, urine only one pound since last report. Pulse 88 and rather oppressed, tongue white but clean, œdema the same. Rept. V. S. ad ℥ xvj. Habeat tinct. digital. min. xxv quater die. Habeat omni nocte pilul. ex calomel. gr. ij, pulv. scillæ gr. iij. 5th. Blood buffy, some relief to breathing but there is still tightness across the chest and respiration is hurried. Bad rest in consequence of being purged, gums white and swollen. Pulse 92, small and rather sharp but easily compressed. Cont. medicament. Spoon diet. Rice pudding. 6th. Urine scanty, ammoniacal with sediment, obliged to sit up in bed, little cough, general uneasiness ascribed to want of sleep, pulse 100, small. Cont. pilul. ter die, et tinct. digital. quater. Cream of tartar ℥ss in the day. 8th. Two pounds of urine made, feels better, slept towards morning. Five stools of dirty greenish brown slimy feces with whitish mucus and a little jelly-like secretion; face less puffy. Cont. medicament. 9th. Improves a little, but if he lies either on right side or back the breathing is disturbed and if he is asleep he is awoke. Cont. omnia. 11th. Urine 1℔ 8 oz. high coloured and clear, was ammoniacal with deposit yesterday, slept pretty well, breathing freer, much swelling of abdomen. Pulse 72, soft. Cont. medicament. 12th. Felt sick and low yesterday and digitalis was omitted, urine high coloured, stools rather pale and slimy, slight griping. Pulse 84, very small and easily compressed. Omitt. digital. Cont. alia. 15th. A good deal purged for several days and a quantity of clear mucus is mixed with the stools, which are thin and greyish yellow, little griping, no straining. Had oil on the 13th. Pulse 80, gums a little tender and white, tongue pale red with thin white fur, foul taste. Omitt. pilul. Ol. ricini ℥ss. Rept. tinct. digital. min. xxv ter die. 16th. Stools from oil pale and feculent, 3 in the night of white mucus passed easily, urine yesterday ammoniacal with deposit, in the night clear and red and without smell, respiration more full. Pulse 88, small and oppressed. Cont. tinct. ℞ Pulv. Doveri gr. vj, pulv. scillæ gr. ij. Fiat pulv. bis die sumend. 17th. Vesp. Many stools of grey thin feces mixed with mucus passed easily. Complains much of weakness. Pulse small. Omitt. med. ℞ Calomel. gr. x, pulv. Doveri gr. xij. Fiat. pulv. h. s. s. 18th. Five pale feculent stools in the night which he passed pretty easily, says he has not been quite well since leaving Masulipatam from liver and pains. Had rheumatism with swelling of joints and shins for which he was salivated, never had venereal disease before that. Had bubo long after to which liver succeeded. Soreness of lower part of abdomen. Rept. calomel. et pulv. Doveri bis die. Infric. hypochond. dextro unguent. hydrarg. camphor. ʒss ter die. 19th. Vesp. Asleep at morning's visit but rested ill, many whitish stools in the night, six to-day of yellow feces with a little mucus, face more puffy, nausea from powder, and brought up that taken to-day with bile. Pulse 100 small and regular, skin soft, foul taste of copper, gums hardly sore. Calomel. gr. x, opii gr. ij, h. s. 20th. An easy night but did not sleep. Three natural stools with a slight mixture of mucus, urine much increased, made 65 oz. since yesterday morning, less puffiness of face and he looks better. Pulse 92, small and pretty firm. Habeat tinct. digital. ℈ss ter die. Vespere. Feels worse. Five stools of scybalous, and pale watery feces and mucus tinged with blood. Pulse quick and small, cold sweats, breathing the same. Rept. calomel. et opii h. s. Enema emollient. statim. 21st. No stool since he had the pill, three before that of yellow feces mixed with muddy coloured dejections and mucus, sweated much but had a good night, urine 2℔ 6 oz. pretty natural. Pulse 92, gums not yet sore, breathes with more difficulty on his back and having turned on it in his sleep felt oppressed. Ol. ricini ℥ss. Rept. tinct. digital. bis die. Milk diet. Habt. h. s. calomel., opii, aa, gr. ij. 23rd. Two small thin pale stools with an irregular spot or two like blood on the surface, urine 2℔, clear. Pulse 80. Much œdema of abdomen; on lying on his back, feels as if a weight were pressed on the pit of stomach, there was formerly tenderness here. Rept. tinct. digital. bis die et pil. h. s. Cont. unguent. 28th. Urine 2℔ 8 oz., gums very sore, spits none, nausea in the evening. Cont. pil. Omitt. tinct. digital. 29th. Urine 3℔ 10 oz. natural, feels much better, rested well, 3 stools. Pulse 80. Omitt. medicament. 30th. Asleep yesterday, stools more natural, less frequent and there is no abdominal pain. Respiration rather freer. Pulse smaller. Feels very weak and sense of weakness and of cold across his loins. Eats very little. Sweats. Urine free. Vespere. Slight headach for two or three days, worse this evening, stools yellowish, frothy with a little slime, slight warmth of skin of head and body. Enema purgans statim. 5th October. Has continued much the same; coughs occasionally and uses ammoniac, tinct. camphor. comp. and squills; liniments and bandages to the legs. 24th. Has taken the treeak farook pills for fourteen days and thinks the swellings are less tense and feels himself lighter and better, respiration freer but part of the change is to be ascribed to the weather which is fine, thighs and legs are tense and greatly swollen and abdomen much distended with fluid. Less œdema of the trunk but it extends to neck, face puffy but less so and there seems no swelling of arms. Respiration not quite free on the back but much more so than some time ago. Bowels loose, stools sometimes white, at others green or brick dust coloured. Pulse 94 to 100, small, tongue red, smooth with irregular sulci, back weak, no deposit in urine, chest sounds pretty well and respiratory murmur distinct, slight ægophony posteriorly; sound on percussion and respiratory murmur natural around the cardiac region. 26th. Feels much worse, frequent purging with nausea and vomiting, signs of effusion into the thorax with acute pain in the lumbar region. Pulse 100. Œdema of face and hiccup, urine free. Omitt. pil. Applicent. hirudin. xij part. dolent. ℞ æther. sulphur., æther. nitric., āā, ℨss, tinct. opii gtt. xxx, mist. camphor. ℥ss. 8 A. M. Vomited the draught. Rept. haust., cum tinct. opii gtt. xxx et sine mist. camphor. Vesp. Retained the second draught, no stool, no urine, pulse rapid, some slight dyspnœa, ℞ Liquor. acet. ammon. ℨj, spt. æther. nitric. ℨj, aquæ ℥ss. 27th. Passed a better night, no vomiting, purging, or pain of loins but a general feeling of acute pain and tenderness over the abdomen, pulse the same as yesterday, passed about half a pint of a dark reddish urine, tongue smooth. 27th. Died at 11 A. M.

Dissection. *Head and spine.* Veins of the dura and pia mater congested. Substance of the brain, especially the cortex and cerebellum, rather soft. About an ounce and a half of water in the ventricles. During the dissection much serous fluid flowed from the cellular substance, which was every where distended with the dropsical effusion; there was also considerable congestion of the veins, from the cut extremities of which the blood flowed. This was most remarkable over the superior vertebræ, and the state of the parts exterior to the theca spinalis could not in consequence be satisfactorily ascertained. A coagulum of blood of a dark colour and slightly elastic, with some deep coloured serum, was found in the lumbar region completely surrounding the cord and a slight appearance of the same kind extended as high as the cervical vertebræ. The cord was not diseased.

Thorax. The inferior portion of both lungs adhered to the diaphragm by recent adhesions, and the veins of the diaphragm were much distended with blood. A considerable quantity of muddy fluid was found in both cavities of the chest. The lungs were rather contracted in size, the inferior lobes were infiltrated with fluid, and the superior and anterior parts were natural. The pericardium and heart appeared to be healthy.

Abdomen. There was a very large quantity of a pretty clear fluid in the abdominal cavity, in which a few fibrinous strings were found lying on the peritoneal surface and amongst the folds of the small intestines, but there were no adhesions. The liver was small and converted into a mass of hard tubercles of different sizes, separated from each other by cellular structure. Its surface was marked by sulci corresponding with the structure surrounding the tubercles. Many of the vessels appeared to be obliterated by the altered structure of the viscus, and others seemed to be enlarged. No bile was found in the hepatic ducts. The gall bladder contained a dark tough mucous fluid. The spleen was of a slate blue colour. The kidneys were large with considerable increase of pale cortical substance, which was most remarkable on the right side where it encroached on the internal structure of the gland, which had also an unusually pale striated appearance. The superficial blood-vessels were enlarged, and in one of the glands there was some appearance of extravasation under the lining membrane of the pelvis. Half a pint of reddish urine in the bladder. The intestines were healthy externally. The whole internal coat of the duodenum was of a milky white appearance and distinctly œdematous. This last appearance was less evident in the other small intestines, but commenced again in the colon and nearly closed up the rectum. On cutting through the mucous surface much clear serum could be squeezed out from the subjacent cellular substance. There were a few slight honey-comb excoriations of the mucous coat of the ileum."

APPENDIX C.

The following extracts from the half yearly reports of Mr. W. Turnbull, garrison surgeon of Bellary, on the health of the prisoners in the jail at that station, confirm the opinions stated in the text, of the connection of many symptoms of beriberi with disease of the heart and pericardium. There is good reason to doubt, however, whether the disease was the same complaint as that we have described. The prevalence of sickness in the jail is ascribed by the superintending surgeon "to the state of the country and population "consequent on the failure of the usual supply of rain. Prisoners crowded "into the jails in proportion as distress and starvation became more and "more pressing. Hunger and poverty naturally engendered crime; and, "as might be expected, the wretched individuals admitted under these cir"cumstances were peculiarly liable to the invasion of disease; more especi"ally when congregated in greater numbers than the jails were originally "calculated to accommodate." In this state of things it has been found, that a great proportion of the deaths has taken place, in every jail, amongst the prisoners who had been recently committed; and that the most fatal diseases were dropsy and diarrhœa, usually attacking the same individual at the same time or alternately. It also appears from the returns of the jail of Bellary for the second half of 1833, that a great proportion of the casualties were caused by the same complaints, and Mr. Smith, the present garrison surgeon, informs me, that the cases returned as beriberi which he had seen had no paralytic or spasmodic affection, and that he did not consider them to be examples of that disease. Through the kindness of Mr. Turnbull and of Mr. Smith I have received a collection of the detailed cases, from which it would appear that the paralytic symptoms of beriberi were in most instances wanting, or only appeared in the latter stages. Mr. Hoskins the apothecary attached for many years to the garrison and by whom the cases were carefully observed, never saw a disease of the kind before the very dry season of 1832-33.

It is, however, remarkable that the decided symptoms of inflammatory cardiac disease observed by Mr. Turnbull were wanting in the jail dropsies of other stations, although a tendency to affection of the heart was detected at Nellore and other places, where the disease had certainly nothing else in common with beriberi. In general, the old, diseased and worn out subjects were the principal victims, the gums were occasionally livid, and the tongue like soaked leather. The appearances on dissection were more or less effusion (not often very extensive) into the cavities of the abdomen, pleura and sometimes into the pericardium. The liver and spleen were often small and pale; the colon was frequently found thickened and ulcerated, the whole intestinal mucous membrane red and pulpy as if covered with red currant jelly, and the intestines full of thin feculent or pultaceous matters such as were passed during life. In other instances, the intestines were uniformly pale and preternaturally transparent and no structural alteration could be detected; occasionally, however, some marks of subacute inflammation of the peritoneal coat of the cæcum and ascending colon were observed. Pain could seldom be detected on pressure, and the patient had in his despondency and hopelessness no other answer to any question but "I am well." Many of these patients died suddenly. Mr. Cooper at Nellore found the valves of the heart red in one or two instances, which he was inclined to ascribe to scurvy; the substance of the heart was pale and attenuated in others, and in some the right cavities were enlarged and this seemed to be indicated by a fluttering sensation experienced on laying the hand over the heart. Benefit was derived from a small bleeding when the state of the pulse admitted of it. A peculiar puffy appearance of the face was usually amongst the first indications of the disease, whether in the abdomen or chest. The cases referred to by Mr. Turnbull had no diarrhœa, and the intestines appear to have been healthy.

Extracts from the half yearly reports of the jail of Bellary.

1st half of 1832. "The sick list during the last six months has been rather "heavier than usual, and a good many casualties have also occurred. From "the circumstance of the Bellary jail having been constituted a general de-"pot, there have been frequent drafts from Chittoor and Salem, and a good "many of them were soon admitted into hospital with dysenteries, seve-"ral of whom died. This may be accounted for by the depressing influence "of a removal from their country and friends, and from some change in the "nature of their food or drink. Old men were the greatest sufferers, and "I constantly observed that when any of this description were seriously at-"tacked either with dysentery or fever, the powers of the constitution were "too feeble to struggle strongly against the disease, a desponding apathetic "state of mind soon succeeded, with indifference to life, and disinclination "to take food or medicine."

2nd half of 1832. "A good deal of sickness has prevailed in the jail of Bella-"ry during the last six months, and more than the usual proportion of deaths, "but for neither of these can I assign any sufficient reason, as no change has "taken place in dieting or working the prisoners; and I can only ascribe it "to a peculiar state of the atmosphere caused by the failure of the N. E. "monsoon. The complaints were those generally met amongst bodies of pri-"soners, but aggravated in fevers, dysenteries and other acute diseases by "despondency and lowness of spirits, and, perhaps latterly, from apprehen-"sion in observing the fate of many admitted with affections similar to their "own. A great many when apparently convalescent lost their appetite, be-"came leucophlegmatic, and eventually anasarcous, which went on to gene-"ral dropsy, ending in death in spite of all treatment, which in fact seem-"ed to have very little effect. Several of these cases resembled in many of "their symptoms *beriberi*, and were treated as such with calomel and squills, "digitalis, active purgation, &c. but without any benefit. As I had long "thought in this complaint that the heart was much implicated, and that "disease of that organ would best account for many of the symptoms in this "formidable and nearly unmanageable complaint, I determined, with the "concurrence of the zillah judge, to make some post mortem examinations "of any well marked cases that should come under observation, and an op-"portunity soon occurred. A patient was admitted on the 25th December

" with well marked symptoms and died on the 1st January, 1833. The body " was examined eight hours after death, in the presence of Mr. assistant " surgeon J. Thomson, 31st regiment and the hospital attendants. General " appearance robust and without much watery distension, except in the up- " per and lower extremities and face. The abdominal viscera seemed ge- " nerally healthy, except the liver, which was enlarged and of a peculiar " mottled greyish appearance. On raising the sternum found it adhering " strongly to the pericardium, which was thickened and adhering to the left " lung and pleura, as also strongly to the diaphragm. More fluid than usual " in the cavity of the pericardium but not that dropsical effusion that might " have been expected. A considerable quantity of fluid was also found in " the cavity of the chest generally. Heart enlarged but this appeared to " be caused principally by distension, as both ventricles were found gorged " with fluid blood. A considerable quantity of an albuminous deposit of the " consistence of boiled white of egg and evidently the product of active inflam- " mation was found in each ventricle, strongly attached to the parietes of the " heart which also bore strong traces of inflammation. These deposits or " masses of coagulable lymph were very peculiar, and no wise resembled the "coagula frequently discovered on opening the heart, were very tenacious, and " of a yellow purulent appearance and as far as this single case and dissecti- " on bears, seems to point to the true source of the disease, and that the pa- " ralysis and weakness of the limbs, the œdema of the extremities gradually " mounting upwards, the general anasarca afterwards, the orthopnœa and " anguish shortly preceding dissolution, may all be traced to impaired and " obstructed action at the source of the circulation, and that the true disease " is inflammation of the substance of the heart."

1st *half of* 1833. " The most fatal disease has been the beriberi from " which no less than twenty-six have died. One half amongst the convicts " and the other amongst those under trial, and as the latter are in the pro- " portion to the former, of scarcely one to three, this may lead to some re- " flections on the cause and nature of the complaint. In my last half year- " ly report I ventured some remarks on this subject, and suggested my im- " pression that inflammation of the heart and its involucra would account for " many of the symptoms of this disease, and in support of my belief gave " the result of one necroscopic examination which appeared to bear me well " out. Since then I have dissected seven more bodies and in every one were " found strong marks of inflammation of the heart and pericardium. The " appearances were nearly all alike and closely resembled the examination " described at some length in my last report. The patients were uniformly " healthy strong looking men with much adipose substance in the cellular " tissue, and as the seizures occurred in a greater proportion amongst the " prisoners under trial who lived a life of indolence with ample food and no " labour, might it not be inferred that the plethora thus induced, produced an " inflammatory diathesis which by some unaccountable or unexplained cause " fell upon the organ at the source of the circulation and terminated in the " train of symptoms usually denominated beriberi, but which I would rather " designate as pericarditis. The treatment has been copious bleeding on " admission generally and locally, free purging with salts and antimonials, di- " gitalis, squills, and calomel, semicupium, frictions and bandages to the " lower extremities, &c.; and though the practice has not been particularly " favourable, still I think it is as much so as might be expected in so formi- "dable a complaint."

It appears from the cases and information communicated by Mr. Smith, that although V. S. and pretty large doses of calomel lessened the symptoms for some days, that they for the most part returned with increased violence and destroyed the patient. Afterwards, free leeching to the region of the heart along with small doses of calomel (half a grain), digitalis and squills were employed with much better effect.

It may not be out of place here to remark, in reference to the observations made at page 230 as to the occurrence of water in the pericardium in the corbutic dropsy of lascars, that Mr. Charles Anderson, surgeon of the free trader Orient in which numerous deaths occurred in 1816 amongst a body of native passengers from England, found water in the thorax and abdomen, the pericardium distended with fluid, and the heart enlarged and full of blood. There were also signs of abdominal inflammation, the intestines were much contracted especially the colon; the stomach was inflamed both externally and internally, and the liver was paler in colour than in the healthy state.

APPENDIX D.

Prosper Alpinus in the 8th, 9th, 10th, 11th, and 12th chapters of the 4th book of his work "de Medicina Ægyptiorum" gives a very particular account of the treeak farook (Tharach faruk), which in his time (1591) was prepared in Cairo under the authority and for the use of the Sultan. "Accedit "etiam, quod id medicamentum apud omnes Ægyptios in frequentissimo est "usu, quando ferè ad omnes morbos ea gens theriaca utatur. Locus, in quo "eam componunt, est templum, urbis Cayri præclarissimum, Morestan voca-"tum. In eo omnes medici jussu præfecti, cum archiatro medicorum, sive "principe, quem Achim—Bassi appellant, simul conveniunt, mense Maio "ferè semper, ut de hac præclarissima compositione paranda consilium "apud ipsos habeatur." Sir J. Smith saw the preparation of the mithridate carried on at Venice with something of the same ceremony, during the present century. Alpinus points out, very particularly, in what the theriak farook differs from the theriak of Andromachi the elder; which consists principally in some difference in the proportions of the ingredients, and in the substitution and deficiency of a few, of which last asphaltum seems to be the most important. He also points out many errors into which he considers the Ægyptians to have fallen, both in the use of simples and in the composition of the pills which enter into the compound; but although these are interesting as containing minute accounts of many articles which have been used in medicine, it is only requisite to refer to the account of the Elchenlimbat or Chian turpentine, to which is to be ascribed the strong smell of spruce by which the treeak is characterixed; "resinam terebinthinam, siccam duram, "lucidam, fovis albam, et intus flavam, odoratam, *quæ linguam aspero sapone* "*ferit.*" It is sufficiently evident however that these preparations differ in nothing material, and it is probable, that the Venetian apothecaries merely add the Arabic designation to secure the sale of theriak of Andromachi in the East. This is indeed stated in the Turkish envelope, of which a translation has been procured through the kindness of a friend, which states "the "teereeak farook" to be "a production of the fortified city of Vendeek; a "famous doctor, named Andromakoo of that place having been its inventor "and manufacturer." On a comparison of the articles contained in each of these compounds with the theriaca Andromachi, as detailed in the Edinburgh pharmacopoias of the last century, and in a translation by Mr. W. Geddes of a formula for its preparation extracted from a Persian work named the Kifeeah Moonsoovie, and a prescription given to me by a native of Bagdad, they appear to be copies of the original recipe, although the difficulty of recognising or procuring some of the ingredients had led to differences in the preparation, and to that of Venice being considered the most genuine.

The most important ingredients are squills, opium, various stimulating resins, Chian turpentine, opobalsamum, myrrh, spices, valerian, gentian, warm tonic herbs and seeds, an astringent extract obtained from the unripe pods of the acacia Arabica, colcothar of vitriol, rhubarb, castor, &c. That this multifarious compound possesses, as Sydenham states, powerful tonic and stimulating virtues cannot be doubted, and that "notwithstanding the ab-"surdity of the original intention of these medicines and their enormity in "point of composition" "the componnds have been found from repeated ex-"perience to produce very considerable effects as warm opiate diaphoretics." (*Edinburgh dispensatory, old edition.*) Hence Bontius recommends the theriac in barbiers. "To complete the cure, medicines which promote sweat "and urine, and strengthen the nerves, should be administered; such as "theriac, mithridate, &c. joined with proper exercise." To these virtues really possessed by it, we must ascribe the obstinacy with which this extraordinary preparation was retained by the British colleges, notwithstanding the absurdity of many of its ingredients, the improvement in pharmaceutical knowledge and the opposition of Heberden and other eminent physicians. Nor have the Edinburgh college been fortunate in the substitute they adopted under the name of theriaca Edinensis, thebaic or opiate electuary.

END OF THE APPENDIX.

OBSERVATIONS

ON

SOME FORMS OF

RHEUMATISM

PREVAILING IN INDIA.

BY ASSISTANT SURGEON JOHN GRANT MALCOLMSON,

MADRAS MEDICAL ESTABLISHMENT.

"Whoever collects and records his facts with care and fidelity, renders some contribution to the advancement of the medical art." *Medico-Chirurgical Review.*

MADRAS:

PRINTED BY ORDER OF GOVERNMENT.

VEPERY MISSION PRESS.

1835.

OBSERVATIONS

ON

RHEUMATISM.

I shall confine myself in the following pages to such practical observations on rheumatism, as it occurs in India, as may not readily occur to a surgeon on his first arrival in the country; to remarks on various disputed points in the history and treatment; and to a few novel observations, which if confirmed by the experience of others will lead to improvement in our knowledge of the disease, and to some valuable practical inferences.

Of the disease called " Burning of the feet" on which no direct information is to be obtained from books, very extensive experience in different circumstances, and much patient enquiry, would be required to enable any individual to draw up a full account, but as every fact contributed to its history is of great importance to the welfare of the Madras army, I shall communicate what I know regarding it, however inadequate to the expectations of the Board this may be.

Rheumatism in Natives.

There is no disease except fever more prevalent amongst the sepoys than rheumatism, and although not often fatal, has been stated, and probably with truth, to be the cause of more men being lost to the service than all other diseases put together.

Neither the general returns ofthe army nor those of particular corps, afford any correct data by which to estimate the loss of life from rheumatism; as it is often confounded with beriberi, to which the greater number of deaths noticed in the "General abstracts of returns" "of Native Sick"* are to be referred, and with various other complaints which supervene more readily in constitutions broken down by this disease; and great numbers are discharged from the service or invalided, whose future history cannot be learned.

It seldom prevails in an acute form, but now and then cases occur, which can often be traced to the direct effects of cold and wet, especially on the setting in of the rains when sultry heat is suddenly followed by storms of rain and wind.

These cases sometimes present the ordinary symptoms of the acute disease in England, as pain and heat in the joints, quick pulse, febrile excitement and foul tongue, and are benefited by treatment of the same kind but more cautiously used.

In a few examples a general bleeding will be advantageous; emetics and purges at the commencement remove the general symptoms; and when the joints are hot leeches never fail to be useful, and if the pain shifts to other joints they are to be repeated in smaller numbers. At first 16 or 24 may be applied, but afterwards not more than 8 or 10. Leeches in India take away an ounce of blood each, and as the effect on a joint is obtained by a few ounces, we must not carelessly order the abstraction of more, as the application will probably be frequently requir-

* Printed at Madras in October, 1831.

ed. Neither general or local bleeding lessen the liability of other parts to suffer, and the natives bear evacuations ill, especially in this disease which passes quickly into its ordinary chronic form, which is always attended with an atonic state of the constitution. Blisters have appeared to be injurious in the acute stage in keeping up fever, and do not remove the pains or they cause them to pass into other joints; and as that is short and more under the power of other remedies, it is proper to defer their use till the second stage, when they are very effectual in removing pain from individual joints. There is less chance of metastasis to other joints in the local affection following acute attacks, than in any other form. The pains are occasionally worse in bed, but whatever may be the case in Europe, it is not the heat of the bed clothes that causes it either in Europeans or natives, as they come on frequently when the sun gets low and continue for the early part of the night, sometimes for an hour or two only. They are not unfrequently attended with some febrile excitement, which is either part of the disease itself, in feverish stations difficult to be distinguished from the intermittent of the place, the fever running into the prevailing form; or it is a complication caused by the same exposure as brought on the rheumatism, or by the great liability of patients in every disease to contract the prevailing endemic. It will be easy to distinguish them, when swelling in the joints take place, when the pains are not confined to the situation of fever pains, and when they are aggravated in the evening while the fever observes a different period. The following case will illustrate some of these remarks.

Case 1st. Meer Hyder, ætat 19, a muscular man; five days before admission had pain and swelling of the knees followed by fever, strong quick pulse and increase of pain. Twentyfour leeches gave little relief on the 2d day, and were repeated on the 3d with no better effect. He was then bled to 24 oz. and this was repeated to 12, which didnot prove buffy and gave great relief to the knees, but the pains soon affected the other large joints and the fingers. Antimonial powder was useless, cold affusion was employed and caused copious sweats but these gave no relief. The tendons of the wrists, hands and arms which he did not complain of at first, were more painful than other parts. He was relieved by anodynes and frictions and discharged the succeeding month.

When there is any fever of an intermittent type, the bark or quinine is usefully combined with other treatment, as without them the fever will often run on for days, keeping up and aggravating the rheumatic affection even when the mouth is sore; and when mercury removes the fever, it is more apt to recur on the ptyalism beginning to subside.

A small number of cases occur, in which the chest is affected with inflammation at the same time and probably from the same cause as induced the acute rheumatism, but others in which pleurisy is a secondary complaint following rheumatism of the parietes of the chest, have been observed.

Case 2. Venketasawmy, ætat. 22. Admitted June 25th. Complaining of pains of hips, back and sides increased on moving, with some swelling and tenderness; chest is now affected with pain increased on full inspiration, short cough and scanty mucous expectoration; pulse quick, skin warm. Leeches were applied, followed by repeated blisters and the chest was relieved. 7th July. Complains only of weakness and of pain of hips. 15th. Has used Dover's powder without benefit. Pains all over him. 27th. Pains gradually left him but returned today in right knee. 5th August. Pain removed by a blister and he is discharged. The explanation of the symptoms in this case, is the same as that given by Baillie of the frequency of pleuritic affection in England; viz. the number of anastomoses between the vessels of the costal pleuræ and the external parts, and " hence whatever may act upon these external vessels, may be supposed capable of exciting an increased action, or of producing an accumulation of blood in the internal ones;" to which I would add, the direct spreading of the rheumatic inflammation from the fasciæ and muscles to their internal investing membrane. As far as a limited number of observations go, this form of rheumatism is most common amongst recruits; but how far it depends on inflammations being most frequent at this period of life; on the change from partial starvation to full feeding, or on the new and, to young soldiers, teasing duties to which they are now subject, I am unable to say. With the exception of well marked benefit derived from the above mentioned measures, from warm baths, and from small doses of calomel combined with antimonials, and in a few cases where one joint only was affected from cold applications; the cases of common acute rheumatism in natives to which I have at present opportunity of referring, are too few to enable me to state positively the effects of the various remedies used, and they may safely be inferred from what is said of them under other heads.

But it is seldom that we are called on to treat these well marked forms of acute rheumatism in sepoys, in whom it is not often characterized by more than its coming on suddenly from cold, and, perhaps, in being apt to shift from joint to joint and being attended with slight fever or a little constitutional disturbance. The important circumstance in particular, of heat in the affected joints, on which so much weight has of late years been laid by Professor Elliotson and others, as indicating active rheumatism requiring free local bleeding and antiphlogistic remedies, is very seldom met with; and the rule of practice confining evacuations to such examples, and to those in which the pain is increased by heat, is not applicable to the Indian forms of the complaint either in Europeans or natives. When the pains are severe and the pulse quick but small, and there is aggravation of the symptoms with fever at night, the case approaches to the acute form, but active antiphlogistic remedies must not be used, and are either inefficacious or injurious. In these cases there is frequently a good deal of disorder in the abdominal secretions; the tongue is loaded, the stools are dark, and there may be pain in some part of the abdomen. Small doses of calomel with antimonials are the best remedies, and the symptoms rapidly leave on the gums getting sore.

But these acute and subacute forms of rheumatism are of little practical importance compared to the common chronic affection, which whether succeeding the acute or arising without evident cause, is a disease of great obstinacy, little under the influence of medicine and lays the foundation of numerous constitutional ailments. When it attacks a healthy person, it may at first be confined to a single joint, which is followed by the affection of others, generally without any relief to the one first suffering. The pain is not generally very acute nor always worse at night, and often is little more than an aching and weakness of the joint.

The parts are most frequently affected nearly in the following order; the knees, ancles, heels, elbows, wrists, hips, shoulders, back and chest. The pain in the knees is always much complained of, and is generally referred to the whole joint, but sometimes a point of the inner condyle is acutely painful and tender, in other instances the patient presses on the patella, or on each side of the tendon of the rectus from the bursæ being principally diseased. There is no heat or swelling and the patients are frequently suspected of skulking and sent to their duty; when, after a month or two of suffering and aggravation of of the complaint by exersise(at this period very hurtful), and the supervention of swelling of the joints, a puffy feel and enlargement of the bursæ, the hands or ancles are tumefied, or the patient wastes, the mistake is seen. The pain in the ancles is usually situated on either side, often a little below the joint, at others in front in the situation of the annular ligament. The heels frequently suffer severely and the pain extends up the tendo achillis and swelling at its insertion is common; but not only does the tendinous substance of this part suffer, but the tendons of the wrists and hands have become painful and in a few instances have swollen, without any reference to the origin of the disease as caused by cold, abuse of mercury, venereal, &c.

The soles of the feet, the calves of the legs or flesh

of the thighs suffer more rarely than the loins or hips. The roots of the toes, the tarsal ligaments, the back of the hands and joints of the fingers are frequently swollen and painful; and the muscular parts of the back, the sides of the chest, the ribs and the sternum often become painful, tender, and swell. And in many rheumatic cases where the patients were ascertained to have had no venereal complaint for years, nor to have taken mercury, the shin bones have suffered from pain and even from swelling. The tissues then, that appear most generally involved in the disease are the ligamentous and tendinous, the periosteum, and more rarely the muscular, and we shall see reason to believe that many others are occasionaly engaged. The complaint is sometimes strictly local, as I have traced it to cold applied to the affected part only, and the liability of other parts to take on the same morbid action depends on the facility with which all morbid actions are propagated from one part of fibrous tissues to another. Those that have least tendency to attack other parts are the puffiness of the bursæ and pain of the bones.

These symptoms may come on without any constitutional affection and remain for a long time, and relapses may attack the patient again and again before his health suffers further injury, but in a very large proportion of protracted cases, the patient loses flesh and strength and a cachectic habit is the consequence: he languishes in hospital or struggles with his duties, and is looked upon as a burden to the regiment and is frequently unjustly supposed to be a malingerer, and because the skill of the surgeon is unable to restore him to health or fully to understand the obscure train of symptoms which afflict him, he often meets with little sympathy, and the repute of European medical science is injured in the eyes of those, into whom it is of the greatest importance to instil different sentiments. The sepoys are very little given to frequent an hospital and malingering is very rare amongst them, except in certain circumstances of harassing service; and those who are supposed most addicted to it, I have usually found to be of the class most subject to low forms of rheumatism. These are most commonly young weakly lads of bad constitution, and often subject from early youth to pains of the limbs, which are induced or aggravated by the fatigue of drill, and depression of spirits from a new mode of life, by which their habitual ails are aggravated, and not uncommonly end in confirmed marasmus. In examining recruits, it is of the greatest consequence both for the good of the service and justice to the individuals themselves, to reject men of this description; but as the best sepoys are frequently, on enlistment, thin meagre boys who have lived on coarse and insufficient food, considerable skill is necessary to distinguish those likely to turn out well from others. The general aspect of the man is the most certain guide, which is only to be learned by experience, but if the abdominal viscera seem healthy, and the skin soft and devoid of minute dry scales or other affections, there is every chance of his constitution improving on his being taken into pay, which will afford him abundance of food. Very tall lads, except they are northern Telingees, are very subject to illness of all kinds, especially to atonic rheumatism, and are seldom effective soldiers. I have seen short but active lads rejected, discharged, or kept back from promotion while those taken in their room or put over them on account of their height, were useless to the service from want both of mental and bodily vigour. The symptoms of a depraved habit, which is sometimes the cause of the rheumatic pains we are considering, and at others follows from their long continuance, are loss of strength, great emaciation, the patient loses his erect position in walking, and all his motions are performed in a languid manner, his countenance is sometimes puffy or pale, he is desponding, indolent and averse to all exertion. His appetite is bad, his bowels costive and the evacuations are often dark. His abdomen is puffy or tympanitic especially after eating, and he complains of indigestion. The tongue is generally swollen and white. In aggravated cases there is a burning sensation in the abdomen, which is extremely distressing and often evidently connected with the other symptoms, and probably depends on chronic inflammation of the mucous membranes. In this form of the complaint the patient gradually sinks, and is too often but little benefited by treatment. A few months leave to return to his native village will in many cases restore him to health; and I have reason to believe, that it is in this form of disease that men who have been always sick, recover on obtaining their discharge from the service; a circumstance which is sometimes ascribed to the patients having imposed on the surgeon, and at others to the efficacy of native medicines. But that the change may be useful, it should be tried early and before the powers of life are irreparably weakened and organic disease has commenced. During the course of these symptoms the skin is dry, rough and is covered with mealy white scales, or an obstinate psora occupies the buttocks, thighs and other parts. These appearances are not uncommon in India, but prevailed to a much greater extent amongst the troops at Rangoon, and were often the first complaints which ushered in the rheumatic pains and marasmus dependent on bad food, moist climate and fatigue. It was sometimes accompanied with spongy gums and other scorbutic symptoms.

The marasmus ends, when fatal, in diarrhœa and dysenteric symptoms, probably depending on intestinal ulceration, like the analogous cases from Rangoon, but the pulmonary symptoms and burning of the feet so frequent in the latter are little if at all known in India. Allied to this, and to an important train of symptoms in Europeans, are a few cases I have met with, of pains in the knees, ancles and soles of the feet being combined with foul indolent ulceration of the legs and feet, foul tongue and irritable bowels. In many cases a scrophulous taint is the apparent cause, and that disease manifests itself in the progress of the disease: in others venereal or mercurial action can be traced to have laid the foundation of the complaint, and it is remarkable that the joints, muscular parts and tendons suffer from these causes, as well as the periosteum and bones.

Rheumatism is especially apt to occur in natives and Europeans after sloughing venereal sores treated by mercury. The dissipation of the Mohurrum, the fruitful source of disease, is also a cause, and in weakly lads the confinement consequent on slight accidents or disease is sufficient to predispose to rheumatism, and this is remarkably the case with fever which often lays the foundation for protracted affections of the limbs. This is sometimes the mere consequence of the debility, but it is also a direct effect of fever, even when no mercury has been taken, and is not unfrequently most severe in the parts in which the pains had been fixed during the pyrexial period; nor can it be wondered at, that the state of parts which give rise to these severe achings in the bones, joints and flesh should, if long continued, lay the foundation of local disease; accordingly it is in cases of neglected fever that these secondary complaints show themselves. The best marked examples I have seen, have been in patients who took no medicine, but continued to go through the routine of their duty for weeks or months with intermittent upon them.

The parts most affected are the shin bones, knees, thighs, and back, and sometimes the head, and these may swell and be worse at night, like mercurial pains. When the complaint is once established it may fix in one limb, which will waste as if the disease were local; and although the pains exist totally unconnected with fever, they are always aggravated by any new paroxysm. The occurrence of this new affection is a powerful inducement to the early and active employment of quinine. The following case of a European serjeant will illustrate these remarks, which apply equally to natives and Europeans. I fear it will prove tedious, but the subject is one of great practical importance, and abridgment would deprive it of the value it possesses not only as illustrating this particular sequela of fever, but also in reference to other important practical subjects. I have every reason to believe that he had had no venereal symptoms for years, and he had undergone no mercurial course, unless the slight one noticed in the reports.

Case 3d. John Jamison, serjeant, ætat. 25. In India 8 years. Admitted 2d April 1832, at 7 P. M. Got severe fever on the Neilgherry hills 9 months ago, and has not been free of it since. At Madras the left hypochondrium became painful, and he says, that he was some days in hospital without benefit. Fever comes on every day at 10 A. M. with a slight cold fit, and is occasionally more severe than it is in general, but he seldom escapes altogether. Pain in the forehead and occiput during the paroxysm, but is now quite free from it. There is a fixed pain of the hollow on the right side of nucha from occiput to the bottom of the neck, increased on motion but not on pressure. Spleen enlarged and tender, and during the fever, particularly the cold stage, the pain is aggravated checking the breathing and shooting up below the ribs. Both shoulders and arms down to the elbows are painful, and he feels the upper extremities weak. A tender and painful spot in centre of epigastric region; pain is dull, constant, and of three or four days standing. Bowels regular, stools said to be dark, urine high in the morning. During the fit the upper part of the abdomen swells and the whole of the cavity is tumid. Tongue smooth with a slight slimy coat on centre, the rest very smooth and rather pale. Pulse now 60, small; skin clammy. The paroxysm yesterday lasted till 9 P. M. and the sweating stage most of the night. Sleeps badly, no appetite, skin sallow, thirst with the fever. Scrophulous marks on the neck, hair auburn, and pupils large. Three stools from cathartic pills. Hirudines xvi hypoch. dextro et epigast. Habt. stat. quinæ sulph. gr. v, et reptr.

q. q. hora ad dosin iv. 3d. Vespr. Took 4 doses of the quinine, no fever, some cold perspiration. Headach from three till five, and has still some pain of right side of occiput. Side and epigastrium much easier. Takes a full inspiration without pain. Four stools said to be dark. Pulse 64. ℞ Calomel. gr. iii, ext. colocynth. c. gr. x, antimon. tart. gr. ½, ft. pil. ii h. s s. Hirudines xii occipit. 4th. Severe headach since 10 A. M., sweating most part of the night and the face, legs and arms are now bedewed with a cold moisture, left side and epigastrium very easy; one stool, not kept; tongue slimy. ℞ Calomel. gr. v, pulv. jalapæ gr. xxv, ft. pulv. stat. sumend : hirudines xx occipit. et. temp. Milk diet. Vesp. Five stools of more natural appearance, not kept. Had 8 grains of quinine at 9 A. M., no fever. Headach continues, no relief from the leeches, no sweating since visit, skin natural, pulse 74, tongue cleaner. Emplast. vesicat. nuchæ. ℞ Pulv. Doveri gr. x, calomel. gr. iii, ft. pulv. h. s. s. 5th. Perspired and felt easier after the powder. Head was shaven with relief to the headach. Blister not applied till morning having fallen asleep, and had a good night's rest, no fever or abdominal pain, one stool. Pulse 68 small, skin cool and moist, Tongue better. ℞. Pulv. rhei ʒss, pulv. jalapæ gr. v, magnesiæ ℈i, conf. aromat. gr. v, aq. menthæ ℥iii ft. haust. stat. sumend.; post horam habt. quinæ sulph. gr. viii, in pil. Bread pudding. 5th. Vespere. One stool. Had 2 doses of quinine. Slight pain wandering about the anterior part of the head; cold sweats at 1 and 5 P. M., skin now natural. To take 12 grains of cathartic extract. 6th. Slept all night; no fever, sweats or headach; neck and pains of shoulders and limbs the same. Spleen tender when pressed on, where it projects beyond the ribs. Some appetite. Tongue less pale. Pulse 68, weak; 2 stools. Hirudines xii hypoch. sinist. ℞ Quinæ sulph. gr. ii ft. pil. q. q. hora sumend. ad dosin vi. Vesp. No stool, no fever, wandering pains of head. ℞ Ol. croton. gtt. i, ext. hyociam. gr. iv, ol. menthæ gt. ii, ft. pil. h. s. s. 7th. Rested ill, no fever but felt as if much tired. Two stools without griping, they are copious, feculent and almost chalky in color. No headach. No pain on strong pressure under the right false ribs or on epigastrium; on full inspiration a little pain in left side. Pulse 70, strong. Appearance improved. Omitt. quinæ sulphat. Habeat calomel. gr. v, in pilul. statim, etiam magnes sulphat. ℥ vj. 8th. Vesp. Much better. Pains particularly severe in right shoulder and arm No stool. Rept. balneum. ℞ Calomel. gr. iv, pulv. Jacobi gr. v, extract. colocynth. comp. gr. viij, fiat pil. ij h. s. s. 9th. Sweated from the bath but complains of its weakening him. Pain in right shoulder worse. Bears pressure under the ribs, neck nearly well, some pains in knees. Pulse 70, soft. One stool said to be dark. Appearance very much improved. Sulphat. magnesiæ ℥iij. 10th. Six stools, still too light coloured. Makes no complaint unless of top of right shoulder which is tender. Pain extends to elbow. No pain of head, neck, or side even on pressure, and the spleen projects less. Tongue cleans and is not now pale, no thirst. ℞ Pil. hydrarg. gr. iij, pulv. ipecac. gr. j, sulphat. ferri gr. iss, fiat pil. mane et vesp. sumend. 12th. Vesp. Asleep in the morning, no rest from the violent pain in right shoulder, otherwise better. One formed stool, light yellow. Tinct. opii min. xxx h. s. 14th. Improved slowly till the 14th. Severe pain of the inner part of right knee since 8 P. M.

Bowels open, spleen subsides steadily. Ammonia liniment and fomentations to the knee. 15th. Relief to pain of knee by frictions, but it increased again and 9 leeches were applied with some relief, but it prevented sleep ; shoulder easy, 2 stools of better color. Contr. pil Fotus frequenter. 16th. Pain of knee came on with violence in the evening, relieved by fomentations. Slept well after the draught. Pains now easier; 2 stools said to be pretty natural in color. Tongue still white, pulse feeble. Fotus. Contr. pil. 17th. Shoulder well, knee better. Pain of right tibia which is in two places a little swollen, since last night. Liniment. ammoniæ. Cont. pil. Madeira 2 measures. 18th. Pain has returned to the knee with some difficulty of moving the joint, and has left the shin. One stool, said to be natural. Emplast. vesicat. parvum genu. 19th. Blister rose with great relief to knee. Slept ill. One stool. Foul taste. Omittr. pil. ℞ Pulv. rhei ℈ii, magnesiæ ʒss, confect. aromat. gr. iv, aq. menthæ ℥iii ft. haust. stat. sumend. 20th. Three stools, spleen has entirely subsided below the ribs. No pain of knee and little of shin where there is still some swelling. Reptr. pil. mane et vespere. 22d. Much pain last night in right knee, two stools a day. Tongue still white and slimy. Thirst in the night, and sweated a great deal. Blister nearly healed. Omittr. pil. Infus. cinchon. c. acid. nitric. Vesp. Habt. tinct opii min. xl h. s. 23d. Much pain in the inner part of the left knee extending down the tibia all night, and slept none till morning. Shin was painful yesterday during a storm and before it (not after). Bowels open. Hirudines x genu sinist. Contr. alia. 24th. No pain in limbs since the leeches were applied; some pain and tenderness of spine between the scapulæ. Contr. omnia. Emplast. galban. dorso. 25th. No pain in knees, soreness along the spine. Nausea in the afternoons, ascribed to the bitters; bowels open and stools are reported to be natural, tongue and pulse the same, felt faint and sweated after the draught, slept ill. Omittr. med. Contr. liniment. ℞ Pulv. columbæ ℈i, gum. guaiac. gr. v ft. pulv. bis die sumend. 26th. Pain in the legs better, sweats freely. Complains more of right shoulder and lower part of arm near the tendon of the biceps. No stool yesterday. Contr. pulv. et liniment. 27th. Was easy yesterday. Much pain of the outer part of the lower extremity of right biceps muscle, no swelling or redness. Arm stiff, legs well. Emplast. vesicat. parv. part. dolent. Contr. pulv. et haust. 29th. No pain of arm. Had pain of left knee yesterday, removed by frictions. The tenderness over middle dorsal vertebræ and some pain between the shoulder blades is increased on moving the arms. Bowels regular, sleeps well, appetite better. Contr. pulv. ter die et haust. h. s. Hirudines vi dorsi part. dolent. 30th. Leeches relieved the back. Knees relieved by frictions, and he slept tolerably. May 1st. Pain in the swelling of the right shin. Emplast. vesicat. part. dolent. 2d. Blister has removed the pain, complains of the border of left knee pan. Did not sleep from pain of blister. Bowels open, appetite good. Contr. med. 3d. Says he is free from pain, but he wishes to go out. Contr. haust. acid. 7th. States that he is free from complaint. There would appear to be some fulness of left side but there is no tenderness. Tongue still white but appearance on the whole pretty good. Discharged to duty.[1] A case in some respects similar, followed by acute hepatitis in a native, will further illustrate the fact and bear on some important questions to be stated by and bye.

Case 4. Mahomed Jacoob after suffering from a very protracted intermittent for which he took no mercury, on its leaving him got pains in the large joints, in the thighs, legs and hams. Leeches were applied with relief to right knee, which was swollen; loins felt weak. He was now seized with severe pain in the right hypochondrium, extending to the axilla and increased on full inspiration and pressure and on attempting to lie on the left side. Easiest sitting up. Pulse 90. Twenty oz. of blood and thirty leeches relieved, and a blister removed the pain. Calomel and antimony were omitted on the symptoms being removed.

Examples of hepatic inflammation are by no means uncommon amongst natives and frequently follow other disease. The following has some features of interest, which will be more clearly understood hereafter.

Case 5. Mahomed Sahib, ætat 23. Admitted 8th August, with pains of the lower limbs ascribed to exposure during the Mohurrum. Has been subject to rheumatism and has now slight evening exacerbations. An emetic, purgative, and frictions removed the pain except from the right leg. Stools changed at short intervals from white to mucous, or yellow and feculent. Sept. 4th. Pains in tibiæ only. 8th. Pain of left side and shoulder, with enlargement apparently of the spleen. No improvement under the use of blue pill, bitters, Dover's powder, mercurial frictions

[1] The fever soon after returned and nodes had formed on the shin, which were only slowly removed. *Original Note.*

to side and baths. 3rd October. Pains severe at night in all the joints, swelling of left clavicle, pulse small and quick, puffy belly in the evening, want of appetite, foul taste, vomits bile occasionally. October 18th. Pain of the side gone. Sternal end of right clavicle swollen. Stools alternately white, green and yellow. Small doses of calomel with antimony were substituted for the blue pill, the mouth was soon affected, and the pains left him, but he was still subject to paroxysms of fever which were at once removed by quinine.

Various anomalous affections of the chest supervene to rheumatism however induced, which I do not possess the means of explaining but which deserve to be carefully studied. One of these cases may be given.

Case 6. Venketaswamy, subidar, ætat. 40. March 8th. Had fever on the march from Hyderabad which was followed by pains of legs especially of tibia, and of shoulders. No fever. April 1st. Has had his mouth made sore with calomel and antimony and used blisters without benefit. Complains of debility and emaciation and of pain in the left leg. May 27th. Improved a good deal when using frictions and bitters, but pain has returned in the left thigh and leg. July 12th. Pain (except when it rains) nearly confined to left ancle which is swollen, pulse quick and weak, appetite good. September 1st. Continues to emaciate, bed ridden. 6th. Suddenly taken with swelling of the abdomen, with great pain of chest and dyspnœa, and soon after expired. The termination resembled that of many cases of beriberi, but the pains in that disease are almost exclusively situated in the muscular parts, and the bones always escape.

The well known affections of the heart so common in rheumatism in Europe are not very common, but are not unknown in India. Two cases have occurred to me in Europeans within the last year, and I find indications of it in natives.

Case 7. Ramanah. Pains in large joints. Dover's powder used without benefit, and after two months unsuccessful treatment he got pain in the left side of chest, increased on full inspiration and lying on the back, at first without dyspnœa, which supervened as the pain increased and struck through to the back, no cough. Pulse quick and small with slight fever. Twenty four leeches to the region of the heart, purgatives and antimony removed the pectoral symptoms. A lad admitted at the same time who had been long subject to rheumatism, got pain in the back of the neck, palpitations and throbbing at the heart, which appeared to depend on permanent disease. In many instances the loins suffer from simple rheumatic action, in no way differing from that affection as commonly described, and relieved by the usual treatment. In one case the affection of the loins was followed by a painful state of the testicles, which was easily removed by a few leeches. But numerous examples of rheumatic affection seem also to be connected with disorder of the nerves of the vertebral canal, which lead to troublesome symptoms very difficult to understand. In the present state of our knowledge the abstracts of a few cases, will usefully direct attention to some of the various affections thus arising.

In several examples of rheumatism, a pain below and to the left of the umbilicus has been accompanied or succeeded by severe and obstinate pain in the loins. A man is taken ill with purging of whitish stools, with pain and hardness of abdomen; pain of loins succeeds and as well as the epigastric hardness is obstinate. Tonics did harm, blue pill, leeches, and a blister and mercurial frictions to the stomach completed the cure. Severe and protracted fever in a sepoy was followed by numbness and pricking sensations in the extremities, and to these pain of the knees and ancles, which swelled, succeeded. Syed Hommed had pains and swelling of the elbows, knees and ancles for twelve days, which were relieved by a slight sore mouth; but pricking sensations below the knees supervened, to which pain of the loins and from the hips downwards succeeded, and were slowly removed by frictions, baths, &c.

Some of these cases, where beriberi prevails, are with difficulty distinguished from that disease, and in a few examples, the two diseases are not only united in the same individual and run their course independant of each other, but the symptoms of one may be so modified by the other, that any line of distinction is impossible. Such examples are rare however. The following seems to be an instance.

Case 8. Shaik Madar, havildar, admitted 9th April with pains of all the joints and swelling of the right elbow, tongue furred, pulse 88, small, debility, and pricking sensations over the body; skin dry except when taking Dover's powder which afforded no relief. Gums were slightly affected by calomel, antimony and opium which aggravated spasmodic twitches of the limbs, particularly of the calves, which had come on at night, and occasionally extended to the body. Irregular fever succeeded, with sensation of internal heat. Bark and carbonate of iron did no good. Symptoms were worse from 9 to 11 P. M. and about day light. In June pains returned from 4 to 6 A. M. and were nearly confined to the knees which were slightly contracted. Oleum nigrum did no good. He was injured by purgatives, and was much emaciated when sent on leave to his village.

The relation of these cases to "burning of the feet" will be noticed in a following page, but to the illustration of these complaints a very extensive experience would be necessary, in more favourable circumstances for the investigation, than often fall to the lot of an Indian practitioner. In native corps, dissections cannot be procured, and in the jails the practice is either very limited, or the circumstances of the patients too different from ordinary life, to admit of successful researches into the pathology of a disease, on which in its best understood forms, a late European authority states, that "dissection has as yet thrown no light."*

I shall now make a few observations on the efficacy of particular modes of treatment, in addition to those scattered through the foregoing remarks, confining myself, nearly, to those about which difference of opinion exists and suggested by the cases before me or notes taken at the time, trusting little to general impressions and recollections. Many early and slight cases soon recover with rest and frictions and require nothing more, nor should medicines, especially active ones, be more employed with natives than is absolutely necessary. In all periods and in every form of the common Indian rheumatism, frictions are necessary and may perhaps be considered the principal means of cure; but European surgeons seldom employ them, in an

* Gregory, chapter on Rheumatism.

efficient manner, nor do the means at their command enable them to do so. A few minutes rubbing by the dresser or common sweeper is by no means sufficient, and men cannot be got from the ranks for purposes of this kind, unless in very particular circumstances. An addition to the hospital establishment of one or two regular rubbers, would be of the greatest importance to the credit of European medical officers, to the welfare of the men, and good of the service. The supply of liniments is also far too scanty, and the common camphor oil usually employed is of little efficacy, and what is worse, the men (both Europeans and natives) have no confidence in it, and will never use it more than they are obliged to do. Turpentine, ammonia, soap liniment or some of those preparations in use amongst the natives, as the dammer liniment should be issued freely to all native corps. Cajaput oil, an essential oil distilled from lemon grass, and other species of Andropogon, are highly stimulating, and have cured very obstinate pains, but they are probably too expensive for ordinary use.

The rheumatism of India is seldom what has of late been called the hot variety, and is almost in every instance benefited by warmth; it is therefore of great consequence to furnish the sepoys, who cannot be kept warmly clothed, with flannel rollers for the affected parts, which are also of great benefit in the puffy state of the joints and bursæ: and as the disease is kept up by the men lying with only a thin carpet between them and the floor of the hospital, cots or straw matresses should be furnished to the sick, especially in the northern division.[2]

[2] At the time this was written, I was not aware that Government had, at the recommendation of the Medical Board, sanctioned the issue of cots to native hospitals.

Blisters are remedies of great value, but are seldom useful when the affection is acute, and when many joints are affected they seem hardly admissible. When any degree of fever was present, or the pain had made its attack suddenly, they seemed to favour the transfer of the pain to other joints, but in ordinary cases, especially when the knees, ancles, heels or smaller joints are painful or puffy, they are far more effectual than frictions and are often the only means by which a cure can be effected; and, fortunately, the natives, notwithstanding their strong prejudice to them in internal complaints, are very fond of them in the rheumatic affections to which they are most adapted. Pains in the loins and hips also readily yield to their use; and if other joints are afterwards affected, their repetition is equally or more advantageous than at first. Blisters and indeed all local remedies have been objected to of late by several writers, from some erroneous notion regarding the constitutional nature of the affection, and perhaps, because they had employed them in the acute stage of active rheumatism: but the practitioner in India is in no danger of being misled by reasoning of this kind, against the every day proofs of their usefulness. Not only do blisters exert a beneficial influence over the joint to which they are applied, but also seem to lessen the pains and the chance of affection of other joints. Much more depends on the counter-irritation they occasion than on the discharge, and a repetition of blisters is therefore to be preferred to keeping them open. No particular advantage has been observed from ointment of tartrate of antimony, or moxas. Mercurial plasters with a little tartrate of antimony rubbed on their surface, have appeared to reduce puffy bursæ, and to ease the pain of the joint. Leeches are not only useful when the joint is hot and recently swollen, but in almost all stages when the pain is local, especially when it is fixed in the hands and condyles of the knees and elbows. They are to be frequently repeated in small numbers if they do good; and blisters will afterwards perfect the cure. When the pains occupy the whole of the long bones, the flesh of the thighs, legs, &c. they are less useful, but swelling of the periosteum of the tibia, clavicles and sternum when circumscribed, are often greatly benefited by their application. Fomentations are very beneficial in all forms of rheumatic pains, but particularly in those of the bones, or from mercury. A favourite remedy of the natives is marking nut (Semecarpus anacardium) applied to the joints, and is often of great service, but is violent and unmanageable, frequently exciting much inflammation and causing troublesome ulcers.

Warm baths where warmth can be secured to the patient afterwards, are generally grateful to the feelings, relieve pain and irritability and are of permanent benefit. If profuse sweating and weakness follow, they are to be omitted; for debility is especially to be avoided in this disease. Dover's powder is often a valuable auxiliary, when given along with the bath, and as directed by Cullen in his materia medica, in a large dose and repeated in smaller quantities at *short* intervals. If the abdominal secretions are unhealthy it is not to be employed alone. I regret to observe, that an eminent clinical lecturer in London congratulates the profession on the neglect into which Dover's powder and baths have fallen in the treatment of rheumatism; but I can state from extensive experience that in recent cases when properly administered, they deserve our highest confidence. Many cases it is true will not be cured; old ones and those where the complaint is fixed in one spot, and painful nodes will derive but a little temporary relief; and if the powder is given in the usual way (8 or 10 grains three times a day) without reference to other circumstances, it merits the ill repute into which it has been endeavoured to cast it. Tincture of opium with antimonial powder is a good substitute, but the latter alone is very uncertain even in the largest doses. Laudanum to procure sleep and relieve the pains, will often require to be given in large doses, and by the ease it procures, saves the constitution from much of that destructive irritation which undermines the powers of life and aggravates the local symptoms. It seldom has any injurious effect not easily obviated. Guaiacum to be used with effect, must be given in large doses; a drachm of the gum three times a day has proved, in a number of instances, of great service. It has like most other remedies often failed; but I am not able to state the circumstances in which it is most useful. The decoction of the wood and the volatile tincture have also been advantageously employed, but they are not remedies of much power. Colchicum is supplied to the hospitals in acetous solution, and whether from the decay of virtue of the medicine, or the form of the disease, it has not been very beneficial. The oleum nigrum has been occasionally prescribed, principally where there was some suspicion of beriberi, but it did not appear to possess anti-rheumatic virtues. In some cases communicated to me, the cold affusion was employed and caused free sweating, but seldom relieved any of the symptoms. Sulphur has removed the pains and cutaneous symptoms together, but whether it did so by restoring the healthy state of the skin, or by its powers over the pains themselves for which it is a popular remedy in Europe, I cannot say; but I have known it useful in common rheumatism where the skin was not diseased. There is a hot spring in the bed of the Godavery, 4 miles below Badrachellum, which has considerable reputation as a remedy in rheumatism. It abounds in sulphuretted hydrogen and has a temperature of 140. The well is a very powerful vapour bath, and the coincidence of its use with the recent investigation by Dr. Bardesley, of the powers of artificial baths of the same kind in rheumatism and affections of the skin, establishes the correctness of the popular opinion. It is in too inaccessible a spot ever to be of much general use.

But of all the remedies used in rheumatism, mercury is beyond comparison the best, and there are very few forms in which that disease is seen in India, in which it is not safe and generally effectual. The cases which have derived no benefit from it, were those affecting the calves of the legs, and attended with pricking, numbness, and other beriberi and neuralgic symptoms; and where there were scrophulous ulcers or other signs of tainted constitution, and some examples of pains following sores and buboes which perhaps had something of a strumous character. In nocturnal pains of syphilic origin it exerted its usual well known powers, and in numerous cases in which pains and swelling of the bones and joints could be clearly traced to mercurial action or to exposure when under its influence, the benefit was marked and sudden. In a few of these examples as well as others of common rheumatism, the patients appeared to be less subject to relapse than when relieved by other means, but more generally, the liability to return was greater. Of these anomalies, the cases suggested the following explanation, viz. that when mercury had removed the diseased state of parts which other treatment had only mitigated, the cure was more permanent; but that by its action on the parts subject to rheumatism, they were rendered liable to take on new diseased actions, or to have the old ones, renewed; and also, that many old and bad cases beyond the powers of other remedies being benefited by this treatment, rendered the proportion of relapses greater. On the whole it is better to try what can be done by other means, but much time must not be lost, as the disease gets more inveterate by neglect. The bones, joints and tendons are more relieved than muscular parts. When the affection was at all active and attended with fever, touching the gums removed the pains; but if the fever is of an intermittent character bark or quinine must be exhibited at the same time, which are also very useful as general tonics in these and other cases, but do not exert, as far as I have observed, any direct power over the discease itself. When blisters relieve the pain of individual joints and general remedies have done good but the cure is imperfect, a sore mouth generally completes it in a few days; and in the most obstinate cases, which have resisted all other plans of treatment, it for the most part restores the patient to health. The cure is, however, not unfrequently imperfect, and frictions, baths and Dover's powder, and blisters to the site of any local pains which may continue after the other symptoms, are to be used as auxiliary measures; and the effect they now produce is remarkable, when compared with their failure before the mercury was prescribed. When there are old pains without swelling, the effect is less decided. It is not in the active forms of rheumatism only, as stated in recent works, that mercury is useful, but also in the old atonic form in which we principally see it in this country. When the abdominal symptoms formerly described, with emaciation and depraved secretions supervene, it is a valuable and indeed the only very useful medicine. Although the pains of beriberi are not relieved by mercury, rheumatism following that disease is as much under its influence as other forms of the complaint.

The form in which it is administered is of considerable importance, and I have therefore made it a particular subject of enquiry. The mouth is easily affected, and as it is necessary to avoid more than very slight mercurial action, and to keep it up for several days, small doses are to be given. Three grains of calomel twice a day have been found too much, and in general one grain and a half two or three times a day is as much as can be given with advantage. It is advantageously combined with antimonial, or, what is better, with James' powder to the extent of three grains; this often opens the skin gently without irritating the intestines, which are liable to take on dysenteric action from more active medicines. For this reason the tartrate of antimony, although a more certain antimonial has been found inconvenient, by inducing purging. When given by itself, it has not caused sweating, when prescribed in less than one grain doses, and even when combined with opium it has not given relief till a grain of calomel was added: and although in this combination it did not often disorder the bowels, it is better to avoid the use of two irritating remedies at one time. When purging takes place from the use of tartar emetic in this or any other form, it is immediately to be omitted, and an anodyne followed by castor oil administered, which at once removes every troublesome symptom. Blue pill is too uncertain; it does not assist the diaphoretic virtues of other remedies, and its long continued use is injurious to the stomach without benefiting the pains. The native practitioners use mercury to a great extent in rheumatism, and their imperfect combinations often cause violent salivation; but I have known men who were long treated by European surgeons with a great variety of medicines, cured by this means even when the ptyalism was so severe as to constitute a troublesome disease. These observations although bearing particularly on the treatment of natives, may be applied to that of Europeans to which they are equally applicable. Mercurial fumigations were strongly recommended some years ago by a Bombay medical officer on the ground of his own experience, derived from his having observed many sepoys discharged the service as incurable, recovering under the native treatment by fumigations with oxide of mercury, and the Bombay medical board recommended it to the service. I made a series of experiments with it, using the common mercurial ointment spread on a piece of an earthen pot, which was placed on a small vessel of charcoal between the patient's feet, who was covered, with the exception of the head, with blankets (cumblies) and the fumes allowed to continue in contact with his body for ten minutes. A cure was frequently effected by this means. A profuse sweat was generally caused and the mouth was often made sore, but the mercurial action sometimes could not be induced at all, in others ptyalism was sudden and profuse, and on the whole, I thought the plan unworthy of general employment. One fact was ascertained in opposition to the prevailing opinion of physiologist's, viz. that the skin, when the cuticle is unbroken, is capable of absorbing; for the fumigation was performed in the open air and precautions taken to prevent the patient inhaling the fumes. The circumstance of the discharged sepoys recovering is explained, in part, by what is said above on the effect of leave of absence, and in others by the mercurial action and the modified vapour bath.[3]

[3] The following observations on rheumatism were drawn up, at my request, by my friend surgeon J. Adam. The remarks apply principally to the disease as it occurs in the circars and although written from recollection and without having access to his journals, are evidently the fruit of close observation; I therefore consider the coincidence of his views with those which had previously been submitted to the Medical Board in this paper and with which he was not made acquainted, a very valuable confirmation of some opinions which are of considerable practical importance. Some of the cases were probably examples of the chronic form of berberi.

After remarking that few diseases are more frequent in their occurrence or more destructive to the constitution and that the pathology is ill understood, he proceeds to state the peculiarities which seem to distinguish rheumatism in India, from that form of the disorder described by authors. "I "have generally observed this complaint to attack those subjects who had "previously been suffering from other diseases, more especially as the se-"quela of fever, or whose constitutions had been impaired by former attacks "of sickness. On a narrow scrutiny of the previous state of health nothing "strikes one more forcibly, than the prevalence of symptoms indicating a "deranged state of the digestive functions, before the patients complained "of the local affection, which was afterwards the chief subject of complaint; "and I have been led to believe that this condition may be looked upon not "only as connected with the disease but as a predisposing cause. It is ne-"vertheless true, that numerous cases occur in which no previous ailment "had been noticed, and wherein there was no evident symptom of deranged "health existing"

"The symptoms which characterize the disease are well marked and con-"sist in pain of the several joints, more especially affecting the articulations "of the elbow, knee, ancles and wrists. Generally speaking there is no ex-"ternal swelling and the other characteristic marks of inflammation, with "the sole exception of pain, are wanting. There is no heat of skin, the "pulse remains unaffected, the tongue is occasionally furred, the appetite "usually defective, but sometimes good. There are, however cases in which "febrile disturbance will take place, more especially towards evening, caus-"ing much restlessness during the night. As the complaint progresses the "patient becomes weak and languid, the digestive organs suffer considera-"bly, a general atrophy succeeds, with abatement of the pains of the several "articulations; and should the lower extremities have been the seat of the "complaint, a tottering of the gait approaching to a paralytic state is observ-"ed. The tongue becomes red and glassy, a diarrhœa the result of long pro-"tracted irritation supervenes, though this is by no means the invariable con-"sequence, and nature exhausted sinks at last under continued suffering.

Burning of the feet.

The disease which has acquired the name of "Burning of the feet" has only come into notice since the Burmese war, and nothing has yet been

"The period when this disease prevails most is during the rainy and cold "seasons, and it often occurs, from the genial influence of the succeeding "hot weather, that an amelioration of the complaint is effected and there "is every seeming prospect of recovery, when a change for the worse takes "place on the first setting in of the rains. Many patients whom I have seen "doing well during the hot weather have suddenly sunk on the approach "of the monsoon, and so unaccountably, as only to be attributed to the shock "produced on their tender frame by atmospherical vicissitudes common at "that juncture. In enumerating the symptoms peculiar to this disease, I "must not omit to mention the harsh, dry, and squalid state of the skin so "prominent in the latter stages of the disease, as well as the total want of "appetite, &c. and I am led, from a consideration of circumstances, to look "upon an intimate sympathy subsisting between the alimentary organs and "cutaneous system and a deranged or diseased condition of these, to be con-"nected with the nature of the disease."

"When local symptoms evidence any degree of inflammation, the appli-"cation of leeches followed by hot fomentations is the most appropriate re-"medy, and to prevent the disturbance to the general system or to regulate "it should such have arisen, a purgative of calomel, colocynth and tartariz-"ed antimony given at night, and followed by aperient mixture is highly use-"ful. When the bowels have been fully opened and the local inflammation "controled, although pain still continues, it becomes necessary to apply "some rubefacient remedy, for which purpose either blisters or tartarized "antimony ointment may be had recourse to, and to determine towards "the surface of the skin so as to keep up a gentle moisture, a diaphoretic "mixture with doses of Dover's powder, was what I was in the habit of em-"ploying with great advantage; and where there prevailed great restless-"ness at night a full opiate occasionally was found highly beneficial, in allay-"ing the general irritation and conducing to a recovery of health. When "debility alone remained afterwards, nourishing diet with the use of wine "or spirits and tonic remedies were recommended, as well as frictions to "the limbs with linimentum saponis; and as much gentle exercise as the pa-"tient could take without fatigue, for on this principally did I rely with a "view of preventing the succeeding atrophy, into which, from their own "passiveness, they are so wont to fall. The warm bath I should deem very "useful, but I have never employed it. When there were great languor and "debility existing from the commencement, I generally employed blisters "to remove the local pain, frictions with strong stimulating liniments, and "the internal use of guaiacum, camphor and ammonia with bark decoction "or sarsaparilla two or three times a day; regulating the stomach and bow-"els as well as the secretion of the liver by means of blue pill and gentle ape-"rients of the warm kind exhibited occasionally. In one or two cases I had "the happiness to see a recovery effected from a most deplorable state, by "means of mild purgatives and the use of the blue pill until the system was "impregnated, after a variety of other remedies had failed. Amongst the "modes of cure recommended, I have tried the plan of mercurial fumigation "extensively, and although I have witnessed beneficial effects to follow from "its use, yet I cannot say that my experience would warrant a reliance on it "excepting as an useful adjuvant. Of all remedies, however, there is none "that ought to be more persisted in, after the local symptoms have been du-"ly controled and nothing but debility or a tendency to marasmus remains, "than *exercise*. *Change of air* to a warmer climate may be ultimately ne-"cessary previous to the expected monsoon, if the patient indicates no ap-"pearance of recovery from his weakness, as this disease chiefly prevails in "those latitudes where atmospherical vicissitudes are most common, and

written expressly on the subject,[4] nor has any opinion been advanced as to its nature, with the exception of the advertisement of the Board, in which it is stated to be a neuralgic affection occasionally a sequela of rheumatism. In some of the cases of disease of the lungs published by Dr. Conwell, this symptom was present, and the dissections he records throw some light on its causes, but rather on the circumstances of general disease of the body in which it occurs, than on the particular pathological state on which it directly depends. In his patients the whole system was diseased; no organ retained its natural functions in a healthy state, the structure of most was altered, and the patients were at once too ill for successful treatment, and for useful enquiry into the history of any particular affection, or the efficacy of remedies. The description both of the symptoms and treatment, is also too concise to be of much assistance. A comparison of these, however, with the disease as it occurred to the Eastward, and with the history of men who returned labouring under it in a milder form, and in whom its progress to recovery could be observed, may be of some use; and with other papers, by persons of more experience, may direct enquiry into the proper channel and save from gross and fatal blunders; which is all that can be expected in so

" where the rains set in at an early period of the year. What particular " state is induced by the application of cold conjoined with moisture to the " affected parts is difficult to determine, but I have thought that from the " great pain generally complained of by the sufferers and the little appear- " ance, frequently, of symptoms of inflammation, that it was more an affec- " tion of the local nerves than of the vessels. In fine, my opinion with " respect to the nature of rheumatism in India as it occurs in natives is, that " it is more an affection of the *nervous system than inflammatory.*"

[4] There is a short paper on the subject, in the 2d volume of the transactions of the Medical and Physical Society of Calcutta by Mr. J. Grierson; and a few valuable observations will be found in Mr. Burnard's paper, on the medical topography of Arracan, page 44 of the third volume. At the time of drawing up the paper, I had no opportunity of referring to books and these remarks were unknown to me.

new a subject of enquiry. On no disease that the Board could have selected is information so much wanted; as I have no hesitation in stating, that an ignorance of the complaint has led to the sacrifice of many lives, and the entailing of great and permanent expence on government. In a disease like this, of which nothing was known, and which had no sensible signs by which it could be recognized; when the patient was not emaciated, as often happened in elderly men of a naturally corpulent habit and in slight cases amongst the young, he was suspected of malingering to avoid harassing duties or to procure leave to return to his own country; an opinion which would naturally lead to the greatest practical cruelty, in refusing rest in hospital, leave of absence and change of climate to men, to whom they afforded the only chance of recovery. Melancholy instances have come to my knowledge where men have died in making exertions above their strength, after having been looked on and treated as malingerers, and others where slow decay and uncontrollable disease have carried them off. This could not fail to lead to the loss of the confidence and respect of the men, amongst whom our practice in this country must lie; and even of the better informed European officers, however much they may be disposed to think, that the "doctor is not aware of the skulking going on," and perhaps disposed to go further and to lead a young medical officer to look on his patients with a suspicion, which takes away all stimulus to exertion; and may induce him, if of a complying disposition, to refuse admission to cases of obscure disease such as that under consideration. My own impression on first meeting with this complaint, on which I possessed no information, and from a dislike to admit men for whose disease I knew no remedy, was the same, but before I treated the disease as trivial or feigned, I fortunately met with it, in men of the best charaoter and little likely to deceive, and without an object to do so. Nor is this impression removed through the service by the experience of the Burmese war, as I have had occasion within these few months to insist strongly, in conversation both with medical and other officers, on the necessisty of the utmost caution in treating this complaint either as one of slight consequence, or in supposing that it was usually unreal. And here it may not be improper to repeat, that malingering is rare amongst the native troops, and when sepoys report sick with trivial complaints when there is much hard duty, they are generally men of broken constitutions, often from hardship on foreign service, or young weakly lads unequal to the constant recurrence of severe bodily exertion. It deserves also to be observed that corps subject to the same causes, have, in many instances, been sickly ever since and the men particularly liable to rheumatism and marasmus; and officers who do not consider this, are apt to ascribe the number of men unable to go through their duties, to disinclination, instead of to inability or indolence arising from indifferent health.

As far as my experience goes "burning of the feet" cannot be considered a sequela of common Indian rheumatism, and is very little if at all known at those stations where that complaint prevails most extensively. To the native practitioners north of the Kistnah it seems to be unknown. A case occured in the jail of Masulipatam after bowel complaint, and was removed by Dover's powder which caused free sweating. This weakened the patient so much that the medicine was necessarily omitted, and the burning in the feet returned. The gentleman to whom the case occurred,*. justly observed, that the sensation was the effect of the skin being dry and the nervous influence imperfectly distributed. But in the following instance at the same place, it evidently arose from diminished power in the nerves.

Case 9th. A paria prisoner ætat. 24, admitted 1st January, came to hospital yesterday complaining of sense of numbness of his body and a burning of his feet, with costive bowels. Pulse at that time frequent and skin was slightly warm. Had half a drachm of compound powder of jalap which operated four times; says to day, that the numbness is better, but the burning of the feet, and he now adds of the abdodomen, is no better; pulse 120, not very strong, skin is natural, tongue pretty clean; in walking moves steadily enough, except that he does not place his feet at once firmly on the ground, and he complains of pain in the calves of the legs. Has been ill 3 days. To take treeak farook pills and a diet of meat and wheat cakes. 2d. Pulse to day 112, skin natural; says he feels better of the heat in his feet and abdomen and that the numbness is quite gone, bowels twice opened. 3rd. Pulse 106, skin natural, one stool; says he has no complaint. 4th. Pulse 96, no heat or numbness. 7th. Pulse 84; no complaint. Omitt. med. 9th. Discharged.

This case was evidently allied to beriberi which was prevailing at the time, and of which burning in the feet is an occasional symptom. It does not, however, often occur in that disease, and is found to affect the

* Assistant surgeon G. Thomson.

soles and the calves of the legs, the back of each side of the spine and occasionally the flesh of the legs, in all of which a connection can be traced with other affections of the nerves of the part. The symptom is not confined to any class of cases, being observed in recent and slight examples, and in old and hopeless ones, but in which I have, in general, found the numbness not very great, and to be combined with other signs of slightly obstructed nervous power Both, then, appear to depend on an affection of the nerves, and their occurring together would suggest that they are modifications of the same disease; which is further supported, by the fatal cases exhibiting many of the graver symptoms of beriberi. The evidence of an occasional correspondence in some of the symptoms and even of the appearances on dissection, are however by no means sufficient to identify two diseases, as these must often run into each other, if similar parts are affected. The general history of the complaints, therefore, affords the only satisfactory evidence; on which I am enabled to communicate the result of extensive observation, in the most favourable circumstances which have ever presented themselves. On the return of the troops from Ava in the middle of 1826, the corps that were sent to the northern division were in general suffering from "burning of the feet", but no beriberi shewed itself till some months after, when the other complaint had almost entirely disappeared; and after this, and the disappearance of the sloughing ulcers and bowel complaints connected with depraved habit which prevailed with them, these regiments were very healthy, until the period of residence and season disposed them to the endemic of the circars. It was also observed, that men with burning of the feet were not peculiarly liable to beriberi, which attacked indiscriminately all new comers whether from Rangoon, or from places in India, although it was true that those men whose constitutions were impaired by this or other disease on foreign service, were rather more liable both to beriberi and fever. This observation was not confined to any particular corps, but was equally true of all those suffering from "burning of the feet" which entered the districts where beriberi prevailed, and also when stationed in towns where other troops were losing men from it. It was perhaps more instructively exhibited in the 4th extra regiment at Ellore than in any other. This corps was raised in January 1826, and was composed of recruits, and of men returned sick from Rangoon who were transferred to it. Amongst the latter, burning of the feet prevailed but did not attack any of the other men, and before beriberi made its appearance, which did not happen till the end of the year when the subjects of it had been exposed to the influence of the place for many months, the former disease had disappeared, except in a few obstinate cases, none of which ran into beriberi. The first instances of beriberi were not of a decided character. A man suffering from fever having lost the use of his limbs in September, and in October a sickly boy had œdema of the limbs and face with swelled belly, but without any affection of the nerves. These facts, observed as they were on the large scale in both diseases, afforded much better evidence of the pathological difference of these complaints, than can be derived from a similarity in the latter stages, with some resemblance in the appearances on dissection.

Having thus shown that the disease called "burning of the feet" is a different affection from any stage of the common rheumatism of India and from beri-beri, and stated as the result of extensive observation on the eastern coast and the interior, that it does not *prevail* as a distinct disease in those parts of India,[5] we are directed to enquire in what circumstances it has prevailed amongst the Madras troops. The only regiments in which the disease has done so, were those employed in Ava and in the straits of Malacca, and it did not occur frequently in these till they had been sometime in the country, and was most severe, when to the ordinary injurious influence of the climate and diet, fatigue and exposure were added. The disease did not disappear after a residence of some duration, as men who had been two years in Ava continued to labour under it. To the moist climate much may be ascribed; the air in all those countries being much loaded with moisture and the rains heavy, compared to those of the Carnatic. The variation of temperature is very slight at Malacca where the disease was very prevalent, but it is not confined to the districts near the coast, many being affected at Pegue, Prome and other places in the interior.

In all the places in which the disease prevails rations are issued to the troops, consisting of rice, two ounces of ghee (not always issued), a little salt fish and spices. Of the first and only part in which much nourishment can be supposed to be found, there was as much as a man could use, and I have seen much of the boiled rice thrown away. The deficiency in the food then consisted in the want of variety, of vegetables, of fresh animal food, of which almost all classes of Madras sepoys use a certain proportion, flour, milk, and various articles with which the natives

[5] Mr. J. Bell informs me, that he has seen several patients at Tanjore who complained of burning sensations of the feet. Pain was felt in the situation of the last lumbar vertebra on rotating the spine, but not on pressure. Local applications to the spine removed the symptom.

vary their diet. It cannot be doubted that food of this description weakens the digestive organs, by its sameness and want of stimulating power, but also would gradually bring on a scorbutic state of the system, as I have known the scurvy to attack men better fed than the sepoys; and can state that rice, however abundant, will not preserve either Europeans or natives from that complaint, and that "burning of the feet" and sloughing ulcers will be aggravated and make their first attack in men on boardship, abundantly supplied with the same diet as is issued to them on shore. It is true, however, that men who had the means of getting better provisions, and who probably did furnish themselves with some addition to their rations, suffered; and on the whole, while we are fully justified in the conclusion that the change from a dry to a moist climate and long continued deficient nourishment, in circumstances otherwise unfavourable to health, predisposes to this disease, much remains to be done to assign to these their limits, and to point out the accessary causes to which the peculiar form of the complaint may be ascribed. If, however, we observe the success that has attended enquiries of the same kind in other diseases, we shall be little sanguine, in expecting soon to arrive at any thing like accurate knowledge on this—so lately noticed, and only to be observed in peculiar circumstances not likely often to occur.

"Burning of the feet," which is the designation usually applied by Europeans, from the distressing sensation being for the most part confined to the soles, is merely a translation of the ordinary expression of a native soldier on presenting himself at the hopital, and has no pretensions to accuracy, but it deserves to be retained, as marking the distinction and importance of the affection, till a more accurate knowledge is acquired of its nature. The burning frequently extends over the surface of the lower extremities which are affected with severe pains, in many instances confined to the fleshy parts, especially the soles of the feet and calves, as in other cases of affection of the nerves at their origin, and the limbs sooner or later emaciate. The hands have partaken of the morbid state, and in a few cases the burning has extended to the whole body and even to the face. The parts are dry and do not feel hot to the touch, but I made no observations with the thermometer; and on this subject, and the distribution of the morbid sensations, and their relations to other symptoms often present, no accurate observations have been made. In some cases the burning is stated to be worse at night, in which it partakes of the nature of those more common sensations which arise from slight nervous derangements common in dyspepsy, menstrual irregularity, and convalescence from severe disease. Nor is there any reason to doubt, that nervous irritability from deranged capillary circulation was occasionally a cause of the morbid sensation in Ava, as it unquestionably was of the analogous complaint in the prisoner, in whom it was removed by the diaphoretic action of Dover's powder, which, conjoined with tonics, Good states to be the proper remedy for sensations of this kind depending on irritable habit.[6] Besides the

[6] A gentleman of robust habit but subject to slight disorder of the bowels, was much distressed with painful scalding sensations in the soles and palms coming on in the evening and lasting most of the night. After some time, the parts became tender to the touch so that walking was painful, and the skin exhibited spots of a reddish tint which were slightly elevated. He was dyspeptic and the skin was usually dry. He derived temporary benefit from bathing the feet in hot water, and from blue pill and James's powder; but he owed his recovery to active exercise by which a free perspiration was excited.

pains in the lower extremities and emaciation, symptoms of a generally depraved habit were present; and in the worst cases extensive organic disease. The skin was dry and harsh, often scaly or covered with itch, the patient was harassed by irregular attacks of fever; he felt weak and was exhausted on slight exertion, to which he often had a great aversion. The tongue was usually pale, swollen, smooth or furred, and only red when the intestinal mucous membrane was excited. The gums were observed by several gentlemen to be swollen and soft, but the symptom was neither common or remarkable in degree. Night blindness was not of unfrequent occurrence as in some forms of scurvy. Cough was more common than in any other complaint to which the natives are liable, and there was distressing dyspnœa in the advanced cases. The pulse was little altered in the early stages, and, when uninfluenced by the organic affections, was small, irritable and easily excited by exertion or irritation of any kind. The digestion was in almost every instance impaired; the appetite was weak and irregular, and the most wholesome food caused uneasiness at stomach, puffy belly or pain. The abdomen was often tympanitic and tender to the touch; diarrhœas, dysentery, pain in the course of the colon or around the umbilicus frequently occurred, and increased the emaciation or destroyed the patient. In some instances, however, both the appetite, digestion, and evacuations were natural. In the worst cases stiffness and numbness of the lower extremities were complained of. Dropsical swellings of the legs were not uncommon and usually the result of debility alone, disappearing on the patient being enabled to keep in the recumbent posture, but also in many instances the effect of organic changes, and complicated with effusion into the cavities. Although in most cases where "burning of the feet" was complained of, careful enquiry could detect signs of general disorder in the tongue, skin, or abdomen, a few had no other symptom and yet the disorder was real, and in time caused emaciation and bad health. In some all the general symptoms and even pain in the calves and soles of feet, numbness, &c. have been present without burning; and in others, the pains in the limbs have left the patient and yet the burning was unrelieved many months after the patient's general health was restored, by his return to his own country. Nor is this surprising, when the different kinds of morbid sensations induced by even local disease of nerves are considered. Neither will the appearances on dissection throw any *certain* light on the cause of the sensation, the same morbid changes having taken place where this symptom was wanting as where it was present; but they point to the lower part of the spine as the seat of the local disorder, and are of the greatest use in leading us to a correct estimate of the formidable nature of symptoms, which end in extensive alterations in the structure of the viscera of all the cavities. It is of great importance however to observe, that these alterations are not essential to the disease, as a very large proportion of the patients if placed in favourable circumstances, may be restored to health in a moderate period of time. I shall select a few cases in which the symptom was present, from Dr. Conwell's work, in which the account of the morbid appearances is very complete, although there is some difficulty in deriving information out of so indiscriminate and lengthy a narrative of ordinary and extraordinary appearances.

Case 10th. Sunnassee, ætat. 22. Admitted 6th September, having been ill 9 months with burning sensation in the feet, which now extends to the knees; he is emaciated, restless, appetite and digestion imperfect, bowels regular, excited tongue, no abdominal pain on pressure. He did not improve at Wallajabad, and on the 1st December the burning sensation continued, with numbness, dyspepsia, irregular fever and diseased skin. In February and March he was more emaciated and complained of cough, debility and pains. Face was puffed. Died 28th March. Three pints of fluid were found in the right, and ten ounces in the left cavity of the chest. The upper part of the right lung a mass of tubercles, the lower hepatised, with scattered tubercles. Lungs and pleura costalis adherent.[7] Heart small and pale. Abdomen contained thirty two ounces of fluid. Kidneys diminished. Irregular vascular spots at the lower extremity of the œsophagus, and a slight appearance of ulceration at the termination of the ilium. Some effusion at the base of the brain derived from the spinal theca. *Spine.* A little gelatinised serum is effused into the cellular substance posteriorly to the theca, the vessels of which are unusually small. Pia mater at the 10th dorsal vertebra on the left side is dark, and the cord at this place is soft. The equinal nerves of a dull bluish blanched appearance.

But this softening of the cord does not appear in any way connected with the symptom, as in the following case it was not present.

[7] I do not notice the air and œdema, as they are mentioned in a way which leaves much doubt as to either having been present. Thus, weight of the lung is not enough to characterize œdema, nor if there had been much gas and 3 pints of water could the lung have remained uncollapsed. The cases are a valuable contribution to pathology, although in their present form of little *general* use. *Original note.*

Case 11th. 28th January 1826. Mahomed Issoph, subadar, ætat. 46, had been five months ill, his complaints coming on in the following order; dysentery, swellings of legs and body, pain of limbs, burning sensation, dyspnœa, wasting and debility. Is now emaciated, feeble, and complains of dyspnœa, œdema, impaired appetite and digestion, sleeplessness, burning pains and partial paralysis of the lower extremities; pulse 60, slight fur on the tongue. Dark spots on the skin. Pain on pressure over the colon, and the lungs are imperfectly traversed. In March there were abdominal swellings; in June, griping about umbilicus, tongue red, was much purged, the stools of mucus, feces, and tinged with blood and he died on the 18th. *Dissection.* Some fluid in the cavities of the pleura and pericardium; cartilaginous tubercles in the lungs. *Abdomen* contained 20 oz. of fluid with jelly like flakes. Peritoneum thickened and milky; some ulceration of the mucous membrane of the ilium; and the colon was thickened and much ulcerated. *Head.* There seems to have been no disease in the brain or its membranes. *Spine.* Much fluid without and in the theca; considerable vascularity; and the cordiform mass healthy.

The same appearances were observed in several other patients, in whom the disease was excited apparently by slight wounds, dysentery or other common disease. How far the effusion in the spinal canal is the cause of the burning and numbness, or the mere result of the general hydropic and cachectic disposition is somewhat doubtful. The former opinion is supported by the following case in which the upper extremities suffered, as well as the lower, and the effusion exterior to the theca extended as high as the first cervical vertebra.

Case 12th. Ramaswamy, sepoy, ætat. 25. Was three months ill, a sloughing ulcer having been successively followed by diarrhœa, dysentery, pains, heaviness of the body and limbs, stiffness, burning of the palms and soles, and numbness of the extremities. He is now emaciated and weak, his legs are œdematous and his appetite and digestion very bad. Has ten serous stools daily, urine scanty, pulse quick, soft and feeble; tongue pale and smooth, skin thick and dry, slight abdominal fluctuation; no pain on pressure. He died suddenly soon after. The lungs were found tuberculated. The liver large and pale; the mucous membrane of the intestines vascular, and that of the colon much ulcerated. There was water in the ventricles, and the cellular structure exterior to the theca was injected with gelatinised fluid from the first cervical vertebra to the sacrum; slight effusion only, into the theca. The cord appears to have been pretty natural, although the lower part was somewhat soft.

It must be observed that burning is by no means a certain consequence of the effusion, although its existence is indicated by other symptoms, and the constitution is in the same morbid state as in other examples. The following case is selected to show this, the connection with scorbutic habit, and the tendency to effusion and tubercular formations, and is in many points of view instructive.

Case 13th. Menthoo, who had suffered from dysentery at Prome was successively attacked with dyspnœa, thoracic pains, sore gums and teeth loosened, œdema, pustular eruptions especially of the extremities, pains, heaviness and numbness of limbs, emaciation, anorexia, indigestion, and watery stools. The transverse colon was tender and was felt enlarged; effusion took place into the abdomen, the thoracic symptoms were aggravated and he died in four months after his return from Ava. *Dissection.* Adhesions of the costal and pulmonary pleura, and of the heart to the pericardium which was thickened and cartilaginous. Much fluid in the abdomen and the peritoneum was thickened, red, and studded in all its convolutions with minute, firm, white tubercles containing a fluid. Liver rounded and irregular anteriorly. *Head.* There was much effusion between the arachnoid and dura and pia maters but very little in the ventricles: the cerebral substance was soft. *Spine.* Much fluid external to the theca and between it and the cord. Cervical and lumbar portions of the cord soft. The cauda equina surrounded by a substance like current jelly and appears blanched.

There can be no doubt of the *general* effect of these effusions in the spine, but in a sepoy who complained only of some abdominal pain and cough, and emaciation with quick pulse and vomiting towards the termination, but no burning or numbness, nearly the same appearances in the spine presented themselves on dissection. The lungs and mesentery were tubercular, adhesions had formed between all the abdominal viscera, and the newly formed false membrane of which they were composed had acquired a tubercular structure; and the mucous membranes were ulcerated and that of the colon had sloughed. In other instances, severe pain in the lower extremities was the only effect of these effusions, observed during life.

The pathological inferences to which these cases lead are of great importance, and demonstrate that the disease is not confined to one part of the body, but appears to be connected with a general depravation of the system and morbid state of the fluids; and that in the progress of these, the functions and structure of the spinal cord and nerves are more or less altered and diseased. The tendency to tubercular formation is in part explained, by the frequency of consumptive complaints in the moist climate of the Straits, and the curious observations of Mr. Baron on the effects of coarse and unnutritious food, in inducing tubercles in the membranes of the animals on which his experiments were made. To say more in the present state of our knowledge would be useless, but as the relations of this complaint to other diseases are so obscure, no fact should be overlooked; and it may therefore be stated, that men labouring under "burning of the feet" appear to have been very subject to sloughing ulcers, of which a melancholy instance occurred to me, in a man who applied marking nut to his foot to remove the former complaint, and died in consequence of the ulcer caused by it becoming immediataly phagedenic, and destroying the foot in a few days. The diseases prevail in similar circumstances, and it is therefore impossible to say how far the one gave rise to the other or were merely accidenttally conjoined [8] These dissections also afford a very important practical lesson, which should be carefully

[8] This observation must not be lost sight of in the treatment, and impresses the necessity of great caution in applying blisters to parts the nervous or vascular powers of which are much diminished. A gentleman who unexpectedly recovered from a most aggravated attack of remittent fever, during which there were unequivocal symptoms of effusion in the spinal canal without cerebral disturbance, nearly lost the use of his legs and arms, and suffered the most excruciating spasmodic pains in the calves of the legs and soles, with burning sensations of the surface of the feet; these were increased in the night. Sinapisms were applied to the feet and, having been allowed to remain too long, vesicated. The serum was discoloured and livid, much of the skin sloughed and he narrowly escaped general mortification of the legs. When the sloughs were removed with the scissars, granulation went on rapidly under the use of hot dressings. Mr. Burnard remarks "that the circulation appears languid in the extremities, and in one instance was so little capable of supporting any increased action, that blisters applied to the calves of the legs to relieve it, produced sores, which went into rapid sphacelus."

attended to, not only by medical officers, but by military authorities who may be connected with future expeditions to the eastward; viz. that the disease of "burning of the feet," and those other affections of an allied character depending on similar causes, although devoid of this symptom, are exceedingly prone to run into irremediable and fatal organic lesions, for the cure of which no medical skill nor the advantages of a return to their native country will be of any avail. It is in vain to recommend the supply of other food, which, in extensive expeditions, cannot be done by any government however liberal. But by allowing of the return of all men afflicted with this malady at an early period of the disease, not only would the real efficiency of corps be preserved in a better state than when burdened with a heavy and hopeless sick list, and the expenditure of passage money more than saved in pensions; but what is of far more importance, the moral effect on the minds of the native troops, which must be produced by the miserable deaths of so vast a part of those employed, would be prevented, and a conviction of the care of the government for their welfare more fully impressed on them. The prognosis is not unfavourable if the visceral affections are slight, the bowels not much disordered, and the emaciation has not proceeded far, and a change of food and climate can be procured: but even then, the cure is likely to take many weeks and months before it is complete, and there is cause to fear that the patient will fall an easy victim to other disease. In other circumstances there is little hope of permanent recovery; I am not, however, able to point out with accuracy the degrees of danger of the various organic changes. None however are so fatal as bowel complaints, which in all circumstances are more frequently mortal in natives than in Europeans, and especially in this disease in which the evils of scurvy and a tubercular disposition are combined.

Of the treatment little can be said. Antiscorbutics have been recommended, and in favorable circumstances may be useful. The treatment by ipecacuan, nitre and small doses of calomel pursued by Dr. Conwell, seemed to do little good. The essential object is change of climate and a return to the usual habits of life and food of the sepoy, with exemption from duty, especially hard drills. This is perhaps best attained by allowing him to return to his village, and if with the regiment, not sending him to duty for a considerable time after his apparent recovery. As the patient gains flesh and strength, the pains and burning leave him, and he recovers without the aid of medicine. Mercury is not beneficial, even in the pains of the legs when the burning is slight or absent.

Case 14th. Paupodoo, ætat. 30, has severe pains in the lower limbs, especially the calves of the legs, which have resisted various treatment. He had irregular fever, headach, his skin was covered with itch, his tongue was parched, he had no appetite and was much emaciated. Mercury was given in small doses but had not the slightest effect in removing the symptoms, which gradually declined and his flesh and strength were restored, after which the pains left him.

Case 15th. Shaik Modinah, ætat. 30. Has weakness, burning in the soles of the feet and pains of the legs, bowels and appetite regular; blisters were applied to the feet without benefit, and calomel and antimony were used with no better success. When left to himself, his strength improved and in a month the pains had nearly left him, and he recovered.

Case 16th. Mahomed Gollib. Burning in soles of feet with pains of the lower extremities, emaciation, dry skin, irregular fever, cough with copious expectoration and dyspnœa on exertion. Treated with mercury which did no good, and may be supposed therefore to have done harm. He was sent to his village for the benefit of his health.

Case 17th. Shaik Mucktoom was admitted with general debility and pains in the legs and soles of the feet; nausea was relieved by an emetic which brought off bile, and he recovered when using bark; but rest and good food seemed the principal means of cure.

Case 18th. Guntaloo, admitted with pains, and a burning sensation in the soles of the feet and "weakness all over the body;" was relieved as he gained strength by rest and bark.

Elderly men are most subject to the complaint and in them the disease is most obstinate, of which the following is a common example. Permaloo, ætat. 54, has had burning in the soles of the feet with pains of limbs, distension at epigastrium and cough for months, and is pensioned as incurable.

There are usually signs of great local debility. Naikloo, ætat. 40, has pains in limbs, burning of soles, œdema of the legs, and feelings of weakness all over him. The œdema subsided rapidly by rest alone, and the burning soon left him when using bark. The restoration of strength and the healthy state of the digestive organs are the indications to be had in view, and for this purpose the mildest laxatives only should be used, such as castor oil, rhubarb and magnesia, &c. Sulphuric acid and ginger have appeared to be useful additions to the bark. If there is local pain a few leeches are to be applied instead of blisters, which are hurtful in constitutions so irritable as those affected with this complaint. The oleum nigrum of Dr. Herklots has been used in a few cases without success, for the pains in the soles of the feet. It deserves a further trial. Of particular remedies of which my experience affords but doubtful evidence it is better not to speak. The various medicines required to obviate the many ails arising in chronic diseases, must be left to the common principles of medical science, except when the good or ill effect of particular drugs have been evident in extended experience.

The complications were often very troublesome and threw the symptom we are considering into the back ground, as in the following case. A man, ætat. 30, had a foul ulcer at the bend of the arm ascribed to a slight wound; it inflamed and the ulcer became foul, he then got irregular fever, tumid spleen with pain in the left hypochondrium and shoulder; after a fit of fever a burning sensation over the body came on (unconnected with fever), and accompanied with severe pains and disordered stomach, from which he did not recover for some time. Another who seemed to labour under the same morbid influence, was admitted with great debility, nearly complete loss of voice and pain extending down the gullet to the stomach on swallowing. To the investigation of these and many cases of the same character, great opportunities and zeal would be required.

I have not seen any case of disease in Europeans which I believe to be of the same nature as that we have been considering; although a burning of the surface has been a symptom of disease of the brain, or other part of the nervous system. Of the first, an example occurred in J. Allan, an artillery man who was severely injured by the explosion of a tumbril. He continued for years to suffer from headach, and I had occasion to treat him several times for violent pain of the left ancle with wasting of the limb. On the 27th May 1829 he was readmitted with great increase of headach, and numbness of the limbs accompanied with sensation of burning, although they were cool to the touch. Leeches and purgatives gave him no relief, headach was attended with soreness of the scalp over the occiput, and was equally painful day and night. His tongue was dry and white and the stomach was irritable. The whole body was affected with the burning sensation, and he was not relieved by bleeding, which was performed at his own request. He then suffered from giddiness and had occasional epileptic fits. He improved a little under gentle laxatives and occasional leeching and cold to the head, and was ultimately pensioned.

The following case occurred at Hyderabad where I believe beriberi is hardly known, but the symptoms were similar in some respects. A sergeant, in India 10 years, had been ill for five weaks after exposure to cold when he had committed excess: the lower extremities swelled and became painful and weak immediately after, with high colored and scanty urine; he had cough and thick ropy expectoration and increased action and uneasiness about the præcordia. The œdema receded, and the lower limbs became almost paralytic with numbness and a most distressing burning sensation nearly to the hips. When I saw him this had diminished, and with the numbness, was confined to the inner side of the legs and to the soles of the feet. The flesh of the calves were tender to the touch, and he complained of pricking sensations of the knees and "creeping" of the legs: there was much pain and stiffness of the soles of the feet, which were exceedingly tender to the touch and the burning heat had not quite left them; the skin was soft and on the slightest motion of the legs, which were much emaciated, they were bathed in perspiration but without feeling cold to the touch. Tongue furred, appetite unusually great, pulse 100, small, rather sharp and weak; urine now copious and of natural color. Had never lived hard,* had venereal or head symptoms, and had been always healthy. No pain or tenderness of the spine. Had at the commencement a little numbness and pain at the extremities of the fingers. Warm bathing of the feet has relieved the pain and stiffness. He derived much benefit from the diligent use of frictions with turpentine, and especially from sinapisms to the inside of the legs and soles of the feet, which rapidly removed the numbness and burning sensations and increased the powers of the limb. Blisters to the lumbar vertebræ and oleum nigrum were used at the same time, and seemed to do good. His recovery in two months was almost complete.

A case in some respects analogous is recorded in the *London Medical and Surgical Journal,* April 28th 1832, under the head of chronic sciatic neuralgia. A gentleman after exposure to cold, had pains of the joints, neuralgia of the sciatic nerves and spasms of the legs and thighs. Pains were aggravated from 4 P. M. to 4 A. M. and were compared to severe scalding. He was much emaciated. Iron, arsenic, quinine and an open blister failed. The cure was effected by issues, but

* It is probable that he had drank a good deal. *Original note.*

erratic neuralgic pains continued for some time.

Rheumatism in Europeans.

The subject of rheumatism as it affects Europeans in India is of the greatest practical importance, and has been entirely neglected, as far as I know, by almost every writer on intertropical disease; probably from a belief that the climate has little influence in modifying its character or treatment. Notwithstanding its general and frequent prevalence over the globe, it has by no means been studied with such success as to render it unnecessary to investigate its history further, and especially, the varieties it exhibits in different climates. At present I shall confine my observations to a few points of considerable interest, the opportunity for laying which before the Indian medical service is my chief inducement to write this paper. Should these meet with the approbation of the Board, I shall have much pleasure in adding the result of my experience in such other points, as may be thought to stand in want of further illustration than is to be found in books.

The common acute rheumatism of Europe is very little known in India, and when cases in some degree resembling it do occur, they are attended with little hardness of pulse, and the skin instead of being bathed in perspiration is usually dry, although instances of the contrary do now and then occur. The joints are then hot and painful, but I have hardly met a case where heat was not agreeable to the patient. Repeated leeching where the pain is not much diffused is of signal advantage. General bleeding has very seldom done good, and the blood is rarely buffy except when the external complaint is complicated with thoracic affections. Warm baths and Dover's powder have been less useful in this form of the complaint than in any other, even when they caused free and general perspiration. Tartrate of antimony in large and frequently repeated doses has been often of great use, and should be more generally employed in this form of the com plaint than I believe it has yet been; one grain or a grain and a half may be given every hour with advantage, and will be found to remove rapidly a complaint, to which other remedies are not adapted or cannot be safely used. Its effects do not depend on its diaphoretic or evacuant virtues, as when none of these have followed its exhibition, the benefit from its general constitutional action has been great. A caution however is necessary against continuing the medicine too long, as it causes considerable debility, and therefore, when the symptoms are relieved it should be omitted, and bark with good diet and a moderate allowance of spirits at dinner prescribed, by which the appetite and strength are rapidly restored. Instances have occurredwhere the internal use of tartar emetic has been greatly assisted by the constitutional effect of camphorated mercurial ointment, but the combination of calomel and the tartrate is apt to irritate the bowels. Blisters are not to be used till the excitement has been removed, as they irritate and excite fever, and do not often relieve the pain. Imperfect cures have been completed by their means. The acetate of colchicum has been useful in this form of the disease, and also in rheumatism of an opposite character but coming on suddenly; nor have I found its beneficial effects confined to cases of affection of the joints and bursæ as mentioned in some recent papers. The wine has failed, principally I believe, from its having been obtained at considerable expence and therefore prescribed to the most obstinate cases only; it is a form better adapted for this country and would, I have no doubt, lead to more successful practice were it supplied from the government stores.* In rheumatic gout in India, it is as powerful a remedy as at home. Caution in its use is necessary, as I am informed by an experienced surgeon on this establishment, that he lost a patient from abdominal inflammation brought on by its use in doses of the usual strength.

The consideration of the varieties of chronic active and passive rheumatism I shall not at present enter upon, but proceed to state the result of my experience on several points which are still undecided by authors, or on which I have found the opinion of practitioners in this country to differ.

It has been stated of late that rheumatism is never a local complaint, and Mr. Lawrence is of opinion that local remedies are of no use; but in India as in Europe examples constantly occur, in which it can be traced directly to a cause acting on a part of the surface, which alone takes on diseased action, and this will frequently exist for a long time with great severity without attacking other parts; and not uncommonly, the whole limb is slowly wasted by the continued pain and inaction before any other parts suffer. In such examples as well as many others, whatever effect mercury and other remedies may have on the local disease, the cure is most certainly and quickly brought about by local means, and they are very important auxiliaries in every case where the pains are at all fixed.[9] The tendency to affect other parts is not, in ge-

* The wine of colchicum is now supplied from the stores.

[9] A few drops of croton oil rubbed on the part, is a useful and economical counter-irritant.

neral, an evidence of constitutional taint, but is merely the result of the easy transference of the diseased action to other structures of the same kind; although in long continued disease the whole habit partakes in it, as is evident by various new parts suddenly and without ostensible external cause, after long intervals of apparent health, taking on the old disease in its original form.

Cold is a very general cause and affects especially those of weakly constitutions, convalescents from other diseases, and men in confinement; the disease also prevails most severely in districts where the variations of temperature are great, especially when these are accompanied with much moisture. Numerous cases however occur in the height of the hot weather, which cannot be traced to any cause, and are often exceedingly obstinate. In feverish districts rheumatism is very prevalent, partly from the moisture and variable climate being exciting causes of both diseases, and partly from the frequent origin of rheumatism in long continued attacks of intermittent and remittent fever. An interesting example of this has already been related, in which even swellings of the periosteum arose from neglected ague, and multitudes of others have been carefully observed. It is true, that in individual cases it is difficult to prove that the affection does not arise from venereal disease, but when the effect is of frequent occurrence, immediately follows the supposed cause, is aggravated by its recurrence, and when in many instances the assertions of the men that they had not laboured under syphilis are corroborated by the hospital records, and when they have no motive to conceal their having had disease and describe with accuracy syphilitic symptoms under which they had laboured years before, I do not think that vague surmise of previous taint can be received as an explanation deserving of much regard. To this I would add, that the comparison of venereal sequelæ in the same body of men, in districts where fever is little known and when treated on the same plan, has fully borne out the opinion, that all forms of rheumatism, and pains in the bones and periosteum, are often induced by fever treated with or without mercury; and I may add, that nodes of the long bones may arise without any syphilitic or mercurial action, and as a simple consequence of rheumatism. Few parts suffer more from rheumatism after fever than the scalp; and the intermittent hemicrania is, in many instances, a form of febrile paroxysm coming on with obscure chills and going off with sweats; and at others a sequela of the fever, but partaking of the character of the idiopathic disease of the scalp, which, though intermittent, is often unconnected with fever and not to be cured by the same means. In both forms of the complaint the periosteum is occasionally inflamed and swollen; and the treatment requires to be carefully varied, till a successful combination of measures is discovered. The diffusion of the pain over the scalp or down the neck takes place in each form of the disease, and when that is most distinctly of a febrile character if it continues long or relapses are frequent, all the joints and the trunk suffer; and in one instance the heart became inflamed and required active treatment, principally by local bleeding and mercury. The internal ear is frequently involved in both these complaints, and morbid sounds, pain and even discharge follow fever and occur in simple rheumatism, and are often obstinate. It is difficult to distinguish some of these complaints from cerebral affection, and they have in my experience been the precursors of very alarming disease.[10]

The intermittent pains of the side of the head are also sometimes of a neuralgic nature, when they prove very obstinate and require the greatest perseverance on the part of the surgeon. They are generally attended with abdominal or uterine disorder, and to these the attention must be directed. The pain often shoots along the jaws and sometimes the teeth ache dreadfully, and if they are diseased the diagnosis is increased in difficulty, as similar symptoms arise from diseased teeth which had been attended with no inconvenience for years. I have seen the whole teeth of one side of the head or of half the lower jaw loosened by the nervous affection, although unconnected with organic disease or any constitutional taint.[11] These cases as well as all others of intermittent headach, are remarkably benefited by change of air, and a return to Europe and residence for sometime there. In other examples no hope of cure can be entertained, but when there are no general symptoms of disease of the brain, I do not know that we can ever determine that these affections are incurable. In the following remarkable case there was no room to doubt; but when we consider how many of the European soldiers are subject to obstinate pain in the head, consequent on fever, mer-

[10] In one, after fever discharge from the ear took place, and caries of the os petrosum and suppuration of the cerebellum terminated a very painful illness. In another the singing in the ears was attended with pains of the scalp and general ill health and wasting; afterwards serous effusion appeared to have taken place on the brain, indicated by inability to *direct* the motions; partial palsy; loss of power to articulate *certain* letters; forgetfulness of certain letters and of common words in writing ordinary sentences and loss of the power of writing distinctly; enlarged pupil and rapid pulse. Bleeding did harm. He was cured by mercury and blisters. *Original note.*

[11] Œdema of the eyelid and other parts may be induced by the pain; and in one case not only was the temperature increased, but a number of small boils was the result of the excited state of the vessels.

cury, excesses and exposure, it is reasonable to suppose that many of them are dependant on minor degrees of organic change.

Case 19th. An invalid artillery man had been long subject to headach. I found him complaining of severe pain in the left side of the head which was most violent after 1 P. M. and during the night, and easiest in the mornings and forenoon; severe pain of the left upper jaw bone and in the teeth of the same side none of which were carious, but the gums were retracted and spongy. He had also occasional epileptic fits and the power of the lower extremities was diminished. The fits became more frequent. The intellect was not sensibly impaired till two days before death when he was insensible, the eyes fixed, pupils contracted but affected by light; pulse frequent, small and feeble; breathing difficult. Died convulsed. The vessels of the pia mater were gorged with blood. The substance of the cerebrum was harder than natural, and the induration extended down the medulla oblongata and to the forepart of the spinal cord. When it was attempted to separate the dura mater from the anterior lobes of the cerebrum, the substance of the brain was torn away with it, and all the parts immediately above the orbits were broken down and had the appearance of an abscess. The membranes were much thickened; the whole hollow space between the left petrous bone and optic foramen was full of round cartilaginous tubercles, some of them as large as a walnut, attached to the singularly thickened membranes. They extended upwards to the transverse spinous process of the os sphenoides, and had caused the partial absorption of the bone leaving a sharp spicula. There was fluid in the ventricles and at the base of the skull. The cerebellum was healthy.

Another very frequent cause of rheumatism is the use of mercury, which deserves the utmost attention, not only from its vast importance in reference to the judicious use of that most valuable remedy, but also from its bearing on many questions of practical importance in all countries. It has been asserted by a large body of the profession, that nodes do not arise from venereal disease, if mercury has not been given for its cure, but I have found this and all other forms of secondary symptoms to follow that disease when carefully treated (as I am in the habit of doing in the vast majority of cases), without the use of a grain of mercurial medicine; but these are far from common, and do not often prove obstinate if a mild mercurial course is had recourse to. On the other hand, I can state from extensive experience carefully recorded, that pains in the limbs, periostitis, and nodes do arise in India very frequently from mercurial action for whatever cause induced, and however carefully, and in whatever form it may be administered. Mr. Lawrence in his valuable lectures on surgery denies that the periosteum is ever diseased by mercury, because it is the best remedy; which cannot be admitted as a proof so long as we are ignorant both of the manner in which the disease is induced and cured, and consequently unable to reason on the subject; and to me it appears that the proof of its activity in disease of the part, affords a probability of its having also a power of bringing on morbid action when the part is in health. Dr. Alison whose philosophic caution is equal to that of any living writer I am acquainted with, admits that with cold mercury may produce periostitis, but I am every day in the way of seeing it induce severe pains of the bones when the weather is equable and hot, and the patient is carefully cased in flannel and protected from the possibility of catching cold. He also thinks mercury an unsafe remedy in inflammation of the periosteum induced by it, a supposition certainly probable enough in theory, but which careful observation has convinced me to be an ill founded rule in practice, although important to be kept in view as a caution in the method of its employment. Dr. Alison is also of opinion that mercury never produces symptoms like syphilis, and reasons from "the ascertained fact" that in tropical climates such never result. On this subject I have reason to entertain opinions somewhat different, as I have observed various cutaneous affections arise from its use, especially an eruption of inflamed pustules over the body and face; and in one man, who there was reason to believe, had not had any venereal complaint for twelve years, repeated courses of mercury for hepatic affections and fever, and subsequent exposure on a march in the wet season, caused severe nocturnal pains, tumefaction of the tibia, an eruption of round dark coloured scaly blotches over the body and very slow ulceration of the throat, of which he died. Dr. Musgrave, whose authority appears to be recognised by the principal medical journals as conclusive, declares he never saw pains such as we are considering in the course of a practice in the West Indies, in which he appears to have abused it beyond measure. Whether there is any way of explaining this I know not, but I have already stated, that pains are thus produced in natives, and I have had more extensive opportunity of noticing it in Europeans. Notwithstanding the high opinion I entertain of mercury as a remedy in most intertropical diseases, I employ it with great caution, never persevering in its use when its effects are not easily induced, or when it does not soon do good, nor are many men severely salivated under my care; yet so common and so immediate is the effect on the limbs in many instances, that mercurial pains are ever a subject of dread and often of expectation, being an evil to which we must submit in preference of greater ills. In proof that these pains are really the effect of the use of mercury, in addition to the remarks made above on the nature of the evidence of rheumatism being caused by fever, it may be observed, that these pains follow *immediately* the mercurial action, at a time when rheumatism from other causes is almost unknown. The nature of the disease for which it is administered does not seem to make much difference in the frequency and severity of the pains, as they follow hepatitis, dysentery, and simple membranous inflammation when treated by mercury. Whether they more commonly occur after venereal diseases, I cannot say, not being in the practice of using it unless in obstinate or old cases. There is no form of rheumatic inflammation and pains that is not caused by mercury, but the lower extremities suffer most frequently, especially the thigh bones and legs. Sometimes the pains are of a neuralgic character affecting the fleshy parts below the loins, which are occasionally tender to pressure, and they gradually leave the patient from above downwards. When the treatment of severe disease is conducted, however cautiously, by large doses of calomel, the patient rarely escapes more or less subsequent suffering from pains. But it is especially in those examples of frequent occurrence, in which salivation does not follow the exhibition of mercury, that pains follow, even when not persevered in to any great extent. This is one reason amongst others which makes it imperative to stop the medicine, whenever it is evident that it will not affect the system, or fails to do good. An opinion still prevails with many, that the mercury is not absorbed in such cases, which is exceedingly injurious in encouraging its continued employment long after it must have acted as a poison, under an idea that its specific virtue is the only thing that can overcome the disease. That this opinion is erroneous I have had abundant proof, not only in the subsequent pains, the occurrence of profuse ptyalism days after the omission of mercury on the disease yielding to other means, and in the paroxysm of an intermittent fever and even the irritation from a blister, stopping the mercurial action while they lasted; but also in the following observation made some years ago, and confirmed by a great number of subsequent observations. *After a moderate quantity of calomel is taken the gums are slightly affected and the mouth runs a little, but while the medicine is continued it gets drier and less sore, and perseverance in its use never fails to be injurious and its ordinary effect on the mouth or on the disease cannot be produced.* This observation I have found of great use in practice, not only in avoiding the production of pains, but in preserving the lives of patients who would otherwise sink from the combined influence of visceral disease and mercurial irritation.[12] The joints do not always escape the pains arising from mercury; but in two cases which occurred to me lately, inflammation and increased secretion into the cavity of the joint itself, appeared to have had some connection with hepatic and intestinal disease; the affection, however, is not very common, and extensive experience would be necessary to ascer-

[12] The observation in the text does not supersede the necessity of careful attention to the appearance of the gums and the character of the ptyalism, caused by mercury when it does not act beneficially.

tain how far this was an effect of the drug taken for the disease of the internal parts.

A stout European suffered from several violent inflammations of the liver, particularly of the left lobe. He was several times successfully treated, but his health was at last broken and he had pains in the knees, &c. In April 1831 I lost sight of him, and met him again in 1832. In the interval he had got worse, the left lobe could be felt hard and enlarged, he had a nearly constant purging of whitish stools mixed with puriform matter, and occasionally alternating with reddish feculent evacuations. He suffered from pains, especially of the knees, which were swollen on each side of the tendon of the rectus, and it was remarked, that the internal pains and bowel complaint and pain of the knees in some degree alternated. The left colon was felt thick and the whole of that gut was tender. He was anasarcous, the belly tumid, and his breathing obstructed in the recumbent posture, and he gradually sunk and died convulsed; he could swallow and his face remained sensible to the last. The brain was healthy. Bloody serum was found external to the theca *anteriorly*. The tongue which was red and smooth during life was now pale. The mucous membrane of the great end of the stomach was red and pulpy, as were the whole of the small intestines, with the exception of spots here and there near the colon. There were some superficial ulcers of the right colon and some marks of others having healed, and the whole gut was irregularly gorged; the sigmoid flexure greatly thickened, its external coats seem cartilaginous, and ulcers were more frequent. The liver was very smooth, enlarged and shapeless, the white matter unusually developed and the edge of the left lobe so much so as to appear devoidofglandular substance,andthewho leliver had a fleshy look and tore like rotten leather. The gall bladder contained only a little pale watery bile. The white secretion passed in such large quantity, appeared to have come from the small intestines and to have passed rapidly and little changed through the colon. The kidneys were vascular,and the urine had deposited a thick white sediment, was of low specific gravity (1012.), and afforded some coagulum with muriate of mercury. There was much swelling of the knee joint on each side of the patella, arising from the distension of the capsule which extended two inches above the knee pan. The bursæ seemed healthy.

The pains in the other case followed on the 8th day of a bowel complaint, at first apparently mild but connected with disordered and deficient biliary secretion, for which he had taken small does of calomel and ipecacuan, without affecting his mouth except on one side: the pains were at first very violent but after some time declined, and puffy swelling on each side of the tendon of the rectus muscles, and of the bursæ of the ancle joints took place, proved exceedingly obstinate, and reduced the patient to a state of great emaciation from which he is not yet recovered. The mercurial action did not appear to be the sole cause of the pains, and the secretions showed the disease to approach in its nature to the preceding case.[13] At one time the pain was most severe in the muscles of the right thigh, and it deserves notice, that in some cases of hepatic disease there is pain in the right knee and thigh or in the groin, and even in the foot. Heberden also describes a case of inflammation of the spleen, which was attended

[13] The patient was transferred to the cantonment hospital at Secunderabad, and sunk under a relapse of the bowel complaint.

with severe pain in the calf.[14]

Notwithstanding my conviction of the frequency of mercurial rheumatism I can assert on the ground of extensive experience, that mercury in small doses and judicious combination, is the most generally effectual remedy in all forms of rheumatism in Europeans in India; and the remarks on its employment in natives apply without any material modification to Europeans. It is especially necessary to give it in small doses, for very little will affect the mouth, and as there is danger of relapse being caused by the peculiar effect of mercury, it should never be given more frequently or continued longer than is absolutely necessary. This caution is the more necessary, as it is stated in some recent works, that mercury affects the system with difficulty in acute rheumatism; and in other cases, ten grains of calomel every night or five grains two or three times a day are recommended, which is far more than I consider safe. Mr. Wyllie, formerly cantonment surgeon at Nagpore, who was averse to the free employment of calomel in other diseases, assured me, that it was the only agent which had any power over the severe rheumatism of that place. The manner of its action is, I believe, little understood, I shall therefore communicate the following case which throws some light on one part of the subject.

[14] Sense of uneasiness and distressing aching pains of the thighs are of frequent occurrence in chronic dysentery, and are of the same nature as those which are so often complained of in the hips. They are of a neuralgic character, and apparently arise from the nerves near the diseased intestine partaking more or less in the morbid actions. When the colon on one side is diseased and the rest of the gut is little affected, the pains are confined to the limb of the same side. The thigh has been observed to be stiff and to be extended with some difficulty, and the surface may be benumbed. The pain, in aggravated cases, has been described as peculiarly severe at the inner side of the knee joint, and its motions are not performed freely. The nerves running along the inner side of the limb have been most affected, causing tenderness down the inner side of the thigh and leg, to the heel and ancle which have been severely pained; and the connection of these symptoms with the abdominal affection is indicated by the pain shooting into the iliac region and round the hip. These pains are least felt from 4 A. M. till evening; they are aggravated before rain but not while it falls.

Case 20th. Joseph Johnston, corporal, ætat. 30. In India 8 years. Was admitted in September 1831, with severe pains in the arms and chest, increased at night, and relieved by warm bathing; the fingers and wrist swelled; pulse quick and small. He ascribed the complaint to cold, and has had no venereal complaint for a considerable time. He was cured by tartrate of antimony and a little calomel, but was too soon discharged.

Readmitted in October with pains in the arms, hip and legs, and also in the chest and left ancle. Pulse 105, rather sharp and small, tongue foul; was treated by a grain, and a grain and half of tartar emetic every hour, which relieved him, but he was not cured till his gums were made a little tender by camphorated mercurial frictions. November 2nd, discharged. Readmitted April 30th, 1832. The general pains had left him and he complained of severe aching at night in the left tibia, which was swollen behind and anteriorly, causing considerable deformity. There were no irregular swellings. Bad appetite and furred tongue. Leeches gave no relief and seemed to increase the swelling, and tension of the soft parts; the pain extended to the foot and the general health was much disordered. His gums were made slightly sore by calomel and antimonial powder, the pain left him and the swelling subsided considerably. He was again ill in June (not under my care) and had irregular bowels and stools of a light or dirty pale green colour, and his recovery was slow and imperfect. He went to duty, and returned to hospital in October: the following is the history of his illness taken from the journal. October 9th. Admitted yesterday with an aggravation of rheumatism under which he has long laboured. Pains in the legs, shoulders arms and hands severe from evening till towards morning and relieved by heat, while any wind distresses him. Abdominal viscera do not show any signs of irritability as on former occasions. Tongue loaded with a yellow fur, and near the root there is a deep sulcus, down the centre it is smooth and red as is the whole anterior part, except here and there where there are spots of white fur; urgent thirst, no appetite, nauseous taste in the mouth. Has pain in the region of the heart with tenderness on pressure between the cartilages; motion aggravates it. About six weeks ago, a spasmodic pain across the hypochondria came on, and after a few hours settled in the breast which had been uneasy before, and had been preceded, for some time, by uneasiness and pain in epigastrium. No palpitation or fainting fits. Breathing rather short but not influenced by position. Has rather more pain in the tip of the right shoulder than elsewhere. Pulse 86, small but harder than natural, sweats much. Urine now pretty natural. Had what appears to have been dropsical swellings after his discharge from hospital a month ago; they went away and left him suffering much from the pains. Hair dark. Much purged by jalap yesterday. V. S. ad ℥xx. ℞ Pil. hyd., pulv. ipecac., āā, gr. iij ter die. Habt. acet. colchici ʒj ter die. Vespere. Bore the bleeding well, blood buffed and cupped; chest is much easier; legs rather more painful. Pulse 96, small, skin moist, three stools. Continue the medicines. Twenty leeches to be applied over the seat of the thoracic pain. Frictions to the limbs. 10th. Free from uneasiness in the chest, sweats much; pains below the knees and in the arm and hands were severe in the night, 36 respirations in a minute. Pulse 92, small. 11th. No uneasiness of chest, pains perhaps a little better; pulse 80, small and a little sharp. 12th. Violently purged. Stools thin but otherwise good, no griping; pains easier. Breast easy, but there is some shortness of breath in the afternoon. Pulse 92, small and weak, sweats freely. Omitt. med. Habt. opii gr j. Vesp. No stool since he took the pill. Pains rather more severe, pulse 88, feels heavy and uncomfortable towards evening, thirst, no appetite. Gums a little tender V. S. ad ℥xij. Balneum calidum h. s. 13th. Blood cupped and buffy. Griped in the night and passed slimy stools with straining. Had an ounce of castor oil with 15 drops of laudanum which relieved the griping, and he has had no stool since. Pains always easier in the morning, abdomen not painful; tongue much loaded; gums tender. Milk 2 pints. Rept. ol. ricini. 14th. Much purged yesterday, stools copious, thin and of a light yellow colour, like eggs and milk mixed together. No griping with the stools. Had an anodyne draught at bed time with relief to purging. Slept better. Pains are easier which he ascribes to the dry weather. Pulse 84, urine brown, gums tender. Habt. calomel., pulv. antimon., āā, gr ij, opii gr. j ft. pil. mane et vesp. sumend. 15th. Had pain extending from the small ribs near the spine round the waist for half an hour yesterday, which was relieved by a draught. Gums tender, pains rather less severe, swelling of the bones of the legs subside, pulse 88, two stools. Hirud. xij lumb. Rept. pil. omni nocte. 16th. No return of pain of back; pains much easier; mouth very sore (and lips swollen) but does not run. Bowels loose and stools light coloured, ascribed to the milk diet; pulse small. Omitt. pil. Rept. haust. acet. colchici, tinct. opii min. x sing. dosi. 17th. Did not feel so well yesterday which he ascribed to some change of the weather, but is easy this morning notwithstanding the clouds, sleeps ill from pain of mouth. Breathing free. Bowels regular, but light coloured and thin stools are passed. Pulse 88 small. Cont. acet. colchici. ℞ Borat. sodæ ʒiss, tinct. myrrhæ, tinct. opii, āā, ℥ss, aquæ ℔iss ft. gargar. 18th. Better. Mouth very sore, slept well. Copious white sediment in the urine which is pale. Cont. 19th. No pain except of mouth. Magnes. sulph. ℥ss. Habt. h. s. tinct. opii min. L. 22d. Complains only of the mouth. 27th. No pains and the swellings on tibia are gone, mouth sore; urine pale with a copious white deposit, it is muddy when passed and smells strongly. Two measures of madeira. ℞ Pulv. ipecac. gr.j, nit. potass. gr. vj ft. pulv. ter die sumend. He was soon afterwards discharged. His recovery was perfect and he has had no complaint since. The deposit was examined and found to consist of a chalky powder nearly free from animal matter, which on being subjected to the usual tests proved to be phosphate of lime. It did not melt before the heat of an ordinary blow pipe. This deserves particular attention as the nodes had disappeared, and after a year of deformity the leg had recovered its natural shape, the morbid deposit of bone having passed off by the kidney. It is probable that the absorbents were excited to increased action in the new parts, but as the deposit continued for some time after the absorption must have ceased, the earthy matter formerly required for the nourishment of the preternatural growth, had probably been separated from the blood by the kidney instead of by the vessels of the tibia; and if this is the case it would indicate the necessity of continuing the treatment for some time after apparent cure, and of retaining the patient under observation. In all recent physiological works it is asserted, and by inconclusive arguments attempted to be proved, that absorption goes on almost exclusively from the *interior* of bones, but this case is a sufficient proof that this is not the fact. Another case analogous to this, also occurred to me lately.

A similar circumstance which I have not found noticed in any author occurs in scurvy. It is well known that in severe cases of that disease, the callus of old fractures has been absorbed, and the epiphises separated from the long bones, and that the urine is fetid; and a recent writer in the *Edinburgh Medical and Surgical Journal* mentions, that the urine is turbid and deposits matter like pus. Connecting these facts together, it appeared probable that the puriform deposit was phosphate of lime. An opportunity soon occurred of examining the urine of an European labouring under severe scurvy, which was at first difficult to distinguish from rheumatic pains of the thighs and calves; and it was found thick, muddy, alkaline and very fetid, and a copious white deposit was found at the bottom of the glass, which on examination proved to be phosphate of lime and mucus. This almost immediately disappeared on his getting oranges and fresh provisions, which is a fact worth much more, than the theoretical chemical objections lately brought forward against the use of lime juice in scurvy by Dr. Stevens. As these facts are new I may be allowed to point out the proof they afford, that absorption goes on more rapidly in bones than is generally supposed, and also, that they are not reduced to their elements in passing out of the body as supposed by Bostock. An opinion has been adopted by some physiologists that the animal body has the power of *generating* the earthy salt, and ingenious and careful experiments have been performed on the chick in ovo, and by Prout on the comparative quantity of lime in the food of fowls and that going to form the eggs, in which he seemed to have proved, the generation of lime and the important geological inferences connected with this view of the question; but in these, the possibility of absorption of the earth of the bones of the animal has been overlooked, which will probably afford an explanation of those curious observations.

In rheumatic ophthalmy which is rare in India, and very difficult of cure by any of the common plans of treatment, mercury is a valuable remedy. The following is a very striking example.

Case 21st. A soldier, aged 26, was admitted January 26th 1833, complaining of rheumatic pains in the left sciatic notch, extending back to the sacrum and unattended with fever. He had never suffered from syphilis, but had gonorrhœa four months before. On the 2nd February the pain left the sacrum and the right eye became inflamed, painful and intolerant of light; the conjunctiva was hardly at all affected, numerous fine straight red vessels ran over the ball to the margin of the cornea, where there was a pink blush. There was latterly, slight sluggishness and tendency to irregularity of the iris and to the formation of an opaque ring round the margin of the cornea. The pain was at first of an aching character and confined to the eyeball from which hot burning tears flowed profusely, but in a few days it was only complained of for a space over the ear of the breadth of the palm, and was very violent at night preventing sleep. He derived but little relief from purgatives, emetics, leeches, lotions of different kinds, fomentations, blisters to the head and nape, quinine and occasional doses of mercury, and the symptoms were worse the beginning of March; when his mouth was made sore with the effect of immediately removing the imflamation, pain and flow of acrid tears. Brownish yellow lines on the sclerotic coat and sluggish pupil remained, and the upper eyelid dropped a little, but he was able to do his duty on the 31st. During the inflammation the bowels were costive and the digestive and hepatic system disordered. I have not met with rheumatic iritis, but have no doubt that it will occasionally occur, as venereal iritic inflammation in India, differs in nothing from the same disease in England following papular eruptions.

Another cause of rheumatic pains is weakness from any acute disease, and in these the cure is brought about by restoring the general health, but still more by exercise, which is of great use whenever the patient can bear it, in almost every form of rheumatism in India. I have not met with cases such as are described in an early paper in the Calcutta transactions, in which the joints were said to be altered in structure and cured by strong exercise in a rough cart; but men who would languish for weeks in hospital often rapidly recover, provided they have resolution to continue their usual employment and recreations. This however should not be recommended without much caution; as when there is any inflammatory affection of the joints or periosteum, it is aggravated by motion; and if the pain is severe, the continued irritation of neglected rheumatism causes great emaciation, and leads to the formation of intractable internal disease. Heberden has remarked that there is no part in which severe pain does not occur without swelling, tenderness, or any sensible symptom, and

I believe this is more commonly the case in India than in Europe, and should be carefully attended to by the intertropical military surgeon, who must meet with many cases of pain of the joints of a nature he may be apt to look on as feigned disease. Many of these I have seen produce *great* wasting of the part, and other signs of real and severe disease.

Disorder of the hepatic system is a cause of painful feelings of the external parts, often existing for long periods, and attended with superficial tenderness not only at the margin of the ribs but over the bones. It is the more necessary to notice this, as Dr. Elliotson states, that the tenderness over the bones to *very slight pressure* distinguishes external from internal disease. The fact seems to be, that the external parts take on diseased actions, and that any diagnostic derived from the nature of the feeling must often be erroneous; In some severe cases of hepatitis the soreness of the skin, bones, and muscles extends over the whole right side of the chest, and gives to the disease much of the appearance of severe pleuritic inflammation, or rheumatism of the chest. In such circumstances, after free evacuations the pain and ordinary symptoms of hepatitis become more distinct, and the diffused pain and tenderness leave the patient. I have found this external tenderness to the slightest touch the *only early general symptom of fatal thoracic disease;* it is therefore necessary to be on our guard in such cases, and to observe their progress with more closeness, than the observations of the professor would lead us to think necessary. Severe injuries have been stated to be a cause of rheumatism, and a remarkable case of this kind occurred to me in a man who had received a beating from one of his comrades, the confinement consequent on which, reduced him to a state of debility and emaciation followed by severe rheumatism: the tibia swelled, and matter, which was afterwards absorbed, formed under the periosteum. The pain extended up the thighs, the ribs of the left side got painful, emaciation increased and the left leg was completely wasted ; hepatic affection with loose greenish white stools seemed to be induced, the tongue was foul, and he had pain in the right side at times. Both the blue pill and mercurial frictions increased the purging; calomel and ipecacuan in ten grain doses were prescribed, and restored the biliary secretion and natural functions of the bowels, the pain of the side was removed by blisters, and his health was gradually restored.

The abdominal affections which occurred in this case were often observed to follow protracted rheumatic symptoms, but it was long before I was convinced that they were a sequela of that disease. At length the known fact of chronic rheumatism seldom existing long without being succeeded by great disorder of the general health, and the frequency of the connection of the same train of very peculiar symptoms with previous severe and protracted rheumatism, left little doubt of the abdominal viscera undergoing some morbid changes. The slow progress of the disease, the necessity of sending many of the patients from the interior to the coast for the benefit of change, and their consequently passing into the care of other surgeons, as well as the uncertainty of the pathology of the white diarrhœa so frequently present, threw great difficulties in the way of obtaining any accurate information, as to the nature of the organic changes or morbid actions on which the affections depended. These are by no means difficult of removal on their first appearance, and are then dependent on mere functional disorder, but they become obstinate if the pains continue long or frequently return, and organic changes sooner or later follow, and a permanent cure is then hardly to be hoped for. As the subject has not so far as I know been noticed in books, and as the nature of the symptoms themselves when arising from other causes is but little understood, it will be necessary to give short abstracts of the very lengthened histories of some cases, the termination of which was ascertained. The first instance occurred in Joseph Concannon an artillery man who had lived hard, and had been long subject to severe pains of the limbs. There were nodes on the tibia ascribed to mercury, and the pains although generally worse at night often came on in severe paroxysms, lasting 12 or 18 hours and attended with fever, in preventing which bark had no influence. An emetic followed by a warm bath, or the bath succeeded by repeated doses of Dover's powder, often removed these severe attacks. In September 1828 my attention was first directed to the abdominal symptoms, when the pains had returned with unusual violence. Diarrhœa was now complained of, and the stools were at first thin and greenish, and then white for a few days, and again green. He also complained of occasional pain at epigastrium which was relieved by leeches, and the tongue was remarkably dry and thickly coated. Purgatives were at this time necessary, and two grains of calomel and antimonial powder twice a day restored the healthy state of the secretions, removed the diarrhœa and relieved the pains. Warm baths and tincture of opium with antimonial powder were also necessary. The relief was only temporary, the diarrhœa became intractable and the stools quite white, with an occasional mixture of disordered yeasty brick coloured secretion. Chalk mixture puffed up the belly, and aggravated the uneasy feelings about the stomach and throughout the abdomen. As these symptoms increased the pains left him. In December the emaciation had become extreme; early in January he could eat nothing and vomiting occurred at intervals; his pulse was rapid and feeble, and he complained of pain below the cartilages of the right false ribs. He died on the 18th January 1829. He stated that he had suffered from similar symptoms some years before, and had recovered on being sent to the sea coast. No venereal disease was known to have existed for years. *Dissection.* Viscera of the thorax healthy although he had suffered from dyspnœa. Liver much enlarged and had pushed down the stomach, so that its lower orifice was on the same line with the superior; its substance was hard and light coloured from white interstitial deposit. The gall bladder very large and distended with a light green watery bile; its ducts small. The mucous coat of the stomach redder than natural. Duodenum rather thickened and adherent to the right lobe of the liver; the intestinal mucous membrane reddish, that of the right half of the colon thickened and of a very deep livid colour, and these appearances extended, though in a less degree, into the rectum. The cause of the white diarrhœa in this case, was evidently deficient secretion of bile and increased morbid action of the intestinal mucous membrane. The morbid action of the intestine probably in part depended, in the first instance, on the liver, as its secretions were irregular before the diarrhœa became troublesome; and it is common in the progress of severe hepatitis, for chalky purging to come on from suppression of the usual action in the liver, and is sometimes so profuse as to lower the patient's strength remarkably in a few hours. An instructive example of this occurred to me lately.

Case 22nd. A man who was thought to be convalescent from a very severe and obstinate attackof hepatitis, was suddenly seized with profuse purging. The stools appeared like pus, the pulse got feeble and rapid and the countenance was a little sunk. Before each stool the head of the colon was felt to be distended with fluid, and it was therefore evident that the matter did not flow into the colon from an abscess in the liver. On examining the stools again, they were found to consist of finely divided mucus, and it was concluded that they were secreted by the small intestine. The purging was checked; for two days the stools continued white, after which the biliary secretion was restored and rapid recovery took place. Had an abscess burst into the intestine, the pus would have reappeared in the stools on the cavity again filling up.

Baillie has described some cases of white diarrhœa in gentlemen from India, and he states that he found it connected with remarkable thinness of the intestinal coats. In the case of Concannon the mucous membrane was thickened, but the accuracy of that eminent pathologist is a sufficient proof that the contrary state of the intestines frequently exists. The following is a very instructive example of white diarrhœa succeeding rheumatism, in which the coats of the intestines were thin and otherwise very remarkably diseased.

Case 23rd. D. B. ætat. 31. In India 3 years. Has been much debilitated by repeated attacks of rheumatism of the upper parts of the body, and on the 10th December 1829, when he was transferred on his corps moving, his appetite was bad and he had thirst; pulse was 100 and soft. He took bark and Dover's powder at bed time. December 22nd. Purging of bloody fluid with shreds, no pain; slight tenderness about the left iliac region. Tongue brown and coated, less thirst. Pulse 76, soft. Omitt. cinchon. Habt. ol. ricini ℥j. 13th. Vesp. Several stools as before, two others of *white* feculent matter. Cont. pulv. Doveri h. s. ℞ Calomel. gr. iv, opii gr. iss, ft. pil. bis die sumend. 23rd. Stools more generally white with spots of puriform matter. 25th. Less blood in the stools, which are clayey. 26th. Stools dark yellow with a little pure blood floating on the surface. Tongue very foul; pulse 84, soft. 27th. No sleep, vomiting, many fluid stools, hiccup distressing, no pain on pressure. Cont. pil.; haust. anodyn. h. s. Empl. vesicat. scrob. cord. 29th. Hiccup at intervals, many scanty fluid stools, partly of whitish feces, gums get tender, takes a little wine and arrow root, dark crust on tongue. 30th. Stools partly dark and watery, or thin, yellow and lumpy with some blood. Less hiccup. He got worse, with hiccup, oppression at stomach, rapid feeble pulse and died at 10 P. M.

Dissection. Lungs adherent to the pleura costalis and diaphragm, but their structure healthy. External appearance of intestine healthy. Liver enlarged and projected beyond the edge of the ribs; convex surface mottled and marked by depressions like old scars, but the substance internally did not appear diseased. Gall bladder large and full of dark bile. Coats of stomach thin, dark brown or black spots on the mucous membrane with ulcers in their centre;

vessels turgid. The commencement of the duodenum was divested of mucous membrane, and there were some ulcers in different parts of the gut, the coats of which were exceedingly thin. The jejunum thin with small ulcers on the rugæ and between them. Further down there was more vascularity, and two large ulcers at the commencement of the ilium and marks of old ulcers which had healed were observed; lower part of ilium vascular and the mucous coat was covered with a minute white papular eruption (like sago grains), some of them ulcerated in their centre. This eruption extended to the rectum. The head of the colon was thin and relaxed, with dark spots ulcerated in the centre. Ulceration extended through the whole gut, but near the rectum the sores were healing.

The aggravated nature of the intestinal affection caused the death of the patient before the liver had passed beyond the first stage of disease, when its functions are not yet permanently obstructed, and the stools exhibited a morbid biliary secretion alternating with a want of that fluid in the stools. The tubercular degeneration of the mucous membrane and consequent ulceration is a curious fact, and when compared with the following case, shows that there is a tendency to tubercular formation in the various abdominal membranes.

Case 24th. Joseph Sweeny had an attack of fever with biliary disorder in July 1829, of which he was cured in a few days, but rheumatic pains followed and distressed him while at his duty till December of the same year, when he was readmitted with severe pain and swellings of the ancles, and pain and tenderness of the tibia. No previous venereal disease or mercurial cause could be blamed for these symptoms.

Warm baths and Dover's powder relieved him at first, but they lost their effect and swellings formed on the tibia. Calomel. gr. iss, pulv. antimon. gr. iij, opii gr. j, were given in pill on the 28th and induced purging, which caused their omission on the 2nd January, but the gums had become tender and the pains were relieved. Walking increased those in the tibia. He rubbed camphorated mercurial ointment on the swellings with benefit. The end of January there was tendency to diarrhœa, the beginning of February he was allowed to go out convalescent and on the 24th returned, having drunk hard. Pains were the same. He was now much purged, his stools watery and composed of white mucus; he vomited much and there was a sense of emptiness in the bowels, but no pain on pressure. His tongue was dry, brown and parched; pulse frequent, bounding and weak. These symptoms were moderated with difficulty, the nodes increased and the pain in the right knee was severe. In April bowels were irregular at intervals, and the pain in the right knee and leg was very violent. He had become emaciated, weak and irritable, and had evening fever. In the end of the month wine of colchicum was prescribed, but in two days the stomach became irritable from its use, it was therefore diminished, and omitted the 4th day. On the 20th May passed light reddish stools. On the 27th he was very low, moaned and was covered with a cold sweat. There was some tenderness along the margins of the ribs on the 30th, vomiting, sensation of cramps in the right leg, and at the heart the action of which was violent. He was relieved by an anodyne. In June he was much better, but the middle of that month complained of soreness of the abdomen mostly to the right of umbilicus; purging returned and stools were white, whitish brown, yellow, and sometimes viscid, dark and mixed with mucus. In July the pains left him, and he had afterwards only some numbness in the legs, but the abdominal tenderness was felt at the bottom of the abdomen, and on lying on the right side had pain of the left lumbar and hypochondriac regions and at the edge of the false ribs on both sides. The face was full, emaciation of the legs extreme, and he got faint and had cold sweats on going to the stool, in which some pus was now observed. A few leeches and fomentations relieved the pain. In August he was much the same, but rain always brought on the purging. In September had œdema of the legs, abdominal fluctuation, pain in the right iliac region, drowsiness and occasional slight delirium. On 2nd October was much purged, stools of various colours, partly of clayey feces, white matter and mucus; abdomen distended in the evenings. October 15th. Many white stools with griping and exhaustion. On 31st abdomen immensely distended with water and flatus; in great distress. There was some obstruction in making his water. He gradually sunk and died on the 27th November.

Dissection. Several gallons of water in the abdomen and some in the thorax. Lungs healthy, marks of scrophulous sores of the neck from which he had lately suffered. Heart small, a white spot on its external covering, but its internal structure was healthy. Liver small, hard and of a grey colour. Gall bladder contained thin bilious fluid; ducts large. The whole of the peritoneum both liningthe cavity and viscera, studded with minute hard tubercles like flat beads of glass of the size of a pin's head. They were easily scraped off the membrane, and in some places they were covered with a red bloody deposition, the peritoneum was very red, and the tubercles were most numerous and the redness greatest in that part of each lumbar region on which the colon lay. The stomach was small and contracted. The mucous membrane of the small intestines was red and vascular, as was that of the colon. Its coats were thick and there were a few minute ulcers on its lower portion. A few of the ulcers seemed to have healed. The small head of the pancreas was large and like white cheese; the glands of the mesentery were hard and white.

While this case was under treatment another in every respect similar, except that there had been no fever before the attack and that the hepatic symptoms were better marked, was in hospital; the patient was sent to the coast in the hope that the change might yet preserve his life, and he was not afterwards heard of.

At the time Concannon was ill, there were several men labouring under rheumatism in whom symptoms of the same kind had appeared, and at the recommendation of the superintending surgeon they were sent from Nagpore to the coast, which is the only measure permanently useful. Several of the milder cases were restored to health and some of them died, *it was supposed*, from the aggravation of the diarrhœa. I lately accidentally met with the history of two of those fatal cases, which are important although no dissection was made.

Case 25th. John Robinson ætat 25, in India 8 years. Had suffered much from rheumatic pains of the extremities especially the lower, tenderness of the sternum and occasional short cough. There was no ground to suspect recent syphilitic taint, and he had not had much mercury except once, three years before when he had hepatitis. In 1829 the pains were aggravated and he was constantly in and out of hospital, they were mostly fixed in the shins and sternum where there was swelling, and in the elbow and occasionally in the head. The appetite gradually became irregular, he had occasional purging of light coloured stools, and evening fever. In October these symptoms had become more severe and permanent, he was emaciated and his sallow dry skin seemed too tight over the attenuated flesh; the dejections were frequent and generally white, although he occasionally passed watery greenish stools; tongue white, thirst, pulse quick, small and rather sharp. In December stools were chalky, frequently preceded by some griping, and *unmixed at any time with bile.* In January 1830 he proceeded to the coast. For six months before, he had laboured under pains and remarkably indolent superficial ulceration of the throat having no tendency to spread, and not at all like venereal ulceration. Great variety of treatment was used with only temporary benefit to the disease, but the throat at length healed. Was admitted into the garrison hospital at Masulipatam on the 11th March with pains, and he had some oppression at the chest and dry cough. Took no medicine but improved from the change of air, and was discharged convalescent on 25th March. Readmitted 13th June with white purging, nausea, irritable stomach, bad appetite and great debility. He took bitters, and on the 21st tinct. camphor. comp. ʒj was added to his mixture on account of short cough; spirits increased the symptoms but wine was beneficial. During this time the pains had nearly left him, but on the 30th July they returned in the knees and shoulders. In August the purging increased, the stools being white and watery with tenderness to pressure about the umbilicus, and extreme emaciation. He died 26th August after nearly three years of ill health. The white diarrhœa probably depended on the same morbid state of the abdominal viscera as in Concannon, the same symptoms being present in each. It is impossible to say that the patient had had no venereal taint, but neither his previous history nor the progress of the symptoms were of that kind which usually follow confirmed syphilis; and if they are to be referred to this head, it will not take from the importance of the observation regarding the internal disease, as the cases in which these occur are an important class of chronic ails, and are in their earlier stages universally considered and treated as ordinary rheumatism. There has been ground to suspect both scrophula and mercurial action as at the root of the evil in some cases, but in others the connection could not be ascertained. The other of the two patients who died after having been sent to the coast, had other symptoms which are intimately connected with the series of diseased actions which we have seen affect the abdominal serous and mucous membranes, the substance of the liver, and the glandular mucous structure of the throat. The skin has in a number of instances taken on diseased action of a slow character ending in ulceration, such as is not uncommonly observed in this country in scrophulous leucophlegmatic subjects, and as is described by Dr. Alison and others as following long continued courses of mercury.[15] In the fol-

[15] I have since met with several intractable cases, in which ulceration seemed to be caused by the action of mercury in scrophulous rheumatic patients. In such examples it is difficult to say what plan of treatment should be adopt-

lowing case they were more immediately connected with the local rheumatic affections, than in any other instance I have witnessed.

Case 26th. Thomas Pearson was admitted in October 1828 with severe pains, and swelling and stiffness of the right elbow which he has had for four months. The tonsils had been painful for a month, the palate relaxed, and superficial indolent ulceration extended slowly from one tonsil to the other behind the soft palate. He had no venereal complaint for two years before the present illness. Had once a sore mouth for an attack of liver, but not recently. His hair and eyes are light and complexion naturally clear, although now sallow. On the 9th November the ulceration had spread, and the arm was worse. A grain of calomel and opium were ordered twice a day and on the 11th the gums were sore, when the pill was ordered every second night and on the 20th omitted, and the ulcer ceased to be painful and began to heal. On the 18th December the throat had again got worse, and no application to the arm or general remedies gave the least relief. The stools were occasionally very dark. From the 22d to the 31st December took half a grain of calomel morning and evening and the throat healed. A white ulcer on the back of the soft palate, only seen by raising it up, disappeared, and the pain in the arm nearly left him, but the joint remained stiff and in a state of semiflexion. On the 2d January 1829, he was allowed to be a convalescent in quarters. In the end of the month ulceration returned in the throat, ulcers were painful, of a livid color little affected by stimu-

ed; it is, however, satisfactory to know that a persevering and judicious employment of local remedies will sometimes restore the patient to health. Numerous chronic ulcers on the hips, thighs, and legs, in a scrophulous patient long subject to rheumatism, healed rapidly under a mild course of iodine and hydriodate of potassa.

lating gargles, and spread along the arch of the palate to the uvula. He had evening fever. The gums were again made sore and he went to his duty the end of February, but the arm was still painful, stiff and swollen. On the 20th March he was readmitted, with severe pain of the inner side of the left knee joint extending to the thigh, and of the elbow and right shoulder. Leeches gave temporary relief, and blisters increased the pain and irritation. The pains extended to the arms, chest, right thigh and fingers, and were increased at night and by thunder storms; his appetite was bad and his tongue white. Various remedies as wine of colchicum, turpentine, guaiac and bark were used with little benefit, and in May his mouth was again slightly affected by blue pill, tartrate of antimony and opium. In August a grain of calomel and opium were given but griped him, and the stools were green. In September, a swelling of the second joint of the third finger of right hand, which had been sometime soft, ulcerated, and left a deep white indolent sore with undermined edges. In December he was emaciated, his general health bad and he suffered from occasional evening irritative paroxysms. On the 12th January he was sent to the coast where he arrived on the 12th March; the pains unrelieved, the elbow swollen, the joint motionless, the right knee was stiff and painful, his nights sleepless and he was much wasted. He improved a little at first, but in April an abscess formed behind the knee which never healed, although it put on a healing appearance, and the right tibia became painful; he used anodynes, sarsaparilla, quinine, &c. On the 24th April vomited in the night; this was relieved by an emetic, but recurred occasionally and proved the first symptom of the fatal disease about to follow;

the bowels were yet regular. The tongue was red and perfectly clean. In May took muriate of mercury in decoction of bark. 14th June. Sore on knee painful, and the painful and swelled part of left elbow above the inner condyle ulcerated, an abscess has formed at the top of the right shoulder, and loose bone was taken from the sore on the finger. July 12th. Purging set in; stools at first dark and watery. 20th. Stomach irritable. August 3rd. Ulcers sloughy. 23d. Right foot swollen and the other knee and hand partook of the diseased actions. 28th. Stools frequent, copious, liquid, light coloured and passed without straining. Pains about the umbilicus increased on pressure and vomiting. Pulse quick and feeble. Urine high. September 1st. Stools scanty, watery *and white*, vomits thick clotted greenish matter. Purging was relieved by opium, chalk, and Dover's powder. 15th. Vomiting, and frequent scanty stools at night; they are occasionally greenish and mixed with mucus. Died exhausted on the 26th September. In a good many instances ulceration of the skin is not, as in the above example, a local disease depending on that of the subjacent parts, but is caused by the constitutional disorder. The ulceration is commonly slow, indolent, superficial, the edges thick and white, and heals at one side or in the centre and extends at the opposite margin or all round the edges. The upper and lower extremities are equally liable, and sometimes the ulcers form over the trunk. In two cases they took on a phagedenic appearance, destroying the muscles, laying open the veins of the inner side of the arm, and killing the patient by repeated hæmorrhage. The following case I saw after the ulcers had healed, and was favoured with a notice of his former history by the surgeon under whom the disease commenced, and by whom he was sent to the coast. The careful enquiries that gentleman* has long been making, into the constitutions in which Indian diseases most prevail and into the succession of these to one another, is a guarantee of the correctness of the opinion he gives, as to the absence of the ordinary causes to which we would be inclined to ascribe the disease.

Case 27th. A very corpulent man of florid habit but without mental energy was subject during 1828 to rheumatism: the end of 1829 the tendency to unhealthy ulceration commenced over the lower extremities, chest and arms; there were also nodular swellings on the bones, irregular febrile exacerbations and tendency to looseness. In January 1832 he was sent to the coast where he arrived in March. Fulness, pain and hardness with tumid belly came on during the journey; the legs were œdematous; the wrist swollen and the pains severe from 7 P. M. till midnight; severe pain shooting through the diaphragm. Ease after eating hot things. Tongue scarlet red, and moist. He was temporarily relieved by blisters, baths and Dover's powder, but they weakened him: the urine was red and scanty and abdominal fluctuation was distinct. Cold sweats towards morning. Bowels costive and stools dark. Liver projects beyond the edge of the ribs. April 11th. Severe pain in the lower part of thorax worse at night, pulse 120, very soft; vomiting, urine muddy, pale or yellow with occasional copious white deposit. 26th. Stools frequent, of various colours, watery, pale, or composed of mucus tinged with blood, or green with clusters of white subtance embedded in transparent mucus. Vomiting. Four ounces of blood were drawn, which coa-

* Surgeon W. Geddes.

gulated firmly and had little serum. He died the end of May. *Dissection.* The brain was healthy, as were the contents of the spinal canal, which contained only a very little fluid such as is often found in chronic disease. Heart small, pale and flaccid. Lungs healthy. Mucous membrane of the œsophagus dark and that of intestines thin, with dark tints and slight excoriation. Great engorgement near the cæcum. Colon livid, with marks of old ulcers. Liver enormously enlarged and all its fissures very deep, the substance having increased without encroaching on them. The great fissure was almost a complete canal into which the finger could be pressed during life, and gave the feel of a collection of fluid, through which the aorta could be felt to pulsate. On the surface of the organ there were some nine or ten deep scarlike irregular fissures, from some of which fibrous processes penetrated into the substance of the liver; but that they were not real scars appeared from some natural hepatic substance being found close to some of them from large healthy vessels passing through them, and from others not penetrating the substance of the viscus, which was seen to be *healthy immediately below them.* The structure of the liver was altered: it was partly changed into a pale white gristly substance, in which minute orange red spots were seen with a magnifier, or numerous white waved lines separated small portions of the natural hepatic matter. The convexity of the organ felt soft like wet sand, but contained no matter; the lower and back part tore like rotten leather. It appeared to me from the examination of this liver, that the marks usually considered as the scars of old abscesses are formed, by the irregular enlargement of the organ caused by its shape, the position of large vessels, and the change of old or deposit of new parts less susceptible of distension. Inflammation may cause this, and the change has also appeared to act as an excitement of the vessels of the peritoneum, thickening it over the depression. Since the notes of this case and the conclusions suggested by it and others were recorded, I have had the pleasure of finding, that Dr. Bright has noticed the appearance and cause of the marks in nearly the same words. The white substance is probably *cholesterine* found in these livers by Dr. Bostock, and the orange deposit was perhaps of the same nature as that found by him in the bile, which was deficient of its usual ingredients. It appears that in chronic disease of this kind adhesions are rarely formed, and the liver protrudes downwards instead of towards the thorax as in acute cases. The kidneys were dark and gorged, and part of the right embedded in the enlarged liver. The coats of the urinary passages were pretty natural. The urine had deposited much white matters. A case hardly differing in any respect from the above was under treatment at the same time; he had laboured under rheumatism, got sores over the body, which had not healed at the inner part of the left arm, his pulse was frequent, feeble and irritable, there was a red patch without fur on the tongue and a red streak in its centre, the urine was pale, copious, generally with white deposit, not coagulable by heat and of sp. gr. of 1012. Some effusion took place in the abdomen, the liver became painful and greatly enlarged, and the pains in the arms and legs were severe. He had profuse sweats at night, and diaphoretics were injurious. He was several times bled, and the blood was buffy and cupped with much serum, apparently from the rheumatic diathesis, rather than the slow hepatic inflammation; accordingly, the evacuations gave no relief, but his health did not seem to be injured by them, although they caused increased paleness of the countenance, and probably did ultimate injury. The stools were at first pale and of natural consistence and frequency; ultimately he was purged, and stools were slimy with traces of blood, there was tenderness about the umbilicus and in right iliac region, enlargement in epigastrium, swelled glands in the neck; and swellings of the bones under the scars of the old sores began to form, when he was sent to another station. I have little doubt that he died soon after.

Abscesses seen rarely to form, notwithstanding the extensive disease of the liver, but in one man who had long suffered from rheumatism of the joints, puffy abdomen, and occasional purging of pale yeasty stools; after recovery consequent on residence on the coast, the liver took on subacute inflammation and ended in extensive suppuration. It was, however, probably a distinct affection, although no doubt the previous disease predisposed to unhealthy action.

Obstruction and chronic enlargement of the liver and disease of the hollow abdominal viscera, are well known to follow long continued gout, and Broussais has asserted it to be a gastro-enterite with a developement "of irritation in the joints;" an assertion which may be reversed, and applied with more justice to many forms of Indian rheumatism. If the conjunction of the external and internal disease had been accidental, it is not probable that so many remarkable cases corresponding in their principal features should have been seen by one individual,[16] in a comparatively

[16] I proposed giving some cases of natives with similar terminations, but the paper is already too long. *Original note.*

short period; and the numerous instances in which the health was broken by long continued rheumatism, in which symptoms evidently of the same nature though in a less degree occured, confirmed the evidence of a pathological connection. It does not seem to be confined to any particular district, although comparatively rare in stations, where simple rheumatism is little prevalent and mild. The very accurate and careful observer who communicated the early history of the last two cases, in allusion to the ulceration succeeding rheumatism observes, "that there is a class of diseases connected with a peculiar cachectic state of the body in this country, which have not as yet been sufficiently pointed out;" which so far confirms my remarks on the subject, by shewing that there has been little attention paid to it. Nor will it appear improbable, that in a climate in which the original affection differs so widely from that of Europe; in which the known complications especially that of pericarditis is so seldom present, and then in a different form; and where the liver and abdominal mucous membrane are so prone to disease, that they shouldbe liable to take on secondary morbid actions. Some remarkable cases have occurred, in which a still greater variety of tissues have in succession been altered in structure or disordered in function, but the details are too voluminous to be introduced at present. A slight notice of two will conclude the subject. A man subject to rheumatism got pain in the cardiac region, tenderness between the ribs to pressure and some other symptoms, which were thought to be caused by chronic pericarditis. He then suffered from cough, viscid expectoration, irritable stomach, rejection of some small dark clots of blood either from the chest or from the œsophagus, on food passing through which there was pain and obstruction.[17] After some months the affection of the heart was aggravated, and a swelling formed in the groin which pulsated violently and had so much the appearance of an aneurism, that it was only distinguished from that disease, by feeling the artery on strong pressure, to be for an inch as if included in a hard cylinder painful to the touch, and probably formed by inflammation of the sheath of the vessel. The loins, right hip, and thigh became violently painful and the latter permanently flexed, a very hard circumscribed moveable swelling which did not appear to be connected with the colon and over which there was tenderness, was detected above Poupart's ligament; on the pains being alleviated, oppression at the chest recurred, bowel complaint, and discharge and violent pain of the ear succeeded, and with aggravation of the original symptoms have completely broken his constitution.[18]

The following is more instructive, as showing the tendency to sudden metastasis of diseased actions, in some respects analogous to those we have been con-

[17] In a man ofthe name of Connors who was long subject to rheumatism, difficulty in swallowing and afterwards loss of power of the right arm occured. Symptoms like those of palsy may arise from and be mistaken for rheumatism, but a mistake of an opposite description is more common. *Original note.*

[18] This patient died on the 2nd May 1833, soon after the paper was transmitted to the Board, having derived no benefit from blisters and moxas to the loins and hips, extract of conium and Dover's powder, iodine, and whatever other means seemed to afford a hope of alleviating his sufferings. The moxas to the hip caused troublesome ulcers, and sores formed over the sacrum. The body was examined 4½ hours after death.

Spine. Fatty matter external to the sheath, from 6th to 11th dorsal vertebræ posteriorly, and a slight deposit of lymph opposite to the 5th lumbar vertebra. Within the lumbar vertebræ there was a quantity of bloody fluid, of which a good deal was also found within the sheath, round the cauda equina. *Head.* Some congestion of the vessels of the brain and red points on cutting into its substance, with slight effusion below the arachnoid and in the ventricles. Considerable vascularity at the base of the cerebrum and cerebellum. *Thorax.* Numerous strong adhesions of the lungs to the pleura costalis, particularly at the upper parts; many minute tubercles in their substance, a few of which contained pus. The pericardium contained a good deal of fluid, but neither it or the heart were diseased. The valves were healthy. A loose cellular substance hung from the root of the aorta, apparent-

sidering. P. Murray had sores on the penis and buboes, followed by eruptions, venereal sores over the body and great debility. In August he was convalescent. In September suffered from pains of the joints. On the 3rd October had fever at noon and again at

ly formed by a doubling of the external coat. *Abdomen.* The peritoneum healthy, as were the stomach and intestines externally. The mucous membrane of the great head of the stomach speckled with red, and slightly thickened; the small end vascular and red. Duodenum empty, jejunum contained a white secretion and its mucous membrane as well as that of the ileum red and getting paler towards the colon, where the secretion is tinged light yellow; coats thin. A few ovale ulcers, evidently of long standing, in the right colon. Some engorgement of the mucous membrane, which is also observed in the transverse colon and in the sigmoid flexure. The liver large, almost entirely white, soft, with the large veins full of thin blood. One scar like mark at the lower part of the convexity of the right lobe; over it the peritoneum is drawn into slight folds and penetrates some way into its substance, but appears to be composed of the natural cellular substance, into which it passes, and also intercepts portions of hepatic parenchyma. Bile of gall bladder thin and of an orange colour. The hepatic substance oily, and a part not dissolved in nitric acid forms a soap with potassa. White flaky substance dissolved by boiling alcohol, and deposited on cooling. Kidneys soft, vascular, and there is much grey substance in their structure. Puriform fluid can be pressed out of the secretory ducts. Bladder large and full of urine. Trachea contains much ropy mucus tinged with blood, inner membrane red. Mucous membrane of the gullet for an inch and a half above the diaphragm spotted with red vessels, and with numerous superficial chronic ulcers running from below upwards. A few vascular and slightly excoriated parts in the upper part of the tube. (See case page 52.) Below the fascia covering the right iliacus muscle a large collection of pus was discovered distending the part, so as to render the extension of the thigh impossible; this extended up along the outer edge of the iliac vessels to the two lower lumbar vertebræ, which were anchylosed, and a round carious cavity four lines in diameter penetrated nearly to the canal. This disease existed opposite to the deposit of lymph in the theca. The matter passed below Poupart's ligament to the groin, and deep between the muscles to the capsular ligament which was diseased externally, with jelly like exudation around it. It was not ascertained if the sinus penetrated the joint, on opening which the head of the bone was found loose, and the femur and acetabulum were soft and streaked with pus; some remains of union may have been broken. The cartilage was lying loose on the head of the bone. The lymphatic glands along the iliac and upper part of the femoral artery singularly altered into a white hard elastic substance; at the top of the thigh they were closely connected with the sheath of the vessels, and a little below the internal iliac, one of them had the size of a small orange; they extended above the bifurcation of the aorta, and several of the same kind, but smaller, were found on the right side.

The patient was scrophulous, and much of the diseased appearances may be traced to this taint, called into action by his long continued suffering from rheumatism. To this cause I am inclined to ascribe the caries of the spine, which could not have existed early in the disease, when the upper extremities suffered even more than the lower. *It is proper to state, that this patient was at one time suspected of exaggerating the symptoms he described himself to labour under.* The extent of disease in the liver gives some support to an opinion expressed by superintending surgeon Adams, in reference to a case of chronic rheumatism which had been under my care, and which terminated in confirmed liver disease; viz. that the great majority of cases of rheumatism arise from derangement of the abdominal viscera.

midnight with severe headach. On the 4th had a paroxysm like ague, that night became violently delirious, but could be made to answer questions. Pain of head was violent, pupil enlarged and sluggish, eyes staring, and shivering ascribed to his being frightened at his own imaginings. Leeches to the crown and a lotion containing æther relieved him; the scalp was observed to be tender, and next day a number of hard tumours (not painful) came out over it, and disappeared on the 6th. On the 7th the left side of the scalp was again swollen, with œdema over the tumefaction; he had purging of various coloured stools mostly pale, and pain and great tenderness of the abdomen. This increased till the 8th, when it left him, and profuse watery expectoration and pain at the lower part of the sternum succeeded. On the 10th violent inflammation of the larynx without affection of the fauces came on, requiring large depletion, and, at one time, I expected hourly to be obliged to perform tracheotomy to prevent suffocation His recovery was ultimately perfect.

THE END.

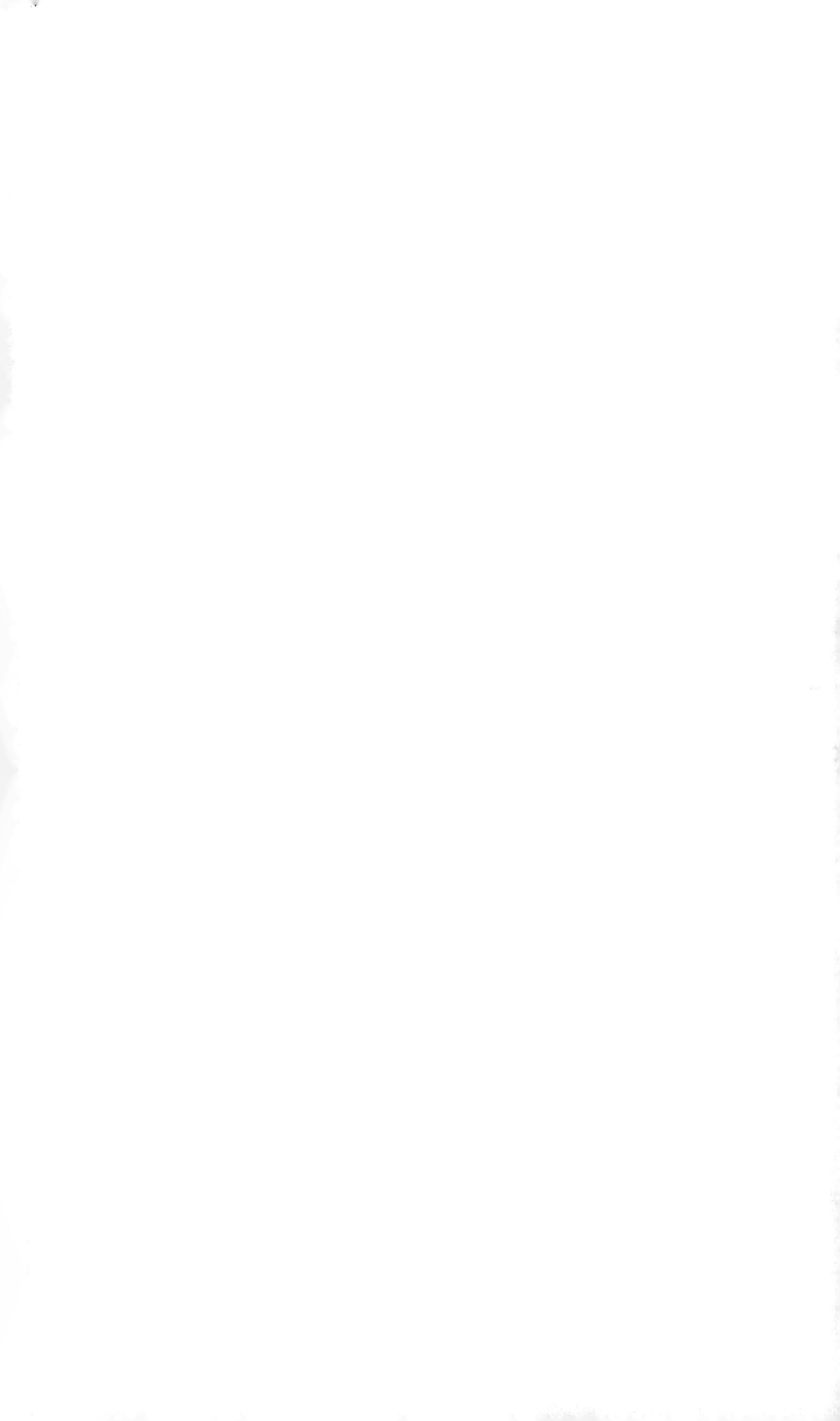